DISTINCTIVENESS AND MEMORY

DISTINCTIVENESS AND MEMORY

EDITED BY

R. Reed Hunt
James B. Worthen

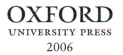

UNIVERSITY PRESS
2006

OXFORD
UNIVERSITY PRESS

Oxford University Press, Inc., publishes works that further
Oxford University's objective of excellence
in research, scholarship, and education.

Oxford New York
Auckland Cape Town Dar es Salaam Hong Kong Karachi
Kuala Lumpur Madrid Melbourne Mexico City Nairobi
New Delhi Shanghai Taipei Toronto
Car

With offices in
Argentina Austria Brazil Chile Czech Republic France Greece
Guatemala Hungary Italy Japan Poland Portugal Singapore
South Korea Switzerland Thailand Turkey Ukraine Vietnam

Published by Oxford University Press, Inc.
198 Madison Avenue, New York, New York 10016
www.oup.com

Library of Congress Cataloging-in-Publication Data
Distinctiveness and memory / edited by R. Reed Hunt, James B. Worthen.
p. cm.
Includes bibliographical references and index.
ISBN-13: 978-0-19-516966-9
ISBN-10: 0-19-516966-2
1. Memory. I. Hunt, R. Reed. II. Worthen, James B.
BF371.D57 2005
153.1'2—dc22   2005015500

1 3 5 7 9 8 6 4 2

Printed in the United States of America
on acid-free paper

Preface

Distinctiveness is a concept that has been invoked either directly or indirectly in nearly every major area of research in psychology. However, in no area of psychological research is the concept of distinctiveness more fully enmeshed than in the area of memory. Laboratory research on distinctiveness began early in the history of formal psychology (e.g., Calkins, 1894) and has continued steadily since. Across that research, the concept has been defined in different ways and applied to a variety of phenomena. Thus, a main objective of our volume was to bring together leading researchers in the area of distinctiveness and memory in an effort to gain insight into the similarities and differences in the application of distinctiveness as a theoretical concept. Toward this end, the present volume includes contributions from researchers doing basic research in the core areas (cognitive, neuroscience, social, and developmental) of empirical psychology.

By providing this forum for leading researchers to share their thoughts and ideas, we hope to achieve two specific goals: (1) to report recent developments in basic research investigating the relationship between distinctiveness and memory and (2) to advance theory related to distinctiveness and memory as a result of this exchange of ideas. To reach these goals, we believed that it was imperative to address the issues that have contributed to variations in the use of the term *distinctiveness* as a theoretical construct. A fundamental issue is the very meaning of the term. What is distinctiveness in the context of memory? Is it a description of the stimulus event or of the psychological processing of that event? Can it be both? Are terms such as *distinctiveness*, *bizarreness*, *vividness*, and *novelty* synonymous with respect to memory? These questions—each seeking a more clear operational definition of distinctiveness—are addressed in the present volume. Additionally, we sought to address the fundamental theoretical issues that have remained unresolved despite years of research in the area: What is the mechanism of distinctiveness effects? Can a theory of distinctiveness help us understand age-related changes in memory as well as various manifestations of memory in social contexts? And a final question of considerable prior interest, what are the neural support systems for distinctiveness?

The first part of the book addresses basic theoretical matters concerning attention. Hunt's chapter discusses two uses of the term *distinctiveness* and the implications of the different uses. In the second chapter, Nairne continues the discussion of the meaning of the term in the context of his theory of distinctiveness. Schmidt also addresses issues of terminology in the context of a distinction between novelty and significance, where he proposes that the two differentially affect memory. McDaniel and Geraci discuss the locus of distinctiveness effects, at encoding or retrieval, and provide an argument that emphasizes the importance of the retrieval process. Schacter and Wiseman describe research suggesting that distinctive processing can be used strategically at retrieval as a heuristic to improve memory accuracy. In the final chapter in this section, Burns raises the issue of measurement and outlines a new method for indexing distinctive processing.

The second part of the book is devoted to research on bizarreness—a topic that is often inextricably linked with distinctiveness. Worthen's chapter provides a thorough review of this research along with a discussion of the relationship between distinctiveness and bizarreness. The chapter also offers a new theory of bizarreness effects on memory. In the chapter by Davidson, additional issues concerning bizarreness are raised in the context of developmental research on memory for bizarre text.

The role of distinctive processing in dissociations between explicit and implicit memory tests is the topic of the third part. Mulligan's chapter reviews literature on test dissociations and the application of the distinction between conceptually driven and data-driven processes as an explanation of dissociation. Drawing heavily on his own important work, Mulligan notes difficulties with that explanation and as an alternative applies the distinction between item-specific and relational processing. In their chapter, Geraci and Rajaram compare distinctiveness effects in explicit and implicit memory and focus on the question of whether the distinctiveness effect in memory requires conscious processing of the prior experience at the time of retrieval. Their work with new implicit test preparations suggests that it does not.

The fourth part of the book considers the role of distinctiveness in memory across the life span. Howe reviews work on distinctive processing in children's memory, both immediate and long-term retention. He considers two alternative theories to explain the development of distinctive processing, and like McDaniel and Geraci's chapter in the first part, he emphasizes the importance of distinguishing encoding and retrieval. Smith's chapter describes research on elderly subjects in which the concepts of relational and item-specific processing have been applied to age deficits in memory. She integrates this work with more recent conceptualizations of distinctiveness.

The next part addresses distinctiveness in the context of social psychology. The chapter by Coats and Smith provides a comparison and contrast between the social and cognitive perspectives on distinctiveness and memory, and then discusses two major social-psychological effects (the incongruency effect and illusory correlation) often attributed to distinctiveness. The authors conclude that both effects can be understood in terms of item-specific and relational processing. Mullen and Pizzuto's chapter discusses social phenomena that are implicitly linked to distinctiveness. Ultimately, they conclude that an approach that links distinctiveness, group composition, and cognitive representations is useful in understanding a variety of social cognition and group processes phenomena.

The neuroscience part begins with a chapter by Fabiani, who discusses multiple neural phenomena that may contribute to the relationship between distinctiveness and memory. Based on the literature reviewed, she concludes that a model that integrates encoding, rehearsal, and retrieval factors might best explain the effects of distinctiveness on memory. Michelon and Snyder's chapter discusses neuroimaging research on memory for bizarre events. The results of this work suggest that the fusiform, prefrontal, and parietal cortices may play a role in determining the effects of extreme forms distinctiveness on memory. The chapter by Kishiyama and Yonelinas makes an important distinction between recollection and familiarity in explaining the effects of novelty on memory. These authors conclude that the effects of novelty on memory are related to processes occurring in the hippocampus and prefrontal cortex.

The final two chapters provide a summary and evaluation of previous chapters as well as new ideas about research on distinctiveness. Tulving and Rosenbaum argue that the distinctiveness effect in memory is the result of poor memory for nondistinctive items rather than extraordinary memory for distinctive items, and they propose a new process to account for poor memory of the nondistinctive items. Craik provides an interesting taxonomy of four cases of distinctiveness, all of which are associated with good memory but for different reasons. Craik then applies this analysis to the research reported in previous chapters as well as to other research on distinctiveness and memory.

In the end, we hope that the work discussed in this volume will serve as a useful description of recent research on distinctiveness and memory and also will stimulate some people to join us in the effort to develop a coherent story about distinctiveness and memory. The authors of the chapters have given us a solid platform from which to launch future efforts, and it is to those authors that we which to express much gratitude. Working with them has been a great pleasure.

We were fortunate to have Catharine Carlin evaluate our initial proposal for Oxford University Press (OUP). As our acquisitions editor, she enthusiastically encouraged us and provided important guidance toward reaching the project's final form. Jennifer Rappaport of Oxford University Press assisted with details of manuscript preparation. The editorial, production, and marketing team at OUP did all one could ask for in taking the original idea for this book to its tangible end point.

Quite candidly, this entire project began as an excuse to go to New Orleans. J. W. proposed a symposium to be co-chaired by R. H. for the 2003 meeting of the Southwestern Psychological Association. The program committee not only accepted the proposal but also provided a generous eight hours of program time. We are especially grateful to SWPA Officers Edward Kardas and Mary Brazier for obliging us to go to New Orleans and for providing the setting that put this volume in motion.

Postscript: As we were editing this work, Hurricane Katrina stormed the Gulf Coast. It is our deepest hope that by the time this book is published we all once again can be welcomed by the gracious citizens of the city of New Orleans.

REFERENCES

Calkins, M. W. (1894). Association. *Psychological Review, 1,* 476–483.

Contents

VII Denouement

Contributors

DANIEL J. BURNS
Psychology Department
Union College
Schenectady, NY
burnsd@union.edu

SUSAN COATS
Department of Psychology
Southeastern Louisiana University
Hammond, LA
scoats@selu.edu

FERGUS I.M. CRAIK
Rotman Research Institute
Baycrest Centre for Geriatric Care
Toronto, ON Canada
fcraik@rotman-baycrest.on.ca

DENISE DAVIDSON
Department of Psychology
Loyola University Chicago
Chicago, IL
ddavids@luc.edu

MONICA FABIANI
University of Illinois
Beckman Institute
Urbana, IL
mfabiani@uiuc.edu

LISA GERACI
Department of Psychology
Washington University
St. Louis, MO
lgeraci@artsci.wustl.edu

MARK L. HOWE
Department of Psychology
Lancaster University
Lancaster
UK
mark.howe@lancaster.ac.uk

R. REED HUNT
Psychology Department
University of Texas at San Antonio
San Antonio, TX
reed.hunt@utsa.edu

MARK KISHIYAMA
Helen Wills Neuroscience Institute
University of California
Berkeley, CA
mmkishiyama@berkeley.edu

MARK A. McDANIEL
Department of Psychology
Washington University in St. Louis
St. Louis, MO
mmcdanie@artsci.wustl.edu

PASCALE MICHELON
Washington University
Department of Psychology
St. Louis, MO
pmichelo@artsci.wustl.edu

BRIAN MULLEN
Psychology Department
University of Kent
Canterbury, Kent
UK
B.Mullen@Kent.ac.uk

NEIL W. MULLIGAN
Department of Psychology
University of North Carolina
Chapel Hill, NC
nmulligan@unc.edu

JAMES S. NAIRNE
Professor of Psychological Sciences
Purdue University
Department of Psychological Sciences
West Lafayette, IN
nairne@psych.purdue.edu

CARMEN PIZZUTO
Department of Psychology
Syracuse University
Syracuse, NY
cjpizzut@syr.edu

SUPARNA RAJARAM
Department of Psychology
State University of New York at
    Stony Brook
Stony Brook, NY
suparna.rajaram@sunysb.edu

R. SHAYNA ROSENBAUM
Rotman Research Institute
Baycrest Centre for Geriatric Care
Toronto, ON
Canada

DANIEL L. SCHACTER
Department of Psychology
Harvard University
Cambridge, MA
dls@wjh.harvard.edu

STEPHEN SCHMIDT
Psychology Department
Middle Tennessee State University
Murfreesboro, TN
sschmidt@frank.mtsu.edu

ELLIOT R. SMITH
Department of Psychology
Bloomington, IN
esmith4@indiana.edu

REBEKAH E. SMITH
Psychology Department
University of Texas at San Antonio
San Antonio, TX
rebekah.smith@utsa.edu

ABRAHAM Z. SNYDER
Washington University School of
    Medicine
Department of Radiology
St. Louis, MO
avi@npg.wustl.edu

ENDEL TULVING
Rotman Research Institute
Baycrest Centre for Geriatric Care
Toronto, ON
Canada
tulving@psych.utoronto.ca

AMY L. WISEMAN
Department of Psychology
Harvard University
Cambridge, MA
wiseman@fas.harvard.edu

JAMES B. WORTHEN
Department of Psychology
Southeastern Louisiana University
Hammond, LA
jworthen@selu.edu

ANDREW P. YONELINAS
University of California, Davis
Center for Mind and Brain
Davis, CA
apyonelinas@ucdavis.edu

I

Basic Issues

1

The Concept of Distinctiveness in Memory Research

R. Reed Hunt

Intuitions often instigate important discoveries in psychology, but left unexamined, intuitions also can become an impediment to progress. Such seems to be the case for distinctiveness and memory, where both the data and theory are intuitive. Everyone knows that distinctive events are well remembered and everyone knows why. A distinctive event attracts attention, and the additional processing enhances memory. The intuitive theory rests on a broad operational definition of distinctiveness as an event that violates the prevailing context. In this definition, distinctiveness is a property of an event; it is essentially an independent variable. The ultimate effect of this independent variable, enhanced memory, results from extraordinary attention. Why would a distinctive event attract more attention than other events? Intuitively, the event is surprising, salient, bizarre, or novel. The subjective experience recruits attention in the form of additional processing that ultimately facilitates memory.

These compelling intuitions have had an impact on the study of distinctiveness and memory. One response is to assume that there is little left to learn. This reaction is reinforced by incorporation of the intuitive theory into explanations of the paradigmatic case of distinctiveness, the isolation effect (Green, 1956; Jenkins & Postman, 1948; Schmidt, 1991), giving one the sense that distinctiveness effects have been explained satisfactorily. Another reaction has been to warn against the use of distinctiveness as an explanatory concept because that explanation would be circular (e.g., Baddeley, 1978; Schmidt, 1991). If, as the intuitive theory has it, distinctiveness is treated as an independent variable, distinctiveness does not explain why distinctiveness affects memory. Taken together, these two reactions to the intuitive approach to distinctiveness question the need for further discussion of distinctiveness and memory.

In answer to that question, this chapter offers an analysis of the term *distinctiveness* as it is used in memory research. Tulving (2000) has noted that the terms used by memory researchers rarely are subjected to careful analysis, which is unfortunate because such analysis goes to the heart of what we mean when the terms are used. The goal of the analysis is to facilitate communication and conceptual clarity. Such an analysis is especially important for *distinctiveness* because the dominant meaning of the term continues to be dictated by the intuitive theory while at the same time a contradictory, secondary meaning has entered the lexicon of memory research. The incongruous meanings of the two uses of the term can hamper communication and stunt theoretical development, the very reasons that Tulving recommended analysis of the terms we use.

The analysis presented here begins with four general points about the term *distinctiveness* as applied to memory. These points are abstracted from two lines of research, both of which use the term with different meanings. Along the way, we shall see that the intuitive theory has not fared well when confronted with empirical evidence. If the intuitive theory is abandoned, the argument proscribing the use of the term as an explanation loses its force, and the way is cleared at least to explore the use of distinctiveness as an explanatory concept. The second half of the chapter outlines one way to think of distinctiveness as an explanation. The value of this latter approach to distinctiveness is illustrated by testing its predictions concerning three separate memory phenomena.

FOUR POINTS ABOUT DISTINCTIVENESS

Two separate lines of research invoking the term *distinctiveness* or a near synonym have produced the data on which this discussion will be based. The first is work using the isolation paradigm, an enterprise with a long history (e.g., Calkins, 1894, 1896). The *isolation paradigm* entails presenting subjects with material to be remembered, a small proportion of which differs on some dimension from the majority of the material. The isolation effect is enhanced memory for the different material. The different material often is labeled "distinctive," and superior memory for that material becomes the distinctiveness effect. With this use of the term, distinctiveness clearly is an independent variable that is a property of the to-be-remembered material.

From the outset (Calkins, 1894, 1896; Jersild, 1929; Van Buskirk, 1932), laboratory data confirmed the intuition that distinctive events are relatively well remembered. With the publication of von Restorff's (1933) classic article, the focus of research shifted from describing the effect of the variable to attempts to explain the effect. Ironically, von Restorff's work yielded some of the most damning evidence against the intuitive theory, which had yet to be formally stated, but this fact went unnoticed probably because von Restorff's paper has never been published in English. Von

Restorff's evidence will be described subsequently. Jenkins and Postman (1948) were the first to explicitly suggest that the isolation effect results from differential attention to the isolate. Green (1956) later would emphasize the importance of subjective experience aroused by the isolate as a cue attracting attention, essentially completing the formal statement of the intuitive theory. These developments were accompanied by substantial empirical work exploring various parametric manipulations on the isolation effect and their bearing on alternative theoretical accounts, most of which is reviewed in the important papers by Wallace (1965) and Schmidt (1991).

A second major line of research invoking the term *distinctiveness* evolved from levels of processing framework (Craik & Lockhart, 1972). In response to research motivated by the original framework, distinctive processing became the progeny of depth of processing as an explanation for the effects of orienting tasks. Distinctive processing was defined as the unique processing of an item at encoding that enhances discriminability of that item at retrieval (Jacoby & Craik, 1979; Lockhart, Craik, & Jacoby, 1976). *Distinctiveness* has a very different meaning in this context than it did in the context of the isolation paradigm. *Distinctiveness* now refers to a kind of processing rather than to the material being processed. In this sense, the term denotes an abstract concept rather than an independent variable. When used as an abstract concept, distinctiveness is in principle a candidate explanation for observed phenomena. Thus, to say that the isolation effect is the result of distinctive processing is not a circular argument. To be of use, however, the concept of distinctiveness must be fleshed out, including at a minimum a description of the conditions under which distinctive processing will occur. The points that follow provide a basis for such elaboration of the concept of distinctive processing.

Point 1: Distinctiveness Is Not a Property of To-Be-Remembered Material

To say that an event is distinctive is to refer to a psychological event, not to the physical object corresponding to the event. Distinctiveness is a characteristic of perception and comprehension but is not an inherent property of the perceived event. At one level, this point is purely definitional. Distinctiveness has as its root the verb *distinguish,* whose definition includes "to separate mentally things or one thing from another; to perceive or note differences between things" (Oxford American Dictionary, 1980, p. 250). Thus, the term *distinctiveness* is defined in reference to psychological processes, not the physical objects on which the processes operate.

The definitional point is readily instantiated by various empirical observations. For example, the proper control condition for the isolation effect is to place the isolated item in a list in which it is no longer isolated. Given that there is better memory in the isolation list than in the control list, any reference to distinctiveness cannot be to a property of the item itself because it is exactly the same physical item in the two lists. As another example, enhanced memory for orthographically distinctive words occurs only when these words are in a list that also contains orthographically common words. Pure lists of distinctive and common words yield no effect of orthography. Indeed, the very perception of orthographic distinctiveness as indexed by ratings depends on the presence of orthographically common words (Hunt & Elliott, 1980).

That distinctiveness is not a property of the environment perhaps is obvious, but the subtle implications of this point are important. If the term *distinctiveness* refers to an independent variable, the variable in question is a psychological representation, not an item in a list. To determine if this variable in fact has been manipulated in any given experiment, some index of the representation must be available (Schmidt, 1991). With the variable having met this criterion, demonstration of enhanced memory for the distinctive (psychological) event then could be followed by a theoretical account proposing concepts to explain the effect, such as salience and attention. This strategy, however, will produce an incomplete account of memory phenomena because it ignores a significant aspect of encoding. There is no provision for explanation of the processes of perception and comprehension that produce the distinctive representation. If the term *distinctiveness* is used to label the processes of perception/comprehension, the distinctive representation is distinctive because it was processed distinctively, an unacceptably circular explanation.

The conundrum can be avoided by reserving the term *distinctiveness* to label abstract (theoretical) processes that are hypothesized to account for certain memory phenomena. That is, distinctive processing yields a kind of representation that, among other things, facilitates memory. In so doing, the meaning of distinctiveness has shifted importantly but subtly from that of an independent variable to an abstract concept that describes a type of processing. The abstract concept of distinctive processing theoretically applies to the operations of both encoding and retrieval, offering a general functional explanation of memory. As we shall see, good reasons exist for adopting this position and abandoning the use of *distinctiveness* in reference to independent variables.

Point 2: Salience Is Not Necessary

The term *distinctiveness* tends to be applied to events that are extremely different from the prevailing context, and in many cases these events are accompanied by a subjective experience such as surprise. Events that elicit such subjective experience often are described as salient. *Salience* refers to an event that is conspicuous; an event that invites further attention beyond its initial perception. Indeed, *salience* and *distinctiveness* sometimes are used interchangeably in psychological literature, a practice that has been encouraged by the isolation paradigm. An isolated item is conspicuous and almost always perceived as different from surrounding items, modeling circumstances outside of the laboratory of extreme violation of context. Consequently, it is understandable that subjective experience became a component of the explanation for enhanced memory of isolated items (Green, 1956). The conspicuous item is perceived as salient and arouses surprise, which draws attention and results in enhanced memory.

In fact, beginning with von Restorff's (1933) widely cited paper, evidence has accumulated against the assumption that salience is necessary for isolation effects. Contrary to most contemporary studies and inconsistent with many secondary accounts of von Restorff's procedure, she did not isolate the critical item in the middle or near the end of the list. Rather, the isolated item appeared at the beginning of the list where "the isolated item was not perceived as unusual and was not particularly salient to the subject" (p. 319). She did so because "we wanted to avoid the situation where the critical item would stand out as perceptually unique" (p. 319). Von Restorff obviously obtained the isolation effect with which her name has become synonymous but did so with a paradigm in which the isolate should not be perceived as salient. Her results have been replicated using the original procedure of isolating the critical item in the second serial position of the list (Hunt, 1995) as well in experiments placing the isolate in the first position in the list (Kelly & Nairne, 2001; Pillsbury & Rausch, 1943).

Dunlosky, Hunt, and Clark (2000) buttressed von Restorff's logical argument that early isolates are not salient by using judgments of learning as an independent index of salience. Current research on how judgments of learning are made suggests that perceived salience of an item inflates the judgment (e.g., Koriat, 1997). Dunlosky et al. presented participants with isolation lists in which the isolate occurred early in the list or halfway through the list. Following each item, the participants gave a judgment of how likely they were to remember the item. The critical results are shown in Figure 1.1 where one can see that judgments for isolates occurring late in the list were indeed inflated relative to proper controls, whereas judgments for early isolates did not differ from controls. The data are consistent with von Restorff's argument that the early isolate is not perceived as salient, but nonetheless the magnitude of the isolation effect on memory did not differ for early and late isolates.

To evaluate the possibility that the early isolate becomes salient as the list progresses, Dunlosky et al. conducted a second experiment in which the participants rehearsed the items aloud. If salience affects memory by recruiting attention to the item, then rehearsal, a prominent candidate for the additional processing in the isolation literature (Cooper & Pantle, 1967; Rundus, 1971), of the isolate should increase as the list unfolds. No such effect was found. Rehearsal of the early isolate did not differ from the pattern of rehearsal of control items. When the isolate occurred late in the list, it did receive reliably more rehearsal than its control item, indicating that rehearsal is sensitive to perceived salience. Importantly, however, the magnitude of the isolation effect was the same for early and late isolates. These data strongly suggest that neither salience nor the additional processing attracted by salience is necessary for the isolation effect in memory.

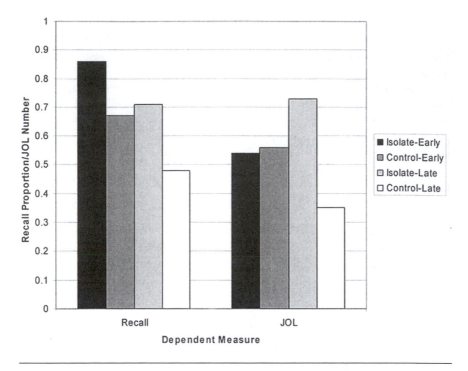

FIGURE 1.1 Proportion correctly recalled and average judgments of learning (scale of 100) as a function of early versus late list position and isolation versus control list (adapted from Dunlosky et al., 2000).

Given that the isolation effect is the prototypic preparation for studies of distinctiveness effects in memory, the data clearly indicate that salience is not necessary for distinctiveness to enhance memory. Disassociating salience and distinctiveness is important for clarification of the term *distinctiveness*. Because intuitions about distinctiveness are drawn from extreme violations of context and because much of our laboratory evidence is derived from the isolation paradigm that models this extreme incongruity, distinctiveness is assumed to cause surprise and salience, which in turn cause good memory. This theory not only is wrong about the necessity of salience but it also implicitly blurs an important distinction between *difference* and *distinctiveness*. These two terms cannot be used as synonyms in discussions of memory, as is illustrated by the third point.

Point 3: Difference Is Not Sufficient

Distinctiveness effects on memory require the processing of differences among items, but difference alone is not sufficient to describe distinctiveness effects. Again, the lesson begins with von Restorff. To make her point, she contrasted the standard isolation list with a heterogeneous control list in which each item is different. Suppose the isolation list consists of nine digits and one nonsense syllable. The difference between the syllable and the digits is substantial, but is it this difference that produces enhanced memory for the syllable relative to the control condition? Suppose we substitute a line drawing for one of the nine digits in the isolation list, giving us two isolated items and the eight digits. The drawing and the syllable are both different from the numbers, but they are also different from each other. We can continue to substitute items of different materials for the remaining digits, but the difference between the syllable (the original isolate) and the other items is just as great as the difference between the syllable and the digits. "In the end, the difference between all other items among themselves and the syllable is equivalent to the initial difference between the syllable and number" (von Restorff, 1933, p. 314). If the isolate were remembered better than the same item in the same serial position of an unrelated list, "then one could argue that other factors besides the difference between one item and other items is important" (von Restorff, p. 314). She, of course, did find that the item was better remembered in the isolation list than in the control list.

Research from the levels of processing tradition converges on the same point. In similar experiments, Epstein, Phillips, & Johnson (1975) and Begg (1978) asked subjects to perform orienting tasks on word pairs that were strongly or weakly associated, e.g., *dog-cat* versus *dog-beer*. The orienting tasks required listing either the similarities or the differences between the words. Subsequent recall of the related pairs was better following difference judgments, but recall of unrelated pairs was better following similarity judgment. The latter result indicates that difference alone is not particularly beneficial to memory, otherwise the unrelated words judged for differences would have yielded superior memory. Likewise, the fact that related pairs were better recalled when rated for difference than when rated for similarity indicates that similarity alone is not optimal for memory. Comparable data from recall of categorized lists were reported subsequently by Einstein and Hunt (1980) and Hunt and Einstein (1981).

Thus, research from both the isolation and levels of processing paradigms converge on the point that distinctiveness effects in memory cannot be captured by reference to difference alone. Differences among materials are an important setting operation for situations that have been described by the term *distinctiveness*, encouraging a strong connotation of difference when the term is used. However, the data suggest that the psychological processing underlying beneficial effects on memory that are described as distinctive involve more than the processing of difference.

Point 4: Distinctiveness Is Relative

The final point, that the term *distinctiveness* is relative, supervenes the preceding three points and consequently has been implicit in their discussion. The relativity of distinctiveness has long been emphasized by those who are serious about using distinctiveness as an explanatory concept rather than as an independent variable (Jacoby & Craik, 1979), and as obvious as the point may be, it is fundamentally important to discussion of what the term *distinctiveness* denotes.

With a paper by Lockhart et al. (1976), distinctiveness began to replace depth of processing as an explanation of differences in retention. In this paper, discriminability of memory traces was argued to be an important determinant of retention, and trace discriminability was the result of qualitative differences in processing. Highly discriminable traces were the result of distinctive processing. Jacoby and Craik (1979) suggested that the memory trace is a functional description of an item. The utility of a trace at retrieval depends on its descriptive contrast with other items. On this view, distinctiveness is inherently relative because a description is necessarily relative to a given context: "Distinctiveness requires change against some background of commonality" (p. 3).

That distinctive processing is relative to the context in which an item occurs is evident from numerous phenomena to which the term *distinctiveness* has been applied. The isolation effect describes better memory for an item in one context relative to memory for the same item in a different context. Orthographically distinctive words are better remembered than orthographically common words only if presented in mixed lists (Hunt & Elliot, 1980). The same holds for bizarre sentences under most circumstances (Einstein & McDaniel, 1987; McDaniel, Einstein, DeLosh, May, & Brady, 1995). Many other examples exist (Schmidt, 1991).

However obvious the relativity of distinctiveness may be, the implications for the use of the term in memory research are instructive. As Jacoby and Craik (1979) argue, relative concepts such as distinctiveness are used differently than are absolute terms such as *strength*. For example, the word *trumpet* is better remembered when embedded in a list of fruit names than when it occurs in a list of musical instruments. This result could be explained by saying that the representation of *trumpet* in the fruit list is "stronger" than is the representation of *trumpet* in the musical instrument list. In so doing, however, the term *strength* merely serves as a description of the data. Explanation of the memory phenomenon requires an answer to the obvious question of why "strength" should differ. One such explanation comes from the intuitive theory of distinctiveness where "strength" of the isolate is enhanced by additional processing attracted by the item's salience. As we have seen, however, the data have not been kind to the intuitive theory.

Alternatively, the relative concept of distinctiveness can be applied to situations in which the qualitative dimensions giving rise to distinctive processing have been described—dimensions including materials, the subject's intent, and the relationship between the study-test contexts. Description of these qualitative dimensions specifies the necessary relative context for distinctive processing. Applied to the preceding example, the dimensions along which *trumpet* in the isolation list is more distinguishable are specified easily, satisfying the criterion for the use of the term *distinctive processing*. When used in these circumstances, *distinctiveness* is a description of processes underlying performance and thus is an explanatory concept, not a term for describing the setting operations (independent variables) or the performance resulting from those operations.

DISTINCTIVENESS AS A THEORETICAL CONCEPT

The use of distinctiveness as an explanatory concept began with refinements to levels of processing, but the development of the concept benefited from a contrast between the literature on levels of processing and the literature on organization. Organization, a prominent topic in the transition from verbal learning to memory (Miller, 1956; Tulving, 1962), was conceived as a process of developing a common code for a set of discrete items. Organization thus places a premium on the relationships among items in explaining memory performance. The focus of levels of processing, in contrast, was on the individual item. Relational processing among the items was not in the purview of levels of processing: "It is now possible to entertain the hypothesis that optimal processing of individual words, qua words, is sufficient to support good recall" (Craik & Tulving, 1975, p. 270).

The gap between the literatures was bridged by a distinction between item-specific and relational processing, first drawn by Humphreys (1976). Relational processing captured the importance of organization in that it refers to the processing of dimensions common to all items within an event. The dimensions can range from semantic to fundamental spatial/temporal commonality. Item-specific processing refers to the processing of properties of individual items not shared by other items within the event. The combination of relational and item-specific processing should potentiate accurate memory because it specifies both the context defining an event and unique properties of a particular item within that event. This prediction was confirmed by research showing much higher levels of memory following combined relational and item-specific processing than following either type of processing alone (Einstein & Hunt, 1980; Hunt & Einstein, 1981). The precise specification (or *description*, to use Jacoby and Craik's term) of an item provided by relational and item-specific processing seems capture the important discriminative function of distinctive processing (Hunt & McDaniel, 1993).

At a fundamental level, the organization and levels of processing literatures, as well as the relational/item-specific distinction, represent contrasting emphases on the importance of similarity and difference. Consequently, research on similarity judgment became important to the development of the concept of distinctive processing. Discoveries about difference judgments were especially informative. In particular, it is now clear that the production of differences depends on similarity. Markman and

Gentner, (1993) report that when participants were asked to produce differences between two items, the number of differences produced and the speed with which they were produced are positively related to the similarity of the items.

Importantly, the differences that were produced differed qualitatively as a function of the similarity of the items. What are the differences between *dog* and *cat*? What are the differences between *gasoline* and *tree*? In the case of related items such as *dog* and *cat*, the differences tend to be conceptually related to the dimension of similarity. For example, one might say that dogs bark and cats meow. These are differences along the dimension of sounds that animals make, and the combination of the dimension of similarity with the differences is highly diagnostic of particular items. Differences between unrelated items, such as *gasoline* and *tree*, are more difficult to produce because there is no obvious dimension of similarity. Thus, one might say that gasoline is a liquid and a tree is solid. This information has little diagnostic value with respect to the particular items because the stated differences correspond to a large number of possible items.

Extrapolating from research based on intentional judgment of similarity and difference, let us assume that the normal course of perception and comprehension involves the processing of similarity among items of an event. The dimension of similarity confers coherence to the event. We label these events at various grain sizes—for example, *lunch, vacation, last year*—but regardless of grain size, the constituent items share one or more dimensions of similarity. The dimensions of similarity do not, however, specify particular items. Precise specification of an item within an event requires processing of differences between that item and other elements of the event. In accord with research on difference judgments, processed differences are dependent on the dimension of processed similarity. The combined processing of similarity and difference yields a precise description of the item. I suggest that this is exactly what we mean by the term *distinctiveness*: the processing of difference in the context of similarity.

This view of distinctive processing follows the precedent established by levels of processing of treating memory as a by-product of perception and comprehension. The perceived dimensions of similarity and the processing of differences within those dimensions are determined by contextual constraints imposed by materials and intentions. At the time of retrieval, perception and comprehension of the memory query reinstate earlier processing. To realize the benefits of distinctive processing, the cue context must reinstate the processing of the original dimensions of similarity and the differences within those dimensions. The retrieval environment is an extremely important contextual consideration for understanding distinctiveness as defined here. In addition to the cues, the demands of the task will influence the probability of distinctive processing at test. The following three examples illustrate the application of the concept of distinctive processing.

The Cause of the Isolation Effect

We have reviewed evidence showing that the isolation effect cannot be explained as the result of differential attention drawn by salience of the isolate. What is the cause of the isolation effect? A plausible answer comes directly from the application of the concept of distinctive processing to the isolation paradigm. In the isolation list, all of the items save one are similar on some dimension. The similarity of the background items exerts two effects that influence memory for the isolation list itself. The first is the obvious effect of establishing a dimension of similarity within which the difference of the isolated items is processed—that is, the isolated item is processed distinctively. The second effect is that the processing of the background items is largely confined to similarity. The background items essentially are a categorized list, and we know that lists containing at least four items from the same category encourage the processing of similarity (Hunt & Seta, 1984). Without processing of differences among these items, distinctive processing does not occur for categorized lists.

The isolation effect is indexed by comparison of memory for the isolated item in the isolation list with the same item in a control list. Control lists can be of two types. A *homogenous* control is one in which the critical item from the isolation list shares categorical similarity with all of the other items in the list. A *heterogeneous* control is one in which there is no obvious similarity among the items. Applying the concept of distinctive processing to memory for the control lists, the critical item in the homogeneous control is not processed for difference, just as is the case for background items in the isolation list. In the heterogeneous control list, no dimension of similarity is available against which to process difference. Thus, distinctive processing does not occur for the items in either type of control list. On this analysis, the isolation effect is due to impoverished processing of the critical item in the control list relative to the isolation list.

According to this analysis, the isolation effect should be eliminated if the processing of control items is properly supplemented. Hunt and Lamb (2001) conducted a series of experiments comparing memory for isolation lists with homogeneous control lists. In the first experiment, subjects studied these lists either under intentional memory instructions or by performing an orienting task requiring a difference judgment between the current word and the previous word. If the failure to process differences hampers memory in the homogeneous control, the addition of the orienting task should remedy the problem and eliminate the isolation effect. The results were in accord with this prediction. Memory for the critical item did not differ in the control and isolation lists for the groups performing a difference orienting task. The groups receiving standard intentional memory instructions showed a typical isolation effect. Importantly, memory for the isolate following intentional memory instructions was comparable to that for the same item in both the isolation and control conditions following difference judgments. This latter finding is important because it suggests that the orienting task was redundant with spontaneous processing elicited by an isolation list.

A second experiment demonstrated that the results were not peculiar to the use of an orienting task under incidental memory instructions. In this experiment, subjects performed either the difference judgment task or a similarity judgment task that required judging the similarity of the current item and the previous item. The similarity judgment task should be redundant with the spontaneous processing of similarity engaged by the homogeneous control list, and thus the isolation effect should persist following similarity judgment. The results are shown in Figure 1.2. Performance on isolation and control lists following similarity judgments showed a standard isolation effect, but as in the first experiment, the difference judgment task eliminated the effect.

The isolation effect has become the prototypical distinctiveness effect in memory, yet as we have seen, the effect has resisted interpretation from the intuitive theory driven by salience and differential attention. The simple experiments reported by Hunt and Lamb (2001) were motivated by the assumption that distinctive processing is the processing of difference in the context of similarity. This concept of distinctive processing predicted the circumstances under which the isolation effect would and would not occur. The data were consistent with these predictions, lending credibility to the use of distinctive processing as a concept.

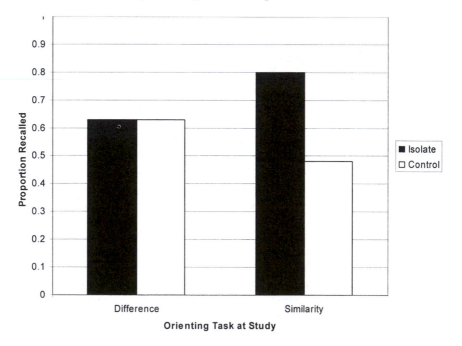

FIGURE 1.2 Proportion recalled as a function of orienting task at study and isolation versus control item from (adapted from Hunt & Lamb, 2001).

Retrieval

In accord with the principle of transfer-appropriate processing, distinctive processing exerts its effect only if the original processing is reinstated at the time of test. That processing is initiated by comprehension of the cue. When that cue corresponds directly to the dimension of distinctive processing, extremely impressive levels of recall ensue as first demonstrated by Mantyla's research (1986; Mantyla & Nilsson, 1988). For example, in one experiment (Mantyla, 1988), participants were asked to generate three attributes of each of 600 unrelated words at study. Subsequent recall cued by the self-generated attributes was 90% correct! Mantyla and Nilsson (1988) provided evidence that cue-target uniqueness was the principal contributor to this effect. Can these findings be explained by the concept of distinctive processing?

Hunt and Smith (1996) applied the concept of distinctive processing to the analysis of cue effects. In experiments inspired by Mantyla's research, subjects were asked to study categorized lists by providing either similarity or difference judgments. The lists were presented blocked by category, with five instances from each category. The orienting tasks required that the subject generate one thing about the first instance in the block that was similar to or different from the other four instances. The reasoning was that the categorical structure would encourage processing of similarity among the five items and that the difference judgment would occur in the context of this similarity. The result would be distinctive processing. The similarity-judgment task was assumed to be redundant with the processing encouraged by list structure and would produce poorer memory than the difference-judgment condition. Following study, subjects were asked to recall the single item from each category on which the judgment had been made. A cue was provided for each item consisting of either the subject's similarity or difference judgment or the similarity or difference judgments generated by another subject. Thus, the experiments allowed comparison not only of distinctive and nondistinctive processing but also of self versus other cued memory.

The results, shown in Figure 1.3, indicated that regardless of cue type, distinctive processing (difference judgment of categorized items) led to better performance than nondistinctive processing (similarity processing of categorized items). Self-generated difference cues produced much higher performance than did self-generated similarity cues; indeed, performance was near perfect with the difference cues. This result is consistent with the idea that subjects in the difference-judgment condition distinctively processed the items and that this processing was reinstated by the difference cues.

The effects of others' cues yielded an informative interaction between the type of study task and the type of cue. Someone else's difference cue led to relatively low levels of recall regardless of how the items were originally processed. The reason that someone else's distinctive cue is of little use for one's own memory lies in the original difference judgment. Very lit-

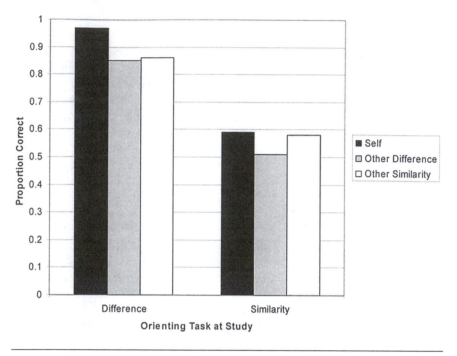

FIGURE 1.3 Proportion recalled as a function of orienting task at study and type of cue from (adapted from Hunt & Smith, 1996).

tle consensus existed on difference judgments across subjects; less than 15% of the judged differences were shared. Thus, perception and comprehension of particular differences can be quite idiosyncratic, and the cue corresponding to that judgment is incapable of reinstating the original processing even though the same cue supports near perfect memory for the person who produced it. On the other hand, the effect of someone else's similarity judgment as a cue depends on how one processes the original list. If one's original processing was through similarity judgment, someone else's similarity-judgment cues yielded levels of recall equivalent to that produced by one's own similarity judgment. This result is not mysterious because, unlike the difference judgments, the similarity judgments were highly consensual. Interestingly, when the original processing was the difference-judgment task, someone else's similarity cue produced the same high level of recall as did a self-generated difference cue. A subsequent study that required within-subject judgments of both similarity and difference showed that the subject's own similarity and difference cues were equally effective when they followed the difference judgment task at study.

Hunt and Smith's (1996) results follow directly from the assumptions in the concept of distinctive processing. The fact that difference judgments on categorized materials lead to better performance than similarity judgments can be understood as the beneficial effect of processing difference in the context of similarity. The advantage of a self-generated difference cue over a self-generated similarity cue is consistent with the expectation that the difference cue reinstated distinctive processing at the time of recall. Note that this effect is not adequately described by simply referring to the cue itself as distinctive because for each cue—similarity or difference—only one item had to be recalled and no cue had multiple target items.

The differential effect of other people's cues offers insight into what could be a rather puzzling situation. Distinctive processing followed by a self-generated difference cue produces very high levels of recall, but the perception of difference as reflected by the judgments is highly variable across people. Someone else's difference judgment does not work for one's own memory. Does this mean that the beneficial effects of distinctive processing are restricted to self-cued memory? The answer clearly is no because someone else's similarity cue produces high levels of memory when one's own original processing was distinctive. Distinctive processing involves both similarity and difference, and a cue corresponding either to the originally processed dimension of similarity or to a particular difference will be effective. Perception and labeling of similarity among familiar events is highly consensual, probably as a function of a shared social and linguistic development. You and I will comprehend the similarity among items defining events such as a lunch, faculty meeting, and wedding in the same way, and cues delineating the dimension of similarity reinstate any original distinctive processing. Through the use of these consensual cues, other people can offer cues that reengage one's own particular, idiosyncratic processing underlying highly accurate memory.

Memory Accuracy

Virtually all uses of the term *distinctiveness* refer to enhanced memory of a to-be-remembered item. Memory accuracy, however, requires not only accepting or producing correct items but also rejecting or withholding incorrect items. Distinctive processing as described thus far has nothing to say about correctly rejecting incorrect items. After all, incorrect items were not present in the targeted event and could not have been processed distinctively or otherwise. Nonetheless, there are two lines of research that have invoked distinctive processing as an important factor for correctly rejecting incorrect items; but the research presents a puzzle for the concept of distinctive processing in that the manipulations of distinctiveness that affect rejection of incorrect items have no effect on memory for correct items.

One of these lines stems from research on false memory using the Deese/Roediger/McDermott (DRM) paradigm. The paradigm entails presentation of a list of words that are all associated with a critical, nonpresented item. The result of interest is that the probability of remembering the nonpresented item is as high as that of the presented items. However, some variables associated with list presentation are now known to reduce false memory for the critical nonpresented item. Smith and Hunt (1998) discovered that visual presentation of the study list leads to fewer false responses to the critical item in both recognition and recall than does auditory presentation of the study list, a result now replicated several times (Cleary & Greene, 2002; Gallo, McDermott, Percer, & Roediger, 2001; Kellogg, 2001). This result was interpreted as an effect of distinctive processing. Smith and Hunt argued that visual processing is less like thought than is auditory processing, which allows better discrimination of studied and nonstudied items in the DRM paradigm. Schacter and his colleagues (e.g., Dodson & Schacter, 2002; Israel & Schacter, 1997) discovered that pictorial presentation of the study items in the DRM paradigm reduces false responses relative to auditory presentation. They proposed that distinctiveness could be used as a heuristic to avoid false responding. The idea is that all of the items of the original event share some property—for example, all studied items were pictures—and memory for items appearing on a recognition test can be examined for evidence of this property. In the absence of such evidence, the item will be rejected. Thus, in studies of false memory, distinctiveness has been invoked to describe the ability to correctly reject incorrect items, but unlike all of the previous discussion of distinctiveness in this chapter, the manipulation of distinctiveness had no effect on memory for correct items in any of these studies.

Similar results have emerged from research on the effects of distracter familiarity in recognition memory. Most laboratory studies of recognition use distracter items that appear only on the test, but we quite commonly are required to make recognition decisions about incorrect items that are highly familiar in the context of the test query. Suppose you sometimes, but not always, have chicken salad for lunch. When asked what you had for lunch two days ago, you might respond "chicken salad" because it is a familiar choice even if you had a hamburger that day. To model this situation, Dobbins, Kroll, Yonelinas, and Lieu (1998) asked subjects to perform an orienting task on a list of unrelated words. The subjects then were given a second list of unrelated words on which they also performed an orienting task. They also were told to remember this list for a later test. Some of the words in the first list were in the second list as well. The recognition test included words from the second list, words from the first list that were not in the second list, and novel distracters. Subjects were instructed to recognize only those words that had appeared in the second list. Distinctive processing was manipulated by requiring either the same orienting task on the two lists or different orienting tasks on the lists. The idea was that performing two different orienting tasks on the list would increase the discriminability of the lists.

Memory accuracy (hits–false alarms) was higher in the condition requiring two separate tasks on the list, but this effect was due entirely to differences in false alarms to familiar distracters. Performing separate tasks on the lists led to fewer errors on items that appeared only on the first list than did performing the same task on the two lists. Dobbins et al. (1998)

interpret their results through Jacoby's (1991) distinction between conscious and automatic processing, but the spirit of the interpretation is much the same as the distinctiveness heuristic. The assumption is that subjects performing two different tasks examine test items with the goal of detecting evidence from memory that the item was processed through the orienting task applied to the second list. In the absence of such evidence, the item is rejected. This strategy obviously would be totally ineffective for subjects performing the same orienting task on the two lists. As with the research on false memory, the manipulation of orienting tasks had no effect on hit rate. This raises the question of whether the term *distinctiveness* refers to the same thing when used to describe acceptance of correct items and rejection of incorrect items.

The concept of distinctive processing advocated here can be applied to both circumstances, but the application requires serious consideration of contextual influences, which in this case are the subtle differences in test demands for acceptance and for rejection. In all of the cited research using the term *distinctiveness* to describe effects of a variable on correct rejection of incorrect items, the correct items have been processed differently from the incorrect items. For example, in the Dobbins et al. (1998) study, *distinctive processing* refers to the use of two different orienting tasks on the two lists. The concept of distinctive processing describes this situation as the processing of differences between the two lists in the context of the similarity conferred by the spatial/temporal similarity of the experiment. The *lists* have been distinctively processed. Importantly, the conceptual analysis implies that distinctive *list* processing does not entail distinctive processing of *items within the list*. The orienting task applied to the target list may or may not encourage processing of differences among items within the context of the list.

Hunt (2003) used this conceptualization in a continuation of the research of Dobbins et al. (1998). The experiments were similar to those of Dobbins et al. in that two lists were presented with instructions to remember the second of the lists, and either the same or different orienting tasks were performed on the lists. However, two important modifications were made to the Dobbins et al. procedure. First, all items (target, pre-exposed distracters, and novel distracters) were drawn from the same set of categories. Second, the orienting tasks were selected to encourage processing of similarity or of difference among the items within a list. The similarity task required a judgment about category membership for each item and the difference tasks was pleasantness rating. These changes from Dobbins et al.'s procedure allowed examination of both list-based distinctive processing and item-based distinctive processing.

The pleasantness rating task should produce distinctive processing because within-list differences were processed in the context of categorical similarity. Thus, correct memory for the second list (hits) was predicted to be higher when the pleasant-rating task was performed on that list than when the category-judgment task was performed on the second list. The particular orienting task used on the second list should have no effect on false alarms to first-list items because the second-list orienting task does not discriminate between first- and second-list items. That discrimination would be controlled by list-based distinctive processing—namely, the use of different orienting tasks on the two lists regardless of which type of task is used on the target list. List-based distinctive processing should reduce incorrect acceptance of familiar distracters that were present in the first list but at the same time have no effect on correct acceptance of second-list target items.

The results are shown in Figure 1.4 as a function of conditions, which were defined by the particular combination of orienting tasks used on the two lists. The data were consistent with the predictions of distinctive processing. The hit rate—correct acceptance of second-list items—was determined solely by the orienting task performed on that list: pleasantness rating led to higher hit rates than category judgment. The false alarm rate to familiar distracters—incorrect acceptance of first-list items—was determined solely by whether the same or different orienting tasks were used on

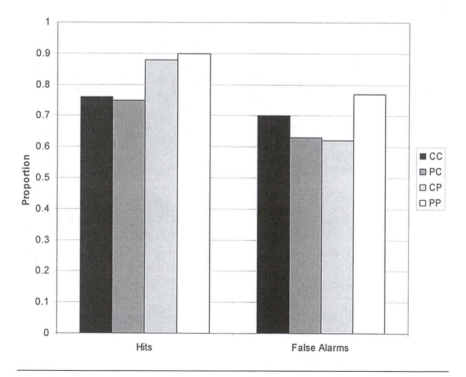

FIGURE 1.4 Proportion of hits and false alarms as a function of orienting task condition (adapted from Hunt, 2003). The conditions are labeled C = category judgment task and P = pleasantness rating task. The first letter is the task applied to list 1 and the second letter is the task applied to list 2. List 2 items were the targeted memory items.

the two lists. As was the case with Dobbins et al. (1998) and the cited research on false memory, the manipulation affecting false alarms had no effect on hits.

One might be tempted to interpret all of these data in terms of source monitoring by assuming that the distinctiveness manipulation reduces false alarms by facilitating correct attribution of the list source. But if this were true, would we not expect the same manipulation to affect hit rates? That is, if I can reject incorrect items because I have access to accurate source information, then I also should be able to accept correct items on the basis of that same source information. On the other hand, if performance is interpreted in terms of processing differences in the context of similarity, processing of differences between lists is not the same as processing differences among items within a list. The former affects false alarms to familiar distracters and the latter affects hits. But both are distinctive processing.

The analysis recommends a corollary distinction between event-based (list) and item-based (item within list) processing. Prior processing can facilitate the decision that an item was not a constituent of the cue-defined event without exerting an effect on the decision that an item was in the event. Like the concept of distinctive processing, the distinction between event-based and item-based processing is totally dependent on context, in this case largely defined by the cues. That is, I am not proposing that perception is parsed into events and items at encoding and stored for subsequent retrieval; after all, we rarely know what we will have to remember from a current experience. Rather, the cues for memory circumscribe some event in the form of a dimension of similarity shared by some set of particular items.

Thus, when applying the concept of distinctive processing, one must keep in mind that the target item and the event in which it is embedded are defined by the cues for memory. The grain size of events and targets can vary with the cue, as illustrated by the following examples:

- *What did you do yesterday?* In this case, the event is yesterday and the targets are anything you did yesterday.
- *What did you do at work yesterday?* Now the event is work yesterday and the targets are things you did at work. Notice that work yesterday could have been a target item for the query about what you did yesterday as well as serving as the event for the things done at work.
- *What did you have for lunch yesterday?* Lunch yesterday now becomes the event for the targeted items. Again, lunch yesterday could have been a target for either of the previous queries.

The point here is that conceptual analysis in terms of distinctive processing begins by identifying the targets and events defined by a particular cue. Then one determines the nature of the original processing for those elements. Distinctive processing will enhance memory accuracy for whatever information is targeted by the cue, but it appears that the effect on accuracy—correct acceptance of correct items versus correct rejection of incorrect items—differs for distinctive processing of cue-defined events and cue-defined items.

CONCLUSIONS

If *distinctiveness* is to be a useful term in memory research, we must attempt an answer to the question "What is distinctiveness?" Obtaining an answer requires analysis of the term by examining definitional and logical nuances as well as how the term is used by researchers. As Tulving (2000) points out, the "what" question is just as important as the "how" and "why" questions that dominate normal research activities. After all, the answer to the "what" question will shape the experiments and their interpretations. Most important, the conceptual analysis required to address the "what" question will add clarity and reduce needless disagreements in our discussions.

The analysis of distinctiveness offered here has yielded two very different meanings of the term in memory discourse. In one case, *distinctiveness* refers to a characteristic of an event. In common usage, the characteristic is attributed to an object in the environment, but analysis of the term indicates that careful application requires *distinctiveness* to refer to a characteristic of a psychological event. Thus the answer to the "what" question is that distinctiveness is a psychological representation that is notably different from other representations. This answer then dictates the approach to the questions "Why is memory affected by distinctiveness?" and "How is this effect accomplished?" On this meaning, *distinctiveness* essentially refers to an independent variable. The traditional explanation of the effect of the variable assumes that the distinctive representation attracts attention and extraordinary processing. Unfortunately, the data raise serious questions about this interpretation. Thus, continued use of the term with the connotation of an independent variable will be fruitful only if a more satisfactory explanation for its effect is forthcoming. In any event, this meaning of *distinctiveness* precludes the use of the term as an explanation for memory phenomena.

The second meaning of *distinctiveness* identified here is an explanatory concept. "What" distinctiveness is is the processing of difference in the context of similarity. Such processing facilitates memory because it precisely specifies items within events—the answer to the "why" question. "How" this happens is that similarity delineates the episodic context of the item and combines with diagnostic differences among items. As an abstract concept, distinctive processing can be applied as an explanation for a range of memory phenomena (Hunt & McDaniel, 1993). The utility of the concept rests with the success of these applications in increasing our understanding of extant issues. To the extent that this success is achieved, distinctive processing can be a valuable explanatory concept in memory research.

ACKNOWLEDGEMENTS

The chapter benefited from the comments of Jim Worthen and Rebekah Smith on a previous draft. The chapter is based on a presentation to the Southwestern Psychological Association, New Orleans, April 2003.

REFERENCES

Baddeley, A. D. (1978). The trouble with levels: A reexamination of Craik and Lockhart's framework for memory research. *Psychological Review, 85,* 139–152.

Begg, I. (1978). Similarity and contrasts in memory for relations. *Memory & Cognition, 6,* 509–517.

Calkins, M. W. (1894). Association. *Psychological Review, 1,* 476–483.Calkins, M. W. (1896). Association: An essay analytic and experimental. *Psychological Monographs, 1,* 1–56.

Cleary, A. M., & Greene, R. L. (2002). Paradoxical effects of presentation modality on false memory. *Memory,* 10, 55–61.

Cooper, E. H., & Pantle, A. J. (1967). The total-time hypothesis in verbal learning. *Psychological Bulletin, 68,* 221–243.

Craik, F. I. M., & Lockhart, R. S. (1972). Levels of processing: A framework for memory research. *Journal of Verbal Learning and Verbal Behavior, 11,* 671–684.

Craik, F. I. M., & Tulving, E. (1975). Depth of processing and the retention of words in episodic memory. *Journal of Experimental Psychology: General, 104,* 268–294.

Dobbins, I. G., Kroll, N. E. A., Yonelinas, A. P., & Liu, Q. (1998). Distinctiveness in recognition and free recall: The role of recollection in rejection of the familiar. *Journal of Memory and Language, 38,* 381–400.

Dodson, C. S., & Schacter, D. L. (2002). When false recognition meets metacognition: The distinctiveness heuristic. *Journal of Memory and Language,* 46, 782–803.

Dunlosky, J., Hunt, R. R., & Clark, E. (2000). Is perceptual salience needed in explanations of the isolation effect? *Journal of Experimental Psychology: Learning, Memory, and Cognition, 26,* 649–657.

Einstein, G. O., & Hunt, R. R. (1980). Levels of processing and organization: Additive effects of individual item and relational processing. *Journal of Experimental Psychology: Human learning and Memory, 6,* 588–598.

Einstein, G. O., & McDaniel, M. A. (1987). Distinctiveness and mnemonic benefits of bizarre imagery. In M. A. McDaniel & M. Pressley (Eds.), *Imagery and related mnemonic processes: Theories, individual differences, and applications.* (pp. 78–102) New York: Springer-Verlag.

Epstein, M. L., Phillips, W. D., & Johnson, S. J. (1975). Recall of related and unrelated word pairs as a function of processing level. *Journal of Experimental Psychology: Human Learning and Memory, 1,* 149–152.

Gallo, D. A., McDermott, K. B., Percer, J. M., and Roediger, H. L. III. (2001). Modality effects in false recall and false recognition. *Journal of Experimental Psychology: Learning, Memory, and Cognition, 27,* 339–353.

Green, R. T. (1956). Surprise as a factor in the von Restorff effect. *Journal of Experimental Psychology, 52,* 340–344.

Humphreys, M. S. (1976). Relational information and the context effect in recognition memory. *Memory & Cognition, 4,* 221–232.

Hunt, R. R. (1995). The subtlety of distinctiveness: What von Restorff really did. *Psychonomic Bulletin & Review, 2,* 105–112.

Hunt, R. R. (2003). Two contributions of distinctive processing to accurate memory. *Journal of Memory and Language, 48,* 811–825.

Hunt, R. R., & Einstein, G. O. (1981) Relational and item-specific information in memory. *Journal of Verbal Learning and Verbal Behavior, 20,* 497–514.

Hunt, R. R., & Elliott, J. M. (1980). The role of nonsemantic information in memory: Orthographic distinctiveness effects on retention. *Journal of Experimental Psychology: General, 109,* 49–75.

Hunt, R. R. & Lamb, C. A. (2001). What causes the isolation effect? *Journal of Experimental Psychology: Learning, Memory, and Cognition, 27,* 1359–1366.

Hunt, R. R., & McDaniel, M. A. (1993). The enigma of organization and distinctiveness. *Journal of Memory and Language, 32,* 421–445.

Hunt, R. R., & Seta, C. E. (1984). Category size effects in recall: The roles of relational and individual item information. *Journal of Experimental Psychology: Learning, Memory, and Cognition, 10,* 454–464.

Hunt, R. R., & Smith, R. E. (1996). Accessing the particular from the general: The power of distinctiveness in the context of organization. *Memory and Cognition, 24,* 217–225.

Israel, L., & Schacter, D. L. (1997). Pictorial encoding reduces false recognition of semantic associates. *Psychological Bulletin & Review, 4,* 577–581.

Jacoby, L. L. (1991). A process dissociation framework: Separating automatic from intentional uses of memory. *Journal of Memory and Language, 30,* 513–541.

Jacoby, L. L., & Craik, F. I. M. (1979). Effects of elaboration of processing at encoding and retrieval: Trace distinctiveness and recovery of initial context. In L. S. Cermak & F. I. M. Craik (Eds.), *Levels of processing in human memory.* (pp. 1–22) Hillsdale, NJ: Lawrence Erlbaum Associates.

Jenkins, W. O., & Postman, L. (1948). Isolation and the spread of effect in serial learning. *American Journal of Psychology, 61,* 214–221.

Jersild, A. (1929). Primacy, recency, frequency, and vividness. *Journal of Experimental Psychology, 12,* 58–70.

Kellogg, R. (2001). Presentation modality and mode of recall in verbal false memory. *Journal of Experimental Psychology: Learning, Memory and Cognition, 27,* 913–919.

Kelley, M. R., & Nairne, J. S. (2001). Von Restorff revisited: Isolation, generation, and memory for order. *Journal of Experimental Psychology: Learning, Memory, and Cognition, 27,* 54–66.

Koriat, A. (1997). Monitoring one's own knowledge during study: A cue-utilization approach to judgments of learning. *Journal of Experimental Psychology: General, 126,* 349–370.

Lockhart, R. S., Craik, F. I. M., & Jacoby, L. L. (1976). Depth of processing, recognition, and recall: Some aspects of a general memory system. In J. Brown (Ed.), *Recall and recognition* (pp. 75–102). London: Wiley.

Mantyla, T. (1986). Optimizing cue effectiveness: Recall of 500 and 600 incidentally learned words. *Journal of Experimental Psychology: Learning, Memory, and Cognition, 12,* 66–71.

Mantyla, T., & Nilsson, L. (1988). Cue distinctiveness and forgetting: Effectiveness of self-generated retrieval cues in delayed recall. *Journal of Experimental Psychology: Learning, Memory, and Cognition, 14,* 502–509.

Markman, E., & Gentner, D. (1993). Structural Alignment during similarity comparisons. *Cognitive Psychology, 25,* 431–467.

McDaniel, M. A., Einstein, G. O., DeLosh, E. L., May, C. P., & Brady, P. (1995). The bizarreness effect: It's not surprising, it's complex. *Journal of Experimental Psychology: Learning, Memory, and Cognition, 21,* 422–435.

Miller, G. A. (1956). The magical number seven, plus or minus two: Some limits on our capacity for processing information. *Psychological Review, 63,* 81–97.

Oxford American Dictionary (1980). New York: Oxford University Press.

Pillsbury, W. B., & Rausch, H. L. (1943). An extension of the Koler-Restorff inhibition phenomenon. *American Journal of Psychology, 56,* 293–298.

Rundus, D. (1971). Analysis of rehearsal processes in free recall. *Journal of Experimental Psychology, 89,* 63–77.

Schmidt, S. R. (1991). Can we have a distinctive theory of memory? *Memory and Cognition, 19,* 523–542.

Smith, R. E., & Hunt, R. R. (1998). Presentation modality affects false memory. *Psychonomic Bulletin & Review, 5,* 710–715.

Tulving, E. (1962). Subjective organization in free recall of "unrelated" words. *Psychological Review, 69,* 344–354.

Tulving, E. (2000). Concepts of memory. In E. Tulving & F. I. M. Craik (Eds.), *The Oxford handbook of memory* (pp. 33–44). New York: Oxford University Press.

Van Buskirk, W. L. (1932). An experimental study of vividness in learning and retention. *Journal of Experimental Psychology, 15,* 563–573.

von Restorff, H. (1933). Uber die Wirkung von Bereichsblidungen im Spurenfeld. *Psychologishe Forschung, 18,* 299–342.

Wallace, W. P. (1965). Review of the historical, empirical, and theoretical status of the von Restorff phenomenon. *Psychological Bulletin, 63,* 410–442.

2

Modeling Distinctiveness:
Implications for General Memory Theory

JAMES S. NAIRNE

The capacity to remember, to use the past in the service of the present, is a highly adaptive component of cognitive functioning. Although one need not reproduce the past, either consciously or unconsciously, in order to benefit from the service of memory, reproduction is clearly an important design feature (Anderson & Schooler, 2000; Nairne, 2005). Telephone numbers, street addresses, medication times, passwords—each needs to be recovered exactly, with the components in sequence, and inferential or reconstructive processing is unlikely to suffice.

To explain the specificity of retention, students of memory appeal often to the concept of distinctiveness, the focus of the present volume. Mnemonic distinctiveness can be defined in various ways—for example, as a property of a stored trace, a retrieval cue, or as a type of processing (see Hunt, Chapter 1 this volume; Schmidt, 1991). I define it here as the extent to which a particular cue (or set of cues) specifies a particular stored event (or target response) to the exclusion of others. Framed in this way, distinctiveness is not a fixed property of a cue, or a target trace, or even of an interaction between a given cue and a given target. It is a property of a cue in context: given a fixed set of alternatives, a measure of distinctiveness can be assigned to a particular cue with respect to a particular alternative. Change the context—for example, by changing how the cue is perceived or the range of possible responses—and the measure of distinctiveness changes as well.

To facilitate our discussion, and to add some formality to the preceding definition, I introduce a simple retrieval model below (borrowed from my feature model of immediate retention; Nairne, 1990a) and show how it helps account for some of the phenomena classically associated with the study of distinctiveness. For example, I show how the model informs us about the particulars of the von Restorff effect (Hunt, 1995;

von Restorff, 1933) and about the paradoxical effects of processing similarity and difference on episodic retrieval (Hunt & McDaniel, 1993). I then consider the role of time in the calculation of distinctiveness and contrast the retrieval model with certain extant models of temporal distinctiveness (e.g., Brown, Neath, & Chater, 2002; Neath, 1993). Finally, I end the chapter by discussing how the retrieval model forces us to reassess some widely held beliefs about memory, particularly the notion that memory is directly related to the match between an encoded cue and an encoded target.

A SIMPLE MODEL

Directed retrieval reduces ultimately to a matter of response selection. There is a vast storehouse of information in the brain; the retrieval problem is to select appropriate content based on information available in the present. When we forget an item from a memory list, we are not really forgetting the item—-we are forgetting that it occurred in a particular space and time defined by the memory list; when we forget where we parked our car, we are not forgetting our car, we are forgetting the position our car occupied today as opposed to yesterday or the day before. Retrieval cues help us solve these kinds of discrimination problems. They provide us with the information we need to pick and choose from the wide variety of responses that are potentially available.

   To formalize the response selection process, I adopt a simple retrieval, or choice, rule of the type often found in categorization and some memory models (e.g., Nosofsky, 1986; Nairne, 1990a, 2001). Under this formulation, an item is chosen for recall by comparing, or matching, the operative retrieval cue(s) to possible candidates in long-term memory (see also Raaijmakers & Shiffrin, 1980). The probability that any particular event, E_1, will be selected as the recall candidate depends on how well the retrieval cue, X_1, matches E_1 to the exclusion of other possible recall candidates (e.g., E_2, E_3, . . . ,E_N):

$$P_r\,(E_1|X_1) = \frac{s(X_1,E_1)}{\Sigma s(X_1,E_i)} \tag{1}$$

The quantity $s(X_1,E_1)$ refers to the similarity of X_1 to E_1, which in turn varies as a function of the number of matching or mismatching features between the two terms (a distance measure). Shepard (1987) recommends relating distance (d) to similarity in the following manner:

$$s(X_1,\,E_1) = e^{-d(X_1,E_1)} \tag{2}$$

This means that nearby items in psychological space (e.g., those that contain few mismatching features) will be deemed the most similar (and thereby produce the largest effects), and similarity will fall off rapidly with increasing distance.

Equations 1 and 2 are not meant to suffice as a complete model of memory. Among other things, one needs to specify how event traces are represented in memory, how probabilities translate into actual output (Nairne, 1990a; Raaijmakers & Shiffrin, 1980), and the similarity and distance measures need to be scaled appropriately as well (Nosofsky, 1986; Shepard, 1987). However, as I demonstrate below, this simple ratio model provides a nice conceptual framework for interpreting the empirical patterns of concern in the distinctiveness literature. Note that equation 1, which expresses the probability that a particular target event will be selected, doubles as our measure of distinctiveness. Distinctiveness is therefore a property of a cue, but only with respect to a particular retrieval candidate. By itself, the measure tells us nothing about whether the retrieval candidate is correct or incorrect, or good or bad from a mnemonic standpoint.

If the goal is to recover event E_1 in the presence of a particular cue X_1, then equation 1 isolates the factors that promote successful sampling. To maximize the probability of selecting E_1, it needs to be similar to the cue, X_1, and dissimilar to other possible retrieval candidates (E_2, E_3, . . . ,E_N). The numerator of equation 1 tells us that retrieval will depend importantly on the match between the retrieval cue and the target (Thomson & Tulving, 1970); the denominator quantifies cue overload, or the extent to which a cue is predictive of many things (Earhard, 1967; Watkins & Watkins, 1975). Successful recovery, put generally, will be proportional to the cue–target match and inversely proportional to the amount of cue overload. Note that because of the ratio form, neither the cue–target match nor the amount of cue overload, alone, will be sufficient to predict successful retention; successful recovery of a target will always depend on both. As I discuss later, this conclusion has a number of implications for general memory theory.

The von Restorff Effect

To illustrate how the retrieval rule works, I begin by applying it to the von Restorff effect—the so-called mother of all distinctiveness effects (Hunt & Lamb, 2001). The *von Restorff effect* (or isolation effect) refers to the memory enhancement that is found for events that differ, or deviate, from their context. In von Restorff's original experiments, participants recalled 10-item lists containing either 10 unrelated items (list 1), nine numbers and one nonsense syllable (list 2), or nine nonsense syllables and one number (list 3). The discrepant items were remembered best (e.g., the number in the list of syllables)—even better, in fact, than the unrelated items occupying similar list positions (e.g., items from list 1), or the "background" homogenous items (e.g., the syllables in list 3).

In experiments of this type, items become distinctive by virtue of their list context; that is, items are "isolated" only relative to particular backgrounds. To consider a specific case, if the number 43 was presented in each of the three von Restorff lists, we would expect its retention to be enhanced only in list 3, where it stands out from the other list items. For the effect to emerge, typically, the nonisolated (or background) items need to share some measure of similarity—that is, the detection of "difference" depends on a background of similarity (see Hunt, Chapter 1 this volume; Smith & Hunt, 2000). As I will discuss later, it is possible to reduce or eliminate the isolation advantage simply by asking people to focus their processing on how items differ from one another in a typical von Restorff list (Hunt & Lamb, 2001).

The isolation advantage also remains robust when the isolate occurs early in the list, even in the first serial position (Kelley & Nairne, 2001; Pillsbury & Rausch, 1943). This is an important finding because it suggests that the locus of the effect should be placed at retrieval. Encoding-centered accounts have been proposed over the years, and it seems reasonable to argue that isolates sometimes do capture more attentional resources (Schmidt, 1991), but encoding-centered accounts have difficulty explaining why the effect is found when the isolate occurs in the first or second serial position. At this point, no list context has been established, so there is no background of similarity against which the item can be considered unusual or especially salient. Instead, as embodied in the retrieval model, it makes more sense to assume that the isolate leads to the encoding of features that potentially help one discriminate its prior occurrence at retrieval, after all of the list items have been presented.[1]

To implement the model, it is necessary to make some assumptions about how items are represented in memory, about how similarity is calculated, and about the nature and generation of retrieval cues. Following Nairne (1990a), one can represent items as lists of features and distance derived by comparing features across each position. The number of mismatching features is summed and the total is then divided by the number of compared features. For example, suppose memory trace A is represented by a vector of five features, [C C 2 3 1], and memory trace B by a second vector, [C X 2 2 1]. A feature-by-feature comparison reveals two mismatching features—in positions 2 and 4. Dividing the number of mismatching features (2) by the number of compared features (5) gives us the distance measure (.40). This distance measure is then plugged into equation 2, yielding a similarity value of .67. (For further numerical examples, see Nairne, 1990, 2001.).

In the retrieval model, the critical similarity comparisons are between cues and viable retrieval candidates stored in long-term memory. Like most memory theorists, I assume that the immediate present is used to recover the past—that is, memories do not spontaneously appear, but rather are cue-driven (Tulving, 1983). In the feature model, which deals primarily with remembering over the short term, the operative retrieval cues are lingering records of the immediate past, which can be accessed directly (from primary memory) or recovered through context. When one is remembering over the longer term, a comparable process occurs: some version of the original encoding record is recovered via context and "interpreted" by sampling from a candidate set of possible responses. Equation 2 specifies how the recovery process proceeds: the record is compared to each possible item in the candidate set and, based on the relative similarity values, a candidate is selected for recall (see Nairne, 2001, 2002a).

A Numerical Example

Table 2.1 shows similarity and sampling probabilities for some hypothetical three-item lists. Encoded list items are represented by trace vectors of five features (e.g., a sequence of letters and digits). The first list, labeled "Control," is meant to contain three unrelated items, although, importantly, some measure of similarity is assumed (e.g., overlapping contextual features). The cue, shown to the left, is an intact version of the second list item; under normal conditions, this cue would presumably be a blurry or degraded record of the encoding, but it is presented intact here for the sake of simplicity. The last two columns show the similarity and sampling calculations based on the comparisons between this cue and each of the three list traces. Correct recall, given this cue, occurs when the second list item is sampled and successfully recovered (see Nairne, 1990a, for details).

The second list, labeled "Isolate," instantiates the isolation manipulation: A new nonoverlapping feature, X, is represented in the trace for item 2, replacing one of the shared contextual features (we might assume, for example, that the second list item was presented in a unique color or voice). In all other respects, items remain the same. Note that the similarity value between the cue and its long-term memory representation remains the same, 1.0, but the probability of sampling that target increases. This is the isola-

TABLE 2.1 Similarity Values and Sampling Probabilities Generated by the Retrieval Model for a Hypothetical Three-Item List

	Cue	Traces	Similarity	Samp. Prob.
Control	[C C 2 3 1]	[C C 1 2 3]	.55	.26
		[C C 2 3 1]	1.0	.48
		[C C 3 1 2]	.55	.26
Isolate	[C X 2 3 1]	[C C 1 2 3]	.45	.24
		[C X 2 3 1]	1.0	.53
		[C C 3 1 2]	.45	.24
Iso/Sim	[C C 2 3 1]	[B B B B 3]	.37	.21
		[C C 2 3 1]	1.0	.58
		[B B B B 2]	.37	.21

Note: All of the calculations are based on a cue vector representing the second item on the list. Sampling probabilties may not add to one because of rounding.

tion effect, and it is caused here by a reduction in cue overload: the correct target is more likely to be sampled because the cue is now less similar to other candidates. The addition of feature X, which is unique to the encoding of the second list item in this list context, reduces the number of matching features between the cue and the target's competitors.

The third list, labeled "Iso/Sim," shows what happens when the control item from the first list is presented against a background of highly similar items. This is the same target representation and cue as in the first list, and the cue–target match remains perfect, but the probability of correctly sampling the target increases substantially. Once again, what determines performance is the overlap between the features of the target item and those of the background items. As the similarity among the background items increases, their match with the operative retrieval cue decreases. Note, however, that it is not background similarity per se that mediates performance; what matters is the overlap between the cue and the nontarget competitors. If the similarity of the background items increases, but in a way that also increases their match with the retrieval cue, then performance would suffer rather than improve.

Of course, recovery of the isolated item in the model also depends on how well the cue matches the relevant target. The cue–target match is held constant in Table 2.1, but it easy to imagine isolation improving the functional cue–target match. For example, by definition an isolated item contains features that are unusual in that list context; consequently, those features, once encoded, are probably less susceptible to interference (i.e., overwriting) from subsequently presented items. This should help guarantee an intact cue at retrieval, one that better matches its representation in long-term memory. Moreover, when the isolated item occurs after the list context has been established, its appearance is surprising, which in turn could enrich the overall encoding (or hurt encoding in some circumstances—see Schmidt, Chapter 3 this volume). Richer or more elaborate encodings tend to be matched better by relevant retrieval cues and more protected from interference. In any given situation, it will be difficult to disentangle the relative contributions of the cue–target match and changes in the amount of cue overload; the presence or absence of unusual features is likely to affect both.

Background Recall

It is also of interest to consider how the presence of an isolated item affects recall of the nonisolated (background) items in the list. In principle, one can conceive of the isolate acting in several ways: enhancing recall of the isolate itself, reducing memory for the background items, or leading to both outcomes. The literature is somewhat equivocal in regard to background recall; sometimes the presence of an isolate hurts the retention of the other list items (e.g., Schmidt, 2002; Schulz, 1971), sometimes recall of those items improves (Farrell & Lewandowsky, 2003), and often there is no effect (e.g., Kelley & Nairne, 2001).

Theoretically, it is easy to justify any of these outcomes. From an organizational perspective, some theorists have argued that the isolate promotes the formation of two list-based categories, one containing the isolated item and a second category comprising the background items (Bruce & Gaines, 1976; Fabiani & Donchin, 1995). Because it is easier to recall items from smaller categories, better memory is expected for both the isolate and the background items. Alternatively, if the isolate captures more attentional resources, or is more likely to be rehearsed, then recall of the background items should suffer because they receive a smaller proportion of the allocated resources. One could argue as well that isolated items, because of their superior mnemonic value, will tend to be recalled early during output, rendering the remaining items subject to more output interference (e.g., Cunningham, Marmie, & Healy, 1998; Schmidt, 1985).

The retrieval model makes no explicit assumptions about encoding, organizational processing, or selective rehearsal; it merely assumes that the recall of an item (isolate or background) will depend on the cue, its match to the relevant target, and the composition of the competitor set. Table 2.2 shows the similarity and sampling values for a background item in our three hypothetical lists. In this case, the cue is for the first list item instead of the isolate, and the correct response is to sample the first of the three list vectors. (Identical values hold for the third item.) Note that the sampling probabilities for this background item change across the three conditions.

Of initial interest is the comparison between lists with and without an isolate. The probability of correctly sampling the first list item in the Control condition is .48 compared to .50 in the Isolate condition. This slight increase, which is predicted by a grouping or organizational account, is caused here by a net decrease in the amount of cue overload (the overall

TABLE 2.2 Similarity Values and Sampling Probabilities for the Background Items in a Hypothetical Three-Item List

	Cue	Traces	Similarity	Samp. Prob.
Control	[C C 1 2 3]	[C C 1 2 3]	1.0	.48
		[C C 2 3 1]	.55	.26
		[C C 3 1 2]	.55	.26
Isolate	[C C 1 2 3]	[C C 1 2 3]	1.0	.50
		[C X 2 3 1]	.45	.23
		[C C 3 1 2]	.55	.28
Iso/Sim	[B B B B 3]	[B B B B 3]	1.0	.46
		[C C 2 3 1]	.37	.17
		[B B B B 2]	.82	.37

Note: All of the calculations are based on a cue vector representing the first item on the list. Sampling probabilities may not add to one because of rounding.

value of the denominator in equation 1 goes down). Because there are fewer overlapping features between the isolate and everything else, the isolate is less likely to be sampled when cued by traces left by any of the other list items. Interestingly, the presence of an isolate actually increases the distinctiveness of the remaining items on the list. The effect is small because the decrease in the denominator is caused only by the comparison between the cue and the isolate; with longer lists, this contribution is less important—it is proportionally smaller—which may help explain why a null effect of the isolate on background recall is often reported.

The same reasoning applies to the third condition, Iso/Sim, although background recall is low relative to the other two conditions. Cues for the background items are less distinctive in this condition because the members of the competitor set (with the exception of the isolate) share lots of features. Despite the low sampling probability, however, background performance is not actually hurt by the presence of the isolated item; in fact, for the same reasons discussed in the preceding paragraph, having an isolate in the list improves the sampling probabilities for background items, at least relative to a list containing all similar items. From the model's perspective, any manipulation that decreases the overlap among traces will increase the likelihood of correct cue–target sampling (assuming the cue–target match remains constant). Consequently, whether background items will show a benefit, no effect, or a loss will depend on the control condition and on other factors such as the length of the lists employed.

Processing Effects

As noted, in its simplest form the retrieval model makes no assumptions about encoding or processing. The isolation effect, as well as background recall, is determined solely by the state of cues, targets, and competitors at the point of recall. However, any encoding manipulation that affects trace composition is likely to influence performance. As discussed earlier, when an isolate occurs late in a list, its surprise value could easily lead to additional processing (or more rehearsal), which in turn could produce a more elaborate memory trace. Moreover, any orienting task that causes participants to focus on common or unique features across to-be-remembered items should have significant effects on performance as well.

In one relevant study, Hunt and Lamb (2001) examined how various orienting tasks affect the isolation advantage. Participants were given lists containing either 10 related items (e.g., a list of vegetables) or 9 related items and 1 item from a different category (e.g., a tool). The standard isolation advantage was produced across the lists—that is, the tool in the list of vegetables was remembered best. Of main interest, however, were several orienting tasks that induced participants to compare item characteristics during presentation. In one condition, participants were asked to state how each item differed from the one immediately preceding it in the list;

in another condition, judgments of similarity were required. Once again, these judgments were made on lists either containing an isolate or not.

Two major findings emerged. First, when participants were asked to focus on item differences, the isolation effect was eliminated; second, when the orienting task was similarity-based, a robust isolation effect occurred. If we assume that the "difference-based" orienting task created list traces with little or no feature overlap, then the results follow nicely from the retrieval model. If traces already contain few, if any, matching features, then inserting an isolate—that is, an item with little or no matching features—should not enhance retention compared to a control. On the other hand, if the orienting task substantially increases the amount of feature overlap, by focusing attention on item similarities, then the isolate should be remembered especially well. It is interesting to note that recall of the background items followed the pattern predicted by the model as well. Difference processing led to a significant increase in background recall compared to the condition requiring similarity processing. Again, difference processing reduces the amount of feature overlap, and therefore the amount of cue overload, for both isolates and background items.

Other empirical patterns in the isolation-effect literature can be explained by reasoning of this sort. For example, it has been reported that the isolation effect is sometimes reduced or eliminated when participants report using elaborative rehearsal strategies during study (see Fabiani & Donchin, 1995). To the extent that elaborative processing leads to richer traces, ones that contain unique individual item information, then the isolation advantage should be reduced for the reasons discussed above. However, the predicted pattern will depend on the type of elaborative processing engaged. If participants relate items together, such as linking them into a cohesive story, then a very different pattern might well emerge. If the net result is an increase in feature overlap, because the processing emphasis has been placed on similarity rather than difference, the isolation advantage could increase.

THE PARADOX OF SIMILARITY AND DIFFERENCE

Our discussion up to this point has centered on the importance of difference. For a given retrieval cue, sampling probabilities are inversely proportional to the amount of cue overload; consequently, manipulations that reduce feature overlap will increase the chances of correct target sampling. However, analysts of memory have known for decades that memory often benefits from the processing of similarities as well. For example, items from categorized lists are usually recalled better than items from unrelated lists (Tulving & Pearlstone, 1966); for unrelated word lists, relational processing, or the processing of commonalities among list items, can benefit recall substantially (e.g., Hunt & Einstein, 1981).

This situation sets up a fundamental enigma or paradox: How can the processing of similarity and difference both benefit retention? From the standpoint of the retrieval model, and the notion of distinctiveness in general, similarity is anathema because it increases cue overload. However, this situation holds only with respect to a particular cue and a fixed set of possible retrieval candidates. Distinctiveness is a property of a cue in context—it merely specifies the likelihood of sampling a target given a specific cue. Left unspecified in this analysis are the variables that determine cue availability and the final composition of the target competitor set. As discussed below, it is here that organizational processing, or the processing of similarities, is apt to leave a positive mark on performance (also see Burns, Chapter 6 this volume).

The virtues of distinctiveness will depend as well on the type of retention test employed. Consider free recall, in which the goal is to recall all of the items on a just-presented list. What is the advantage of using a distinctive cue—one that specifies a single item—as opposed to an overloaded cue that is associated to a variety of items on the list? From a mnemonic standpoint, the goal is to sample any item as long as the item comes from the relevant memory list. Overloaded cues actually seem beneficial from this perspective because they promote the sampling of many list items. Of course, the situation is quite different in serial recall, which requires one to recall list items in their exact positions of original occurrence. If the cue for the second list item leads to the sampling of the third item, the response will be incorrect. Not surprisingly, similarity typically has strong negative effects on serial recall performance.

The Benefits of Relational Processing

To unravel the enigma, we need to focus more closely on the processing consequences of relational and item-based processing. In relational processing, typically participants are asked to process commonalities among to-be-remembered items, such as sorting the items into categories (Hunt & Einstein, 1981). Noting commonalities is likely to increase the amount of feature overlap across encoded traces because common features are encoded, but it can produce a very salient retrieval cue as well: participants know that the to-be-remembered items come from a particular category. Relational processing, as a result, effectively reduces the size of the long-term memory search set, increasing the probability of correct item sampling (see Burns, Chapter 6 this volume; Hunt & McDaniel, 1993; Neath, 1993).

A decade or so ago, my laboratory conducted a number of experiments to illustrate the paradoxical effects of similarity on memory (Nairne, 1990b; Nairne & Neumann, 1993). Each of these experiments tested memory for order: List items had to be placed in their exact within-list positions of occurrence at the point of test. As mentioned above, similarity usually has a strong negative effect on order retention, presumably because any given list cue tends to match lots of items from the list (e.g., the phonological similarity effect). In our experiments, however, rather than testing memory immediately following each list, researchers assessed order retention at the end of the session, after a number of lists had been presented. There were two main conditions: one in which lists were drawn from unique categories (e.g., birds, furniture) and one which contained lists of unrelated words. The surprising finding was that the categorized lists were ordered better than lists containing unrelated items. In this case, similarity helped order memory despite the fact that the within-list traces presumably contained more overlapping features than those from unrelated lists.

The unique feature of our experiments, of course, was the fact that testing occurred after the presentation of multiple lists. Compared to the normal case, in which testing occurs immediately following each list, participants faced a more difficult discrimination problem: they needed to locate not only the item's within-list position in memory but also the list representation in which the item occurred (e.g., it was the second item in the third list). With categorized lists, it should be difficult to recover an item's correct within-list position because the items share semantic features and are easily confused; however, it should be easy to identify the correct list representation because all members of a particular category come from the same list (e.g., if it is a robin, it must come from the bird list). With unrelated lists, the opposite is the case: it should be relatively easy to determine within-list position because the items are unrelated, but difficult to assess the correct list representation (there is no salient category cue to identify list membership). The net effect of similarity, therefore, will depend on a trade-off between ease of access along the list and within-list dimensions (also see Hunt, Chapter 1 this volume).

For example, suppose the probability of accessing an item's correct within-list position from memory is .30 when the list items share features and .50 when the items are distinct. If the list representation is easily available, as in the typical immediate memory context, similarity should impair performance. Further assume that when multiple lists have been presented, the probability of accessing the correct list representation in memory is .80 when the lists are categorized but only .40 when the lists contain unrelated items. If participants access their knowledge about list and within-list positions independently (see Friedman, 1990; Nairne, 1991), and both are required for correct performance, then better overall performance would be expected in the similar condition:

Probability correct for similar = .30 × .80 = .24
Probability correct for unrelated = .50 × .40 = .20

The point here is that the mnemonic effect of similarity, induced either by relational processing or by inherent item characteristics, will depend on the discrimination problem facing the individual. When the task requires discrimination among a fixed set of alternatives, embodied by equation 1 in the retrieval model, processing commonalities among items should lower the probability of sampling the correct target (i.e., there will be an increase in the amount of cue overload). In other environments, however, processing similarity eases the discrimination problem by restricting the search space, enabling one to sample from a smaller set of alternatives (e.g., sampling only from the list containing birds). As the size of the competitor set decreases, the denominator of equation 1 decreases as well. Whether relational processing will produce a net benefit or loss, as a consequence, will depend on the trade-off between the positive effects of delineating the search set and the negative effects of reducing within-set discriminability (see also Nairne & Kelley, 1999).

It is also conceivable that relational processing makes it easier to generate appropriate cues. Again, the retrieval model assumes that all instances of remembering are cue-driven: we use information in the present to decide what happened in the immediate and distant past. But such a model requires a mechanism for generating retrieval cues. In the feature model (Nairne, 1990a), which has been applied primarily to immediate memory, it is assumed that degraded records of prior processing remain available after list-processing for interpretation. To handle cue generation after delays, one commonly appeals initially to context; contextual information, which is assumed to evolve systematically over time, is used either as a cue or as a mechanism for generating cues-to-be-interpreted (e.g., Brown et al., 2002; Raaijmakers & Shiffrin, 1980). Because it induces the processing of similarities among items, relational processing is likely to augment the cue-generation process. Once a cue is generated and interpreted, it becomes a source for the generation of additional cues, either by virtue of simple associations or by fine-tuning the contextual information that is available.

The Benefits of Item-Based Processing

If the primary benefit of relational processing is to restrict the target search set, then the primary benefit of item-based processing is to ease the discrimination of items within that set. Processing "difference" presumably leads to traces with unique attributes—that is, traces with fewer overlapping features—which in turn makes it easier for the cue to access its appropriate target. Item-based processing reduces the amount of cue overload, or the extent to which any given list cue is predictive of many things, lowering the denominator of equation 1.

However, as discussed earlier, cue overload is not always a concern—it depends on the demands of the retention test. In free recall, the task is to recall all of the items from a just-presented list and output order is irrelevant. If relational processing successfully restricts the search set to items from the list, then a cue matching any or all of the list items is likely to be beneficial. A given cue, such as a degraded remnant of the third list item, does not need to sample its appropriate target (the third list item); any list item will do. Under such conditions, at least in principle, enhancing within-list distinctiveness may help one sample a particular item but not improve retention overall.

In most cases, however, relational processing is unlikely to restrict the search set entirely to list items. For example, knowing that a prior list contained "birds" may constrain the search set to birds, but nonlist category members are apt to be included as well. One needs item-based processing, as a result, to discriminate the "list" birds from the "nonlist" birds. Item-based processing, and the encoding of idiosyncratic features, also probably helps keep potential cues intact by lowering the likelihood of interference from subsequent material. Once again, the mnemonic effects of any kind of processing (relational processing, item-based processing, or their combination) will depend on a complex interplay among the cue–target match, the composition of the search set, and the availability of intact cues. As Hunt and McDaniel (1993) argue, it is probably best to encourage both relational and item-based processing to ensure good recall.

Models of Temporal Distinctiveness

Sampling in the retrieval model is based on relative comparisons between cues and possible targets in long-term memory, but the dimensions of comparisons are left unspecified. In principle, event A could differ from event B along a number of dimensions—orthographic, acoustic, semantic, and so on. Over the years, a number of theorists have suggested that time—specifically an item's temporal position of occurrence—is an important feature of an encoded trace: events can be remembered to the extent that they occupy unique or discrepant positions temporally. In this section, I briefly discuss some models of temporal distinctiveness and consider their relationship to the retrieval model proposed here.

The idea that temporal position is a crucial cue makes logical and empirical sense (see Brown & Chater, 2001). Logically, as noted earlier, recovery from episodic memory usually involves remembering that a well-known item occurred at a particular time and place; moreover, in most laboratory-based research, list items do not vary systematically along any dimension other than their time of presentation. Empirically, it is well established that temporal schedules of presentation affect recall probabilities in systematic ways. In free recall, for example, one can increase or decrease end-of-the-list recall (recency) by varying the amount of time that passes between each list item given a constant retention interval (e.g., Neath & Crowder, 1990). Alternatively, one can produce nearly equivalent recency effects across widely spaced retention intervals simply by holding the ratio of the interpresentation interval to the retention interval constant (Glenberg, Bradley, Kraus, & Renzaglia, 1983; Nairne, Neath, Serra, & Byun, 1997).

One of the more interesting properties of temporal variation and memory is scale invariance. Many of the classic phenomena of free and serial recall, such as recency, the shape of the serial position curve, and error distributions, retain their basic form across widely different time scales. Standard bow-shaped serial position curves, including the characteristic recency slope, have been detected for lists presented in under a second, as well as for lists presented over minutes, hours, days, or even months (see Baddeley & Hitch, 1993). What matters is not the absolute passage of time but, rather, the relative temporal positions of items sharing an episode. As discussed below, similar notions fall naturally out of the ratio-based retrieval model.

Models of temporal distinctiveness generally assume that memory traces are represented along a psychologically scaled (usually logarithmic) temporal dimension. A target trace is retrievable to the extent that its remembered position stands out, or is distinctive, along this temporal dimension. To calculate distinctiveness formally, for a given item one simply sums the distances between it and the remembered positions of all possible competitors. Because relative temporal position is what matters, the distinctiveness values are normalized: An item is especially recallable to the extent that it is distinctive compared to the other items on the list (Murdock, 1960; Neath, 1993). This last step, by design, helps to produce the property of scale invariance. As long as items occupy the same relative positions along the temporal dimension, their distinctiveness values will not change (despite changes in the overall passage of time).

There are actually a number of ways to determine temporal distinctiveness (see Brown et al., 2002, for a review). The methods differ primarily in terms of how relative temporal position is calculated. For example, the method just described is a *global* distinctiveness measure because all of the items in the competitor set contribute to the calculation. More *local* distinctiveness measures might consider only an item's immediate neighbors along the temporal dimension (e.g., Baddeley, 1976) or weight the distance values in such a way that psychologically distant neighbors play a less important role (Brown et al., 2002). All of these measures share the insight that distinctiveness is a relative concept; what matters is how the item differs from other items along a perceived dimension of similarity (temporal position).

The retrieval model of equation 1, of course, also stipulates that distinctiveness is a relative concept. Cues will sample particular targets to the extent that they match those targets better than other viable competitors. In this sense, the retrieval model embodies a kind of scale invariance. It is not the absolute cue–target similarity that matters, but the relative cue–target similarity. As long as the relative similarity values remain constant, the absolute cue–target match can change without changing the final distinctiveness values. (I return to this point briefly in the next section.) In fact, one current model of temporal distinctiveness, SIMPLE (Brown et al., 2002), relies on essentially the same ratio rule employed here to determine recall probabilities. In this case, however, the similarity dimension is temporally based: in attempting to recall an item that occurred t seconds ago, one computes the similarity between this duration and the remembered durations associated with each of the list items.

There is little question that time-of-occurrence information can serve as an important cue for retrieving and reconstructing the past. Temporal distinctiveness models have successfully accounted for a number of interesting empirical phenomena, including changes in the shape of the serial position as the length of the retention interval increases (e.g., Brown et al., 2002; Neath, 1993). Moreover, in stressing relative rather than absolute time, these models easily handle data that falsify traditional time-based decay models (see Nairne, 2002b, for a review). For example, psychologists have known for decades that retention sometimes improves with the passage of time (e.g., Turvey, Brick, & Osborn, 1970). Such a finding is clearly inconsistent with decay-based theories, but is easily explained by distinctiveness models. The relative discriminability of traces along the temporal dimension can remain the same with time, or even improve, depending on how the items in the competitor set are situated along the temporal dimension.

SUMMARY AND CONCLUSIONS

Mnemonic distinctiveness, as defined here, is a property of a cue in context. It refers to the ability of a cue to access a particular target in a particular context. As implemented in the retrieval model, correct target sampling depends on two factors: (1) the functional match between the current retrieval cue and the target trace, and (2) the functional match between the cue and the remaining members of the target competitor set. Neither of these factors, by itself, is sufficient to explain target recall—retention performance will always depend on both.

As shown throughout, the retrieval model can account for a number of benchmark phenomena in the distinctiveness literature. The prototypical distinctiveness effect, the von Restorff (or isolation) effect, was attributed primarily to cue overload: cues that match unusual events will tend not to match other events in the same context. Assigning a retrieval locus to the phenomenon, among other things, helps to explain performance levels for both isolated and background items, and accounts for why the effect remains strong for isolated items occurring early in a presentation sequence. The retrieval model also provides a nice conceptual framework for understanding the effects of processing similarity and difference on retention. The net advantage of processing similarity and difference can seem paradoxical, but not when the full discrimination problem facing the individual is considered. Correct target sampling depends not only on one's ability to discriminate among the items in the retrieval set but also on the ability to restrict the set of items to be considered. Processing similarity may impair within-set discriminability, but it can limit the search set by restricting its contents to items that vary along the similarity dimension.

The retrieval model has implications as well for general memory theory. Students of memory have a proclivity for making broad statements about what is best for retention, and the retrieval model places some important constraints on such statements. For example, I have written in detail elsewhere about the commonly accepted "principle" that memory depends directly on the similarity, or match, between retrieval cues and targets, as encoded (e.g., Nairne, 2002a). Although the model specifies that correct target selection is directly proportional to the cue–target match, consideration of the match alone cannot predict performance. In fact, under the right circumstances, increasing the cue–target match can improve performance, produce no effect, or even lower performance.

Suppose that people are shown a list of homophones for study (e.g., *pare, pair, pear*), presented both visually and aloud. At test, the task is to recall the item that occurred in third serial position. In the first condition, no retrieval cues are provided; in a second condition, the sound of the third item (*pear*) is given as an additional retrieval cue. The similarity, or match, between the retrieval cue and the encoded target is clearly increased in this second condition (assuming that people encoded the sound of the item during initial presentation), but it is doubtful that performance will improve. The sound of the item provides no distinctive information about which item occurred—all of the items on the list share the same sound. It is not the absolute cue–target match that matters, but the relative discriminability of the cue.

It is also easy to imagine situations in which adding to the cue–target match might hurt subsequent retention. Suppose, for instance, that we add an "overloaded" feature to the cue—that is, we add a feature that is shared by recall candidates that would not otherwise have been considered. (The addition of a salient rhyming or categorical feature, for example, might recruit new members into the competitor set.) Again, we have increased the similarity, or match, between the retrieval cue and the target trace, but the difficulty of the discrimination problem has been increased as well. To improve performance, it is not matching features per se that are needed (although the retrieval model requires some minimal cue–target match in the numerator); it is the presence of features that help one discriminate the correct target trace from incorrect competitors.

Similar arguments apply as well to proposals about the benefits of relational and item-specific processing (Hunt & McDaniel, 1993) or levels of processing (Craik & Lockhart, 1972). Encoding manipulations, by themselves, cannot be used to predict performance, nor can one speak of distinctive processing outside of a particular fixed retrieval environment (one in which both the cue and the members of the competitor set are specified). The processes of encoding, by definition, determine the variety and quality of trace features, but trace characteristics by themselves do not determine memory. It is the ability of the operative retrieval cue to access that trace that determines retention and, as argued throughout, it is the relative predictability of the cue that matters.

Of course, the idea that remembering is based on the relative predictability of cues is not new in the memory literature (e.g., Jacoby & Craik, 1979), although its implications have often been overlooked. In particular, it speaks to the proper definition of distinctiveness. As noted in the chapter opening, *distinctiveness* has been defined in various ways over the years—for example, as a property of a stored trace, a retrieval cue, or as a type of processing (Hunt, Chapter 1 this volume; Schmidt, 1991). Yet, to the extent that distinctiveness is considered to be a measure of memory, it can be none of these things. Distinctiveness cannot be a fixed property of a cue, or of a target trace, or even of an interaction between a given cue and a given target. It is best considered to be a property of a cue in context: Given a fixed set of alternatives, a measure of distinctiveness can be assigned to a particular cue with respect to a particular set of alternatives.

ACKNOWLEDGMENTS

Thanks to Ian Neath for useful discussions, and the editors, Reed Hunt and Jim Worthen, for their comments on the chapter text. Correspondence about this chapter can be addressed to the author: nairne@psych.purdue.edu.

NOTE

1. Placing the locus of the isolation effect at retrieval does not imply that encoding is unimportant, only that the mnemonic value of the encoded record depends on the retrieval context. Obviously, how an item is encoded will determine its ultimate discriminability within any given retrieval environment and, therefore, cannot be ignored.

REFERENCES

Anderson, J. R., & Schooler, L. J. (2000). The adaptive nature of memory. In E. Tulving & F. I. M. Craik (Eds.), *The Oxford handbook of memory* (pp 557–570). New York: Oxford University Press.

Baddeley, A. D. (1976). *The psychology of memory*. New York: Basic Books.

Baddeley, A. D., & Hitch, G. J. (1993). The recency effect: Implicit learning with explicit retrieval? *Memory & Cognition, 21,* 146–155.

Brown, G. D. A., & Chater, N. (2001). The chronological organization of memory: Common psychological foundations for remembering and timing. In C. Hoerl & T. McCormack (Eds.), *Time and memory: Issues in philosophy and psychology* (pp. 77–110). Oxford, UK: Oxford University Press.

Brown, G. D. A., Neath, I., & Chater, N. (2002). *SIMPLE: A local distinctiveness model of scale-invariant memory and perceptual identification.* Manuscript submitted for publication.

Bruce, D., & Gaines, M. T. (1976). Tests of an organizational hypothesis of isolation effects in free recall. *Journal of Verbal Learning and Verbal Behavior, 15*, 59–72.

Craik, F. I. M., & Lockhart, R. S. (1972). Levels of processing: A framework for memory research. *Journal of Verbal Learning and Verbal Behavior, 11*, 671–684.

Cunningham, T. F., Marmie, W. R., & Healy, A. F. (1998). The role of item distinctiveness in short-term recall of order information. Memory & Cognition, 26, 463–476.

Earhard, M. (1967). Cued recall and free recall as a function of the number of items per cue. *Journal of Verbal Learning and Verbal Behavior, 6*, 257–263.

Fabiani, M., & Donchin, E. (1995). Encoding processes and memory organization: A model of the von Restorff effect. *Journal of Experimental Psychology: Learning, Memory, and Cognition, 21*, 224–240.

Farrell, S., & Lewandowsky, S. (2003). Dissimilar items benefit from phonological similarity in serial recall. *Journal of Experimental Psychology: Learning, Memory, & Cognition, 29*, 838–849.

Friedman, W. J. (1990). *About time: Inventing the fourth dimension.* Cambridge, MA: MIT Press.

Glenberg, A. M., Bradley, M. M., Kraus, T. A., & Renzaglia, G. J. (1983). Studies of the long-term recency effect: Support for a contextually-guided retrieval hypothesis. *Journal of Experimental Psychology: Learning, Memory, & Cognition, 9*, 231–255.

Hunt, R. R. (1995). The subtlety of distinctiveness: What von Restorff really did. *Psychonomic Bulletin and Review, 2*, 105–112.

Hunt, R. R., & Einstein, G. O. (1981). Relational and item-specific information in memory. *Journal of Verbal Learning and Verbal Behavior, 20*, 497–514.

Hunt, R. R., & Lamb, C. A. (2001). What causes the isolation effect? *Journal of Experimental Psychology: Learning, Memory, and Cognition, 27*, 1359–1366.

Hunt, R. R., & McDaniel, M. A. (1993). The enigma of organization and distinctiveness. *Journal of Memory and Language, 32*, 421–445.

Jacoby, L. L., & Craik, F. I. M. (1979). Effects of elaboration of processing at encoding and retrieval: Trace distinctiveness and recovery of initial context. In L. S. Cermak & F. I. M. Craik (Eds.), *Levels of processing in human memory* (pp. 1–21). Hillsdale, NJ: Lawrence Erlbaum Associates.

Kelley, M. R., & Nairne, J. S. (2001). Von Restorff revisited: Isolation, generation, and memory for order. *Journal of Experimental Psychology: Learning, Memory, and Cognition, 27*, 54–66.

Murdock, B. B., Jr. (1960). The distinctiveness of stimuli. *Psychological Review, 67*, 16–31.

Nairne, J. S. (1990a). A feature model of immediate memory. *Memory & Cognition, 18*, 251–269.

Nairne, J. S. (1990b). Similarity and long-term memory for order. *Journal of Memory and Language, 29*, 733–746.

Nairne, J. S. (1991). Positional uncertainty in long-term memory. *Memory & Cognition, 19*, 332–340.

Nairne, J. S. (2001). A functional analysis of primary memory. In H. L. Roediger, III, J. S. Nairne, I. Neath, & A. M. Surprenant (Eds.), *The nature of remembering: Essays in honor of Robert G. Crowder* (pp. 283–296). Washington, DC: American Psychological Association.

Nairne, J. S. (2002a). The myth of the encoding-retrieval match. *Memory, 10*, 389–395.

Nairne, J. S. (2002b). Remembering over the short-term: The case against the standard model. *Annual Review of Psychology, 53*, 53–81.

Nairne, J. S. (2005). The functionalist agenda in memory research. In A. Healy (Ed.), *Experimental cognitive psychology and its applications: Triple festschrift in honor of Lyle Bourne, Walter Kintsch, Thomas Landauer* (pp. 115–126). Washington, DC: American Psychological Association.

Nairne, J. S., & Kelley, M. R. (1999). Reversing the phonological similarity effect. *Memory & Cognition, 27*, 45–53.

Nairne, J. S., Neath, I., Serra, M., & Byun, E. (1997). Positional distinctiveness and the ratio rule in free recall. *Journal of Memory and Language, 37*, 155–166.

Nairne, J. S., & Neumann, C. (1993). Enhancing effects of similarity on long-term memory for order. *Journal of Experimental Psychology: Learning, Memory, & Cognition, 19*, 329–337.

Neath, I. (1993). Distinctiveness and serial position effects in recognition. *Memory & Cognition, 21*, 689–698.

Neath, I., & Crowder, R. G. (1990). Schedules of presentation and temporal distinctiveness in human memory. *Journal of Experimental Psychology: Learning, Memory, & Cognition, 16*, 316–327.

Nosofsky, R. M. (1986). Attention, similarity, and the identification-categorization relationship. *Journal of Experimental Psychology: General, 115*, 39–57.

Pillsbury, W. B., & Raush, H. L. (1943). An extension of the Köhler-Restorff inhibition phenomenon. *American Journal of Psychology, 56*, 293–298.

Raaijmakers, J. G. W., & Shiffrin, R. M. (1980). Search of associative memory. *Psychological Review, 95*, 93–134.

Schmidt, S. R. (1985). Encoding and retrieval processes in the memory for conceptually distinctive events. *Journal of Experimental Psychology: Learning, Memory, and Cognition, 11*, 565–578.

Schmidt, S. R. (1991). Can we have a distinctive theory of memory? *Memory & Cognition, 19*, 523–542.

Schmidt, S. R. (2002). Outstanding memories: The positive and negative effects of nudes on memory. *Journal of Experimental Psychology: Learning, Memory, and Cognition, 28*, 353–361.

Schulz, L. S. (1971). Effects of high-priority events on recall and recognition of other events. *Journal of Verbal Learning and Verbal Behavior, 10*, 322–330.

Shepard, R. N. (1987). Toward a universal law of generalization for psychological science. *Science, 237*, 1317–1323.

Smith, R. E., & Hunt, R. R. (2000). The effects of distinctiveness require reinstatement of organization: The importance of intentional memory instructions. *Journal of Memory and Language, 43,* 431–446.

Thomson, D. M., & Tulving, E. (1970). Associative encoding and retrieval: Weak and strong cues. *Journal of Experimental Psychology, 86,* 255–262.

Tulving, E. (1983). *Elements of episodic memory.* New York: Oxford University Press.

Tulving, E., & Pearlstone, Z. (1966). Availability versus accessibility of information in memory for words. *Journal of Verbal Learning and Verbal Behavior, 5,* 381–191.

Turvey, M. T., Brick, P., & Osborn, J. (1970). Proactive interference in short-term memory as a function of prior-item retention interval. *Quarterly Journal of Experimental Psychology, 22,* 142–147.

von Restorff, H. (1933). Uber die wirkung von bereichsbildungen im spurenfeld (On the effect of spheres formations in the trace field). *Psychologische Forschung, 18,* 299–342.

Watkins, O. C., & Watkins, M. J. (1975). Build up of proactive inhibition as a cue overload effect. *Journal of Experimental Psychology: Human Learning and Memory, 1,* 442–452.

3

Emotion, Significance, Distinctiveness, and Memory

Stephen R. Schmidt

Two kinds of stimuli appear to attract special attention and cognitive resources: the novel and the significant. However, these two categories are
rarely mutually exclusive. Before September 11th, few of us had ever seen
a building collapse after being struck by an airplane. When most of us first
saw the videos of the planes crashing into the World Trade Center, it was
quite a novel experience. In addition, the events of that day had an immediate and longlasting impact on our society. That is, they were very significant. The terrorist attacks and the events surrounding them thus provide good examples of occurrences that are both novel and significant. Both
in and outside the laboratory, novel events are quite often significant, and
significant events are often relatively novel, leading researchers to routinely
confuse the impact of these variables on memory and cognitive processes.
In the following pages, I will explore the relation between novelty and significance. I will begin by defining each of these terms and demonstrate how
they have been confused and confounded in memory research. I will then
review an appraisal theory of emotion as a means toward understanding
the impact of significance on cognitive processes. Finally, I will present several research findings that help to clarify the distinction between novelty
and significance, and I will argue that their respective impacts on memory
and other cognitive processes are very different.

Novelty versus Significance

Gati and Ben-Shakhar (1990) proposed a feature-matching model to describe how novel and significant stimuli lead to the physiological orientation response. Within this approach, the novelty of an item is a positive
monotonic function of the number of new features in the item and a neg-

ative function of the number of features shared between the item and preceding items. This definition of novelty is directly related to the definitions of distinctiveness offered by Eysenck (1979) and Nelson (1979) in which distinctiveness is defined by reference to feature overlap. That is, the distinctive item shares few features with other items presented in the same context. Similarly, in Chapter 1 of this volume, Reed Hunt defined distinctiveness as "a psychological representation that is notably different from other representations" (p. 12). In contrast, the significance of an item is determined by comparing the item to one that is "relevant." Presumably, long-term memory contains a storehouse of representations that are particularly important or relevant to the individual. According to Gati and Ben-Shakhar, the degree of significance of a stimulus is a linear combination of the number of features shared between the stimulus and a relevant item, and the number of features not shared between these two items. The magnitude of the attention response is proportional to the combined impacts of novelty and significance (Gati & Ben-Shakhar, 1990; Ben-Shakhar, 1995).

If novelty is defined relative to a lifetime of experience, then a truly novel stimulus cannot be significant. That is, there will be no match between the truly novel input and anything found in the memory system. However, novelty can be defined both more and less inclusively than in reference to information accumulated in the lifetime of an individual. We can reasonably assume that we are prepared, because of a lengthy evolutionary process, to find some stimuli significant. The sucking and startle reflexes exhibited in newborns come to mind as examples. Thus, certain stimuli unknown in the life of an individual are not novel with respect to our genetic heritage, and these stimuli match information genetically coded as significant. Novelty can also be defined much more narrowly than in relation to our genetic heritage. Schmidt (1991) coined the terms *primary distinctiveness* and *secondary distinctiveness* in an attempt to segment the range of contexts used to define novelty. *Primary distinctiveness* was defined relative to information active in working (primary) memory, whereas *secondary distinctiveness* was defined relative to information stored in long-term (secondary) memory. Wolff (1993) made a similar cleaving when he discussed the contextual probability and the absolute probability of a symbol. Contextual probability referred to the probability that a given symbol followed another in a particular input string. Absolute probability was defined with respect the completely history of previous symbols. Hunt also addressed this issue in his discussion of item-based and event-based distinctiveness (Chapter1, this volume). That is, definitions of distinctiveness must consider the "grain size of events."

Whereas increasing novelty is defined with respect to decreasing feature overlap, increasing significance requires increasing feature overlap. In this sense, significance is the converse of novelty. However, significance requires more than just the recognition of repetition. The significant stimulus is one that is recognized (as a result of conscious or preconscious processing) as relevant. Significance is a value judgment. Certain kinds of experiences have consequences for us as individuals and for society. Through genetic predispositions, classical conditioning, and culturally transmitted values, features of consequential and relevant experiences are coded in long-term memory. Experiences that contain a substantial number of features that match these consequential memories should be judged as significant. Like novelty or distinctiveness, one might guess that context or recency, in addition to feature overlap, influences the impact of significance on cognitive processes.

The role of context in determining the significance of an experience is nicely illustrated in experiments concerning memory for "high-priority events" (Schulz, 1971; Tulving, 1969). For example, Schulz (1971, Experiment 2) asked participants to view lists of words that contained names of famous people (e.g., Columbus). Half of the participants were told to be sure that they remembered the name of any famous person that appeared in the list, whereas no mention of the famous names was made to the other participants. The author argued that these uninformed participants were in "essentially a von Restorff situation" (p. 325). The results demonstrated good recall of the famous names and poor recall for words immediately following the famous names. However, the magnitude of both of these effects was greatly increased when participants were given the priority instructions. In terms of the present framework, the significance of the famous names increased by virtue of the specific instructions to be sure to remember them.

Because both novel and significant events attract attention, both effects are sensitive to contextual manipulations, and because significant events are often novel, it seems natural to conclude that the novel and the significant have similar effects on memory and cognitive processes. I will argue that this conclusion is inappropriate. Ohman, Flykt, and Esteves (2001) provided a startling contrast between the processes involved in the detection of difference and the detection of significance. They employed the "pop-out" procedure to study pre-attentive visual processing. Participants were asked to identify the discrepant stimulus in 3×3 matrix of pictures. The discrepant picture was either a fear producing stimulus (a snake or a spider) or a neutral stimulus (a flower or a mushroom), and the background pictures were either fearful or neutral. Thus, for example, the participants were asked to find a snake in a set of pictures that contained mostly flowers or a flower in a set containing mostly snakes. The participants were able to find a discrepant fearful stimulus more quickly than a discrepant neutral picture. Additionally, search time for fearful but not neutral stimuli was independent of position of the stimulus in the matrix, and independent of the size of the matrix. One interpretation of these results is that evolutionarily significant stimuli "pop-out" of visual displays as a result of pre-attentive perceptual processing. Stimuli that are merely "different" or distinctive do not engender this kind of processing, and do not pop out.

SIGNIFICANCE AND MEMORY

The distinction between novelty and significance begins to blur when one turns to research concerning memory processes. Numerous researchers have investigated memory for significant events and concluded that the results demonstrated a von Restorff effect, or explained their results by invoking distinctiveness (e.g., Christianson & Loftus, 1987; Detterman & Ellis, 1972; Loftus & Burns, 1982; McCloskey, Wible, & Cohen, 1988). Consider, for example, the Loftus and Burns (1982) investigation. Participants viewed a film of a bank robbery that was violent in one condition (a boy is shot in the face) and nonviolent in a comparison condition. The violent version resulted in poorer recognition and recall of details than did the nonviolent version. The authors concluded "that our effects are more accurately described as von Restorff effects (see Wallace, 1965), situations in which an 'outstanding' item is embedded within a list of otherwise homogeneous material" (p. 322). They reached this conclusion even though they also found that the memory impairment occurred only when the event was upsetting and not when it was merely unexpected. It is ironic that the researchers used the relatively poor memory for an isolated event as evidence for the von Restorff effect. Typically, the argument runs in the other direction— the von Restorff effect is invoked as a description of *good* memory for isolated events. Nevertheless, it is easy to see why Loftus and Burns made this attribution. For most us, in most contexts, a picture of a boy shot in the face is distinctive. It is probably also significant.

As a second example of the confusion between distinctiveness and significance, consider a series of experiments conducted by Detterman and Ellis and their colleagues (Ellis, Detterman, Runcie, McCarver, & Craig, 1971; Detterman & Ellis, 1972). In these studies, a picture containing nudes was presented in a series of line drawings of common objects. Not surprisingly, the nude picture was remembered by nearly 100% of the participants. However, when compared to a control list containing only objects, good memory for the nudes occurred at the expense of several pictures preceding and following the nudes. Because there was only one picture in each list that contained nudes, one might conclude (as did Detterman and Ellis, 1972) that the good memory for the nudes was due to the picture's distinctiveness. That is, this picture contained features that were novel in the context of the list. Similarly, in the terms employed by Hunt in Chapter 1, this volume, the picture containing nudes may have encouraged the processing of difference in the context of similarity.

However, it is not difficult to argue that pictures of nudes are significant stimuli. In support of this argument, one could discuss the evolutionary significance of sexual stimuli, or simply cite the ample research demonstrating physiological arousal to nude pictures (e.g., Bradley, Greenwald, Petry, & Lang, 1992; Greenwald, Cook, & Lang, 1989). Schmidt (1997, 2002) conducted a series of experiments designed to untangle the roles of distinctiveness and significance in supporting good memory for nude stimuli. Lists were constructed from 15 full-color photographs of people engaged in easily identifiable activities (e.g., working at a computer, drinking coffee, picking fruit). A target picture, a person reclining on the floor with an open book, was placed in either position 7 or position 8 in the lists. In the control lists, the person in the target picture was clothed, and in the experimental lists the person was nude. Across different groups of participants, both male and female nude pictures served as targets, and both male and female participants were tested. Following the list presentation, the participants engaged in five minutes of arithmetic and then attempted to recall the set of pictures. A summary of the serial position curves from three experiments, differing in only minor details, is presented in Figure 3.1.

The results clearly demonstrated good memory for the nude pictures and relatively poor memory for the three pictures following the nudes. These results replicated the Detterman and Ellis (1972) findings of anterograde amnesia following a delayed memory test. However, the Schmidt (2002) study ruled out several uninteresting interpretations of the original Detterman and Ellis investigations. For example, in the original Detterman and Ellis studies, the target was a photograph and the rest of the pictures were line drawings. This potential confound between nudity and picture types was removed in the Schmidt (2002) study. In addition, one should not attribute the original Detterman and Ellis results to the fact that the target contained people whereas the rest of the pictures contained objects. Schmidt (2002) concluded that the impact of the target picture on memory was tied the participants' response to nudity per se. Another new finding reported by Schmidt (2002) was that whereas the gist of the nude pictures was well

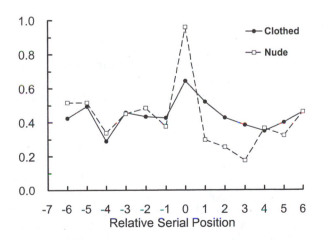

FIGURE 3.1 Recall as a function of serial position. This graph summarizes the results of three experiments. Serial position is graphed relative to a single target picture placed near the middle of the list (position 0). The target was either a picture of a clothed or a nude person.

retained, picture details were not. In fact, picture background details were more poorly remembered from the nude pictures than from the clothed control pictures. There were no differences in either the recall or the recognition of person details (e.g., hair color, age, height) between the nude and clothed versions.

Nonetheless, some may interpret the Schmidt (2002) results within a distinctiveness framework. That is, each experimental list contained exactly one nude, providing difference within the context of similarity. To address this issue, Schmidt (2002, Experiment 3) constructed lists that contained 14 nude pictures and 1 clothed picture appearing in position 8. Memory for this list was compared to a list containing 15 pictures of nudes. As one might predict from a distinctiveness perspective, the isolated clothed picture was recalled better than the comparable nude picture from the all-nude list. However, there was no evidence for anterograde amnesia. Apparently, distinctiveness supports good memory for a picture that contrasts with the surrounding pictures, whether the picture is clothed or nude. However, only an isolated nude picture led to anterograde amnesia.

One might guess that the nude pictures captured and held the attention of our research participants. If this is the case, then a set of nude pictures should be retained better than a corresponding set of clothed pictures. On the other hand, after viewing several nude pictures, participant's interest in the pictures may wane. Similarly, any physiological arousal in response to the nudes may habituate with repeated exposure. These hypotheses were tested in an unpublished experiment conducted with the help of my research team. Nine photographs were prepared that contained women engaged in everyday activities. In one series, all the women were nude and in another series the same women, engaged in the same activities, were clothed. Nine different presentation orders were tested, completely counterbalancing picture with input position. The rest of the procedural details were the same as those followed in Schmidt (2002). We predicted that recall of the nude series would exceed recall of the clothed series, and this effect would be most apparent early in the serial position curve. Much to our surprise, recall of the clothed and nude lists was nearly identical, with the mean proportion recalled equal to .43 in both conditions. In addition, there was no evidence of an interaction with input position. Apparently, when the nude stimuli are not distinctive they were not particularly well remembered.

Based on this research, I have reached three tentative conclusions. First, distinctive stimuli are well remembered, but do not "steal" attention from following stimuli (see Schmidt, 1991, for a summary of additional evidence in support of this conclusion). Hunt's argument in Chapter 1, this volume, discrediting an "increased attention" explanation of distinctiveness, reached the same conclusion. Second, significant stimuli (nudes) are also well remembered, but only when they are distinctive. Thus, mixed lists designs, or designs in which a single significant stimulus is embedded in a series of less significant events, are needed to reveal the effects of significance on memory. Third, isolated significant stimuli steal attention from background material and subsequent stimuli. Further support for this conclusion can be found in several experiments. Both Detterman and Ellis (1972), and Tulving (1969) demonstrated that the anterograde amnesia effect diminished as presentation rates slowed. Schmidt (2002) demonstrated that a short interval between successive pictures removed the anterograde amnesia effect.

If these three conclusions are valid, the effects of distinctiveness and significance on cognitive processes are very different. Whereas distinctiveness supports good memory for material, significance impairs memory for background material and material immediately following a significant stimulus. However, many questions remain unanswered. Why do significant stimuli capture and hold attention? If significant stimuli capture attention, why do we not remember significant stimuli better than neutral stimuli? Why do the effects of significance depend on the context of the stimuli? And when should we expect to see the impact of significance on memory? The answers to these questions may lie in an appropriate theory of emotion.

APPRAISAL THEORY OF EMOTION

In early theories of emotion (e.g., James-Lang; Schachter & Singer, 1962), emotion emerged from an interpretation of physiological arousal. For example, if I encounter a bear in the woods my heart may start to pound and I may run away. I may interpret these reactions as indicative of fear. In contrast, in appraisal theory, emotions are the result of evaluations, or appraisals, of events and situations (see Scherer, Schorr, & Johnstone, 2001, for a summary). Scherer (2001) developed an appraisal view of emotion that seems particularly pertinent to memory processes. I will employ his theory to illustrate appraisal theory in general. As we shall see, this theory has some interesting implications for memory research.

In Scherer's (2001) model, emotional processing involves a sequence of Stimulus Evaluation Checks (SECs). These occur in a fixed order and can be placed into the following four groups: relevance (will it affect me?), implications (how will it impact my goals), coping potential (how can I adjust), and normative significance (importance to my social group). The results of the SECs lead to activation of neuroendocrine, autonomic, and somatic nervous systems, as well as the potential activation of action tendencies. So, for example, if I were to encounter a bear in the woods, the bear would be detected as relevant because it is both novel and dangerous. I might then determine that there is a reasonable probability that the bear could do me great harm. I should then consider if and how I should cope with my current situation. I may also look toward my companions to see how they are reacting to the event. Based on these evaluations I might wisely choose to discreetly, and quickly, withdraw. In the meantime, my heart rate and respiration rate have increased, making a hasty retreat physically possible. This series of computations and bodily reactions are part and parcel of the appraisal process.

Scherer's (2001) framework provides some insightful answers to the questions I raised earlier. Why do significant stimuli capture and hold attention? Significant stimuli are detected as "relevant" and engage the appraisal machinery. This machinery determines how we react to the relevant stimuli. Whereas some of the reactions within the appraisal process are automatic, some will require working-memory capacity. Working memory may be engaged in planning how to react to the situation, and in a search of the environment and long-term memory for relevant information to aid in the planning process. The commitment of working memory may steal attention from the processing of less relevant aspects of the situation. As a result, loss of memory for background details and anterograde amnesia may arise from the engagement of the appraisal machinery.

Why do we not remember significant stimuli better than neutral stimuli? In Schmidt (2002) the participants who viewed nude pictures did not have more detailed or accurate memories for the nudes than did participants who viewed clothed models. I suggest that the cognitive resources elicited by a nude stimulus were not directed at the stimulus per se. Instead, attention was directed to the appraisal processes and to action plans associated with the appraisal. For example, when a person sees a nude, he or she has to decide how to react. The person may ask: "How are the other students reacting?" "What does the experimenter expect me to do?" "Do I have a silly grin on my face?" Determining the answers to these questions does not require a detailed analysis of the nude picture. However, answering these questions requires that we devote some of our limited cognitive resources to the appraisal machinery, stealing resources from the processing of surrounding material.

Why does the impact of significance on cognitive processes depend on the context in which a significant stimulus appears? "Given the constant barrage of stimulation, the organism must decide which stimuli are sufficiently relevant to warrant more extensive processing" (Scherer, 2001, p. 95). To accomplish this, the relevance evaluation begins with a novelty check to determine the familiarity or suddenness of the stimulus. The appraisal process will not be engaged by highly familiar or predictable stimuli. Presumably, one already knows how to react to a highly familiar stimulus. Similarly, a stimulus that is very similar to one that has been encountered very recently will not need to be reappraised. Perhaps the earlier appraisal is still available in working memory for these recently evaluated stimuli. For example, one should not expect the presentation of the third or fourth nude in a series of nude pictures to engage the appraisal processes.

The appraisal view of emotion helps us understand the impact of significant stimuli on memory processes. It also provides a framework from which to make several novel predictions. When should we expect to see the impact of significance on memory? The impact of significance on memory should be in direct proportion to the engagement of the appraisal machinery. The engagement of the machinery should be evident through measures of emotion (e.g., rating scales, physiological responses) and attention (e.g., "pop out," and the emotional Stroop effect). Loss of memory for unimportant background details and anterograde amnesia should be in direct proportion to the level of engagement.

EMPIRICAL EVALUATIONS

These ideas were recently evaluated in two experiments. In the first, Kramer and Schmidt (2004) investigated the impact of alcohol cues on memory. Several kinds of research suggest that alcohol cues are significant stimuli in heavy drinkers. For example, alcohol cues produce significant physiological reactions in alcoholics (Carter & Tiffany, 1999). In addition, there is an "emotional Stroop" effect with alcohol words among heavy drinkers (Stetter, Ackermann, Bizer, Straube, & Mann, 1995). That is, heavy drinkers name the ink color of words like *booze* and *bar* more slowly than the color of alcohol-neutral words. Dennis Kramer and I integrated his research on cognitive processes in heavy drinkers (Kramer & Goldman, 2003) and my research on memory for significant stimuli (Schmidt, 2002). We reasoned that if alcohol cues are significant stimuli, then a picture of an alcoholic beverage presented in a series of common objects should capture and hold the attention of heavy drinkers.

To test this idea, undergraduate students viewed a series of slides containing pictures of common objects (an umbrella, a jar of peanut butter, a coffeemaker, etc.). The procedures from Schmidt (2002), outlined above, were closely followed. A target picture was presented in position 8 of a 15-item list. For one group of participants the target was a picture of a bottle of Pepsi, and for the remaining participants the target was a picture of a bottle of Jack Daniels. After viewing the pictures, the participants engaged in a five-minute distractor task, followed by a free-recall test. They then completed a questionnaire addressing their drinking habits. Based on their answers on the drinking questionnaire, the students were placed into either a high drinker groups ($M = 63.42$ drinks/month) or a low drinking group ($M = 1.44$ drinks/month). Recall of the target picture and the three pictures following the target, broken down by picture type and drinker group, is summarized in Figure 3.2. For the high drinkers, but not the low drinkers, good recall of the bottle of Jack Daniels occurred at the expense of the succeeding three pictures.

The Kramer and Schmidt (2004) results have important implications for memory researchers. The picture of Jack Daniels was a significant stimulus for the high but not the low drinkers. But unlike many previous studies, significance and distinctiveness were not confounded. That is, it is difficult to argue that the alcohol cue was distinctive for one group of participants and not distinctive for another. In terms of shared features within a given context, the picture sequences were identical. One might argue that the alcohol cue encouraged the processing of difference in the con-

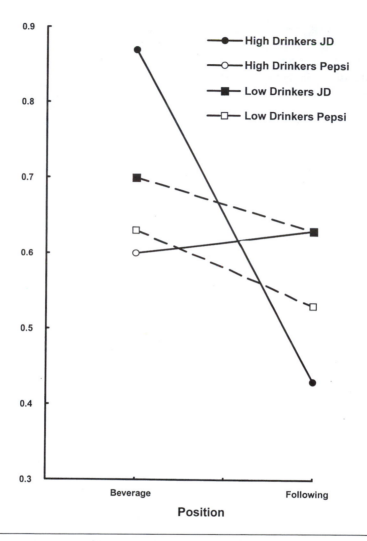

FIGURE 3.2 Summary of the Kramer and Schmidt (2004) results. The target picture was either a bottle of Jack Daniels or a bottle of Pepsi. The recall of the three pictures following the beverage was average for ease of presentation.

text of similarity. For example, perhaps the bottle of Jack Daniels led to associations in the high drinkers but not the low drinkers, and these associations were incongruent with the remaining pictures. As a result, the high drinkers were processing a difference between the pictures not processed by the low drinkers. How was the Jack Daniels bottle different in the context of the pictures in a way that the bottle of Pepsi was not? The only difference was that the Jack Daniels bottle matched something important to a particular type of observer—it was judged as relevant. Similarly, some might argue that relevant stimuli encourage distinctive processing. From this perspective, what I have been calling significance is just a variant of distinctiveness. However, this argument potentially confuses the concepts of novelty and significance. The terms *novelty* and *distinctiveness* should be reserved for situations in which the features extracted from an experience are different from those in a particular frame of reference. By contrast, significance is defined in terms of shared features. In Hunt's terminology, distinctiveness is the processing of difference in the context of similarity; significance is the processing of relevance. Furthermore, the argument that significant stimuli encourage distinctive processing seems to rely on a circular definition of distinctiveness. That is, distinctive processing is inferred from the observation that the material was well remembered, and good memory is explained by distinctive processing. By contrast, significance can be inferred from measurements of emotion and attention that are independent of measures of memory.

If alcohol cues capture and hold the attention of heavy drinkers, a whole range of "special" stimuli may capture and hold the attention of groups of people whose cognitive apparatus is peculiarly dedicated to the special stimulus class. Perhaps the mascot of a football team would capture and hold the attention of fanatic devotees. Perhaps the latest action figure, promoted in the newest movie release, captures and holds the attention of our children. Perhaps Lance Armstrong astride a new Trek "tricked out" with the latest components would capture and hold the attention of an avid bicyclist. Previous researchers have noted that processing the relevance of material can improve memory performance (the so-called self reference effect; Roger, Kuiper, & Kirker, 1977). Self-reference processing appears to encourage both elaboration and organization of the material (see Symons & Johnson, 1997, for a review). I am suggesting that self-reference processing occurs automatically for stimuli that are significant for a participant, engaging the appraisal machinery and leading to interesting mnemonic consequences.

To test the generality of the Kramer and Schmidt study, my students and I attempted to extend the results to cigarette smokers. There is a "smoking Stroop" effect (Gross, Jarvik, & Rosenblatt, 1993) that is similar to the emotional Stroop effect found with alcohol cues. In addition, there is evidence that regular smokers exhibit an "attentional bias" toward smoking cues in visual probe tasks (Bradely, Mogg, Wright, & Field, 2003). Based on these studies, I thought that smoking cues would serve as significant stimuli, would be well recalled in a series of nonsignificant stimuli, and would cause anterograde amnesia.

In order to provide a definitive test of our ideas, we needed to create a homogeneous set of pictures within which to present our significant stimulus. To accomplish this goal, a pilot group of participants was asked to generate objects likely to be found in a typical college student's room. A second group of participants viewed pictures of these items, along with a picture of a pack of cigarettes. This group was asked to rate how likely the items were to be found in a student's room. We used these ratings to select a set of 15 pictures, plus the pack of cigarettes, that all received similar typicality ratings. One picture, that of a package of ramen noodles, was selected as a control item. Students rated the ramen noodles and the pack of cigarettes as equally likely to be found in a student's room, and the packaging of these items were similar in color and shape.

We constructed four lists of 15 pictures from this full set. In two lists the ramen noodles appeared in position 8, and in two other lists the pack of cigarettes appeared in position 8. The remaining 14 pictures were placed into two different orders to create a 2 (presentation order) $\times$ 2 (target picture: noodles versus cigarettes) factorial. The procedures followed the Kramer and Schmidt (2004) paradigm. Introductory psychology students ($N = 183$) viewed the pictures, performed a distractor task, took a free-recall test, and then completed a smoking questionnaire. Based on the students' answers to the smoking questionnaire, each cell of the 2 $\times$ 2 was further subdivided into a smoking and a nonsmoking group. The data from some of the participants were then randomly discarded to balance the number of participants in each experimental condition. The final design consisted of 20 participants in each cell of a 2 (order) $\times$ 2 (target picture) $\times$ 2 (smoking status) factorial.

The results of this study were very disappointing, especially considering the amount of effort that went into selection of the materials. There was a main effect of serial position, $F (14, 1064) = 4.40$, revealing the typical primacy effect, but the serial position by target picture interaction, $F (14, 1064) = 1.07$, and the three-way interaction between serial position, target picture, and smoking status, $F (14, 1064) = .87$, did not approach significance. A summary of the results for just the smokers, focusing on memory for the target pictures and the three pictures following the target, is presented in Figure 3.3. The smokers did remember the package of cigarettes better than the ramen noodles, $t (38) = 1.46, p < .08$, but there was no evidence to suggest that good memory for the cigarettes occurred at the expense of the three pictures following the cigarettes.

There are several possible interpretations of these results. One possible conclusion is that the cigarette pack was distinctive for the smokers but not the nonsmokers. One could point to the good memory for the cigarettes in the absence of anterograde amnesia to support this view. I think this conclusion would be inappropriate, however, because it invokes the tautological use of the term *distinctiveness* alluded to earlier. Another potential conclusion is that the cigarettes were not significant stimuli because they did not produce anterograde amnesia. This conclusion is problematic for two reasons. First, just as we need to avoid circular definitions of *distinctiveness*, we need to avoid a tautological definition of *significance*. *Significance* in the above studies was defined as the presentation of a stimulus that was thought to be particularly important to a group of our participants. We were trying to determine the impact of significance on memory. Second, this conclusion leaves us wondering why the cigarettes were well remembered by the smokers. It seems more parsimonious to conclude that the cig-

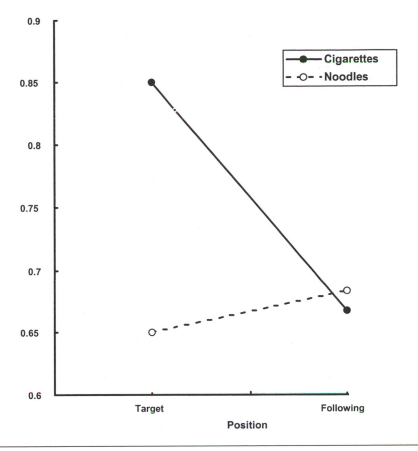

FIGURE 3.3 Summary of the smoking study for smokers only. The target picture was either a package of ramen noodles or a pack of cigarettes. Recall of the three pictures following the target was averaged.

arettes were significant for the smokers, but that significant stimuli do not always cause anterograde amnesia. The anterograde amnesia effect is actually rather difficult to obtain. For example, Schmidt (2002) demonstrated that a short time interval following the presentation of a nude eliminated the anterograde amnesia effect.

Several explanations can be offered as to why anterograde amnesia was not observed in the smoking study. Perhaps a picture of a pack of cigarettes was not a strong enough smoking cue in the experimental context to fully engage the appraisal process. Research with smokers has revealed the presence of event-related brain potentials associated with attention (the P300) in response to pictures of people smoking (Warren & McDonough, 1999). Similarly, smokers exhibit physiological reactions (e.g., heart rate response) in response to the presence of a confederate smoking a cigarette (Niaura et al., 1998). In addition, imagining or seeing a person smoking produces smoking urges in abstinent and nonabstinent smokers (Drobes & Tiffany, 1997). Based on this research, I guessed that a picture of a person smoking would be a stronger cue than a picture of a pack of cigarettes. Perhaps this stronger cue would be well remembered and produce antero-grade amnesia.

My students and I tested the impact of a stronger smoking cue on memory. We inserted a picture of a person smoking in a series of pictures of people engaged in other common daily activities. The experimental design and procedures were similar to those employed in the Kramer and Schmidt (2004) study. Once again, we found good memory for the smoking cue, but no evidence for anterograde amnesia.

Another possibility is that the anterograde amnesia effects following drug cues (e.g., alcohol or cigarettes) may occur only when participants are abstinent. In the Kramer and Schmidt (2004) study, all the students were sober. In contrast, the participants in the smoking studies may still have had nicotine in their blood stream. Using the Stroop task, Gross et al. (1993) found that abstinent smokers took longer to color-name smoking-related words than neutral words, however nonabstinent smokers took longer to color-name neutral words than smoking-related words. Like the Stroop ef-fect, the anterograde amnesia effect to drug cues may require a certain level of craving in participants. Perhaps the attention-hogging appraisal processes engaged by drug cues are drug-use action plans (Tiffany, 1990) that are evoked only by strong physiological craving. Evidence for this conclusion might be found if the smoking studies described above were repeated with abstinent smokers.

CONCLUSIONS

Researchers investigating the impact of distinctiveness on memory need to be careful not to confuse novelty and significance. Both novelty and sig-nificance are defined in terms of feature overlap. These concepts are simi-lar in that they are both context dependent, requiring a specific frame of reference. Both novel and significant stimuli lead to the physiological ori-enting response. Additionally, in many real-world examples and laboratory manipulations, novelty and significance are confounded. However, novel stimuli are those that are unlike information represented in memory, whereas significant stimuli match important memory representations. In-formally, the subjective response to a distinctive event might be a muted "This is different." In contrast, the response to a significant event should be "This is important!" As a result, the impacts of novelty and significance on memory may be quite different.

Significant events may engage cognitive resources as part of appraisal processes. However, attention may be directed to emotional appraisal rather than to the significant stimulus per se. This leads to relatively poor mem-ory for background details contained in an emotional setting and poor memory for events following the significant event. The Detterman and El-lis paradigm, originally designed to study the von Restorff effect, may thus provide a useful tool to investigate the engagement of attention and the processing load of emotional appraisal. Whenever good memory for a tar-get stimulus is accompanied by poor memory for stimuli immediately fol-lowing it, then there is support for the idea that the target captured and held the attention of the participants. Anterograde amnesia thus provides a useful diagnostic for separating the impacts of distinctiveness and signif-icance on memory.

What happens when distinctiveness and significance are not con-founded? There are, unfortunately, only a few experiments that address this issue, including the Kramer and Schmidt (2004) study and the smok-ing studies described here. Apparently, significant stimuli are well remem-bered (when presented in isolation), and sometimes they cause anterograde amnesia. I suggest that the anterograde amnesia results from a shift of at-tention to appraisal processes. But, what supports good memory for significant stimuli when they are not distinctive? There are at least two possibilities.

Perhaps the concept of *emotional distinctiveness*, described by Schmidt (1991), may explain good memory for significant stimuli. That is, a single emotional stimulus embedded in a series of neutral stimuli may "stand out." The emotional content provides for a difference in the context of similar-ity. However, great care should be taken before invoking distinctiveness to explain good memory for an isolated emotional experience. The argument may be inherently circular, in that good memory for the event may be taken as evidence for its distinctive character, and distinctiveness is then used as an explanation for that good memory.

A second explanation may be of greater theoretical value. Perhaps the appraisal processes entail a form of elaboration that supports good mem-ory for the gist of emotional events. As noted above, appraisal may not support detailed analysis of a situation, but the engagement of the appraisal machinery may itself support good memory for the event. The very process of appraising a situation requires one to relate the situation to past expe-riences. That is, appraisal requires self-reference processing that supports good memory performance. These elaborative processes determine how we react to an emotional event and ultimately determine how we remember the event. This idea is similar to what Christianson (1992a, 1992b) de-scribed as "post stimulus elaboration." Because appraisal processes are evoked only by novel or unpredictable events, the isolation of a significant stimulus is required before we can see good memory for the significant event and a shift in attention from background details and subsequent material.

Novelty or distinctiveness may encourage the processing of difference in the context of similarity. Under the right conditions, such processing can be of great benefit to memory, creating rich memory traces that are easily retrieved. The impact of significance on memory is quite different. Significance can also encourage the processing of difference and promote elaboration of an event. However, unlike novelty, significance may evoke emotional processing. Appraisal processes supporting emotion can be complex and resource intensive. As a result, significance can impair memory, disrupt the processing of background material, and lead to poor memory for material immediately following the significant event.

ACKNOWLEDGMENTS

I wish to thank the many students who have assisted me in this research, including Joanna Boucher, Amie Chandler, Mark Gerken, Heather Hill, and Mary C. Powers. I also wish to thank Theresa Schmidt for her comments on an earlier draft of this chapter. The chapter is based on talk delivered to the Southwestern Psychological Association, New Orleans, 2003.

REFERENCES

Ben-Shakhar, G. (1995). The roles of stimulus novelty and significance in determining the electrodermal orienting response: Interactive versus additive approaches. *Psychophysiology, 31,* 402–411.

Bradley, M. M., Greenwald, M. K., Petry, M. C., & Lang, P. J. (1992). Remembering Pictures: Pleasure and arousal in memory. *Journal of Experimental Psychology: Learning, Memory, and Cognition, 18,* 379–390.

Bradley, B. P., Mogg, K., Wright, T., & Field, M. (2003). Attentional bias in drug dependence: Vigilance for cigarette-related cues in smokers. *Psychology of Addictive Behavior, 17,* 66–72.

Carter, B. L., & Tiffany, S. T. (1999). Meta-analysis of cue reactivity in addiction research. *Addiction, 94,* 327–340.

Christianson, S.-A. (1992a). Remembering Emotional Events: Potential Mechanisms. In S.-A. Christianson (Ed.), *The handbook of emotion and memory: Research and theory* (pp. 307–340). Hillsdale, NJ: Lawrence Erlbaum Associates.

Christianson, S.-A. (1992b). Emotional stress and eyewitness memory: A critical review. *Psychological Bulletin, 112,* 284–309.

Christianson, S.-A., & Loftus, E. F. (1987). Memory for traumatic events. *Applied Cognitive Psychology, 1,* 225–239.

Detterman, D. K., & Ellis, N. R. (1972). Determinants of induced amnesia in short-term memory. *Journal of Experimental Psychology, 95,* 308–316.

Drobes, D. J., & Tiffany, S. T. (1997). Induction of smoking urge through imaginal and in vivo procedures: Physiological and self-report manifestations. *Journal of Abnormal Psychology, 106,* 15–25.

Ellis, N. R., Detterman, D. K., Runcie, D., McCarver, R. B., & Craig, E. (1971). Amnesic effects in short-term memory. *Journal of Experimental Psychology, 89,* 357–361.

Eysenck, M. W. (1979). Depth, elaboration, and distinctiveness. In L. S. Cermak & F. I. M. Craik (Eds.), *Levels of processing in human memory* (pp. 89N118). Hillsdale, NJ: Lawrence Erlbaum Associates.

Gati, I., & Ben-Shakhar, G. (1990). Novelty and significance in orientation and habituation: A feature-matching approach. *Journal of Experimental Psychology: General, 119*, 251–263.

Greenwald, M. K., Cook, E. W., & Lang, P. J. (1989). Affective judgment and psychophysiological response: dimensional covariation in the evaluation of pictorial stimuli. *Journal of Psychophysiology, 3*, 51–64.

Gross, T. M., Jarvik, M. E., & Rosenblatt, M. R. (1993). Nicotine abstinence produced content-specific Stroop interference. *Psychopharmacology, 11*, 333–336.

Kramer, D. A., & Goldman, M. S. (2003). Using a modified Stroop task to implicitly discern the cognitive organization of alcohol expectancies. *Journal of Abnormal Psychology, 112* (1), 171–175.

Kramer, D. A., & Schmidt, S. R. (2004). *Alcohol beverage cues impair memory in high social drinkers*. Manuscript in preparation.

Loftus, E. F., & Burns, T. E. (1982). Mental shock can produce retrograde amnesia. *Memory & Cognition, 10*, 318–323.

McCloskey, M., Wible, C., & Cohen, N. (1988). Is there a special flashbulb memory mechanism? *Journal of Experimental Psychology: General, 117*, 171–181.

Nelson, D. L. (1979). Remembering pictures and words: Appearance, significance and name. In L. S. Cermak & F. I. M Craik (Eds.), *Levels of processing in human memory* (pp. 45–76). Hillsdale, NJ: Lawrence Erlbaum Associates.

Niaura, R., Shadel, W. G., Abrams, D. B., Monti, P. M., Rohsenow, D. J., & Sirota, A. (1998). Individual difference in cue reactivity among smokers trying to quit: Effects of gender and cue type. *Addictive Behaviors, 23*, 209–224.

Ohman, A., Flykt, A., & Esteves, F. (2001). Emotion drives attention: Detecting the snake in the grass. *Journal of Experimental Psychology: General, 130*, 466–478.

Rogers, T. B., Kuiper, N. A., & Kirker, W. S. (1977). Self-reference and the encoding of personal information. *Journal of Personality and Social Psychology, 35*, 677–688.

Schachter, S., & Singer, J. (1962). Cognitive, social, and physiological determinants of emotional state. *Psychological Review, 69*, 379–339.

Scherer, K. R. (2001). Appraisal considered as a process of multilevel sequential checking. In K. R. Scherer, A. Schorr, & T. Johnstone (Eds.), *Appraisal processes in emotion: Theory, methods, research* (pp. 92–119). New York: Oxford University Press.

Scherer, K. R., Schorr, A., & Johnstone, T. (Eds.) (2001). *Appraisal processes in emotion: Theory, methods, research*. New York: Oxford University Press.

Schmidt, S. R. (1991). Can we have a distinctive theory of memory? *Memory & Cognition, 19*, 523–542.

Schmidt, S. R. (1997, Nov.). *In search of paradoxical effects of arousal on memory*. Paper presented at the annual meeting of the Psychonomic Society, Philadelphia, PA.

Schmidt, S. R. (2002). Outstanding memories: The positive and negative effects of nudes on memory. *Journal of Experimental Psychology: Learning, Memory, and Cognition, 28,* 353–361.

Schulz, L. S. (1971). Effects of high-priority events on recall and recognition of other items. *Journal of Verbal Learning and Verbal Behavior, 10,* 332–330.

Stetter, F., Ackermann, K., Bizer, A., Straube, E. R., & Mann, K. (1995). Effects of disease-related cues in alcoholic inpatients: Results of a controlled "Alcohol Stroop" study. *Alcoholism: Clinical and Experimental Research, 19,* 593–599.

Symons, C. S., & Johnson, B. T. (1997). The self-reference effect in memory: A meta-analysis. *Psychological Bulletin, 121,* 371–394.

Tiffany, S. T. (1990). A cognitive model of drug urges and drug-use behavior: The role of automatic and non-automatic processes. *Psychological Review, 97,* 147–168.

Tulving, E. (1969). Retrograde amnesia in free recall. *Science, 164,* 88–90.

Wallace, W. P. (1965). Review of the historical, empirical, and theoretical status of the von Restorff phenomenon. *Psychological Bulletin, 63,* 410–424.

Warren, C. A., & McDonough, B. E. (1999). Event-related brain potentials as indicators of smoking cue-reactivity. *Clinical Neurophysiology, 110,* 1570–1584.

Wolff, J. G. (1993). Computing, cognition and information compression. *AI Communications, 6,* 107–127.

4

Encoding and Retrieval Processes in Distinctiveness Effects: Toward an Integrative Framework

Mark A. McDaniel and Lisa Geraci

A consistent and common theme in memory research and theory is that unusual or bizarre information is well remembered, typically more so than information that is usual or commonplace (e.g., Hunt & Lamb, 2001; Schmidt, 1991; see Graesser, Woll, Kowalski, & Smith, 1980, for linkages of this idea with text memory). Indeed, this idea has existed for at least 3,000 years, as a series of scrolls known as the *Ad Herennium*, which advocated the formation of bizarre images to support potent mnemonic techniques. The *Ad Herennium* suggested that images should be "active . . . as striking as possible," with striking later specified as "ridiculous, unusual, rare" (see Wollen & Margres, 1987). Couched in the terminology that gives rise to the title of this volume, the emergent empirical principle is that distinctiveness enhances memory. This principle is so engrained in contemporary work that it is not unusual for researchers to explain superior memory in one condition over another as a function of the relative distinctiveness produced in each condition. For instance, distinctiveness has been invoked to explain superior memory for atypical category members (Schmidt, 1985), words with unusual orthographies (Hunt & Elliott, 1980; Hunt & Mitchell, 1978, 1982; Hunt & Toth, 1990), the generation effect (Slamecka & Graf, 1978; better memory for items that were generated than items that were read at study), and the levels of processing effect (Stein, 1978), among many other phenomena (see Geraci & Rajaram, Chapter 10 this volume).

As a number of contributors to this volume have consistently argued, however, the varied applications of the term *distinctiveness* as both an explanatory construct and an empirical description (see Hunt, Chapter 1 this volume; Hunt & Lamb, 2001; Schmidt, 1991) and the varied and inconsistent patterns described as distinctiveness effects (Schmidt, 1991) have diminished the value of the term as an explanatory construct. What remains a challenge for contemporary researchers is to understand why distinctive information is associated with better memory performance. That is, what are the memory processes and dynamics that produce a mnemonic advantage for unusual or "distinct" information?

In this chapter, we attempt to forge a partial answer by considering two general classes of processes: encoding processes and retrieval processes. We first briefly present these two classes as explanations of distinctiveness effects (Schmidt, 1991). We then review the contemporary experimental work directed at competitive tests of encoding versus retrieval explanations. The upshot is that no clear conclusion seems evident from the existing literature. We attempt to reconsider the findings within an organizational framework that considers encoding and retrieval processes orthogonally with two categories of distinctiveness—primary and secondary distinctiveness (adapted from Schmidt). We suggest that under the lens of this analysis, some informative patterns begin to emerge. Finally, we describe several testable hypotheses using the encoding/retrieval distinction and suggest that primary and secondary distinctiveness effects may be mediated by different memory processes.

ENCODING VIEWS OF DISTINCTIVENESS EFFECTS

Views of differential encoding propose that unusual items are remembered well primarily because they receive differential processing at the time of encoding. In this chapter, we use differential encoding processes to refer to any processing that occurs at the time the individual item is encountered. The most basic and seminal encoding view suggests that distinctive items are remembered better than common items because they receive more attention than common items (Jenkins & Postman, 1948; Green, 1956). Depending on the view, increased attention can have several possible consequences that produce superior encoding of the "distinct" item. The item can receive a greater amount of processing (e.g., Wollen & Cox, 1981; Slamecka & Katsaiti, 1987; Watkins, LeCompte, & Kim, 2000), evaluative processing (Geraci & Rajaram, 2002), or greater elaboration (Waddill & McDaniel, 1998). In the expectation-violation view, unusual items violate expectations regarding the nature of the stimuli that will be encountered and accordingly stimulate more extensive processing of the general context in which the item appears (Hirshman, Whelley & Palij, 1989). This greater contextual encoding contributes subsequently to memory performance when retrieval cues are impoverished (as in free recall).

Somewhat related to the expectation-violation view is Schmidt's (1991) incongruity theory. According to this theory, distinctive items are those that are incongruent with, or contain salient features relative to, conceptual frameworks that are active when the items are being encoded. The incongruency prompts several processing activities. First, the incongruent item attracts increased attention in an automatic fashion. Subsequently, more controlled memory processes are engaged toward the incongruent item that might include elaboration and rehearsal.

RETRIEVAL VIEWS OF DISTINCTIVENESS EFFECTS

An alternative view is that distinctiveness effects are primarily a consequence of processes operating at retrieval. There are two prominent formulations within this theoretical class. One general idea is that the unusual features of the "distinct" items provide highly diagnostic information that benefits memory performance (Hunt & McDaniel, 1993). The benefit may be related to enhanced discriminability of the target from possible candidates generated at recall or provided at recognition (Hunt & McDaniel, 1993; Hunt & Mitchell, 1982), or the advantage may reflect the use of these unusual features to guide access or direct retrieval to the "distinct" items (Knoedler, Hellwig, & Neath, 1999; Waddill & McDaniel, 1998). To empirically illustrate the potency of diagnostic information at retrieval, Peynircioglu and Mungan (1993) examined the generation effect for familiar and unfamiliar categories. They reasoned that people should be able to generate more retrieval cues for the familiar categories than for the unfamiliar categories, but the cues they generate for the unfamiliar categories should be more diagnostic. The results supported the benefit of diagnostic cues: the generation effect was biggest for items from less familiar categories (for example, music words given to sports experts and sports words given to music experts).

Another idea is that distinct items make up their own mnemonic category containing a small set of unique cues (Bruce & Gaines, 1976). Bruce and Gaines suggest that for each mnemonic category, distinct and common, the probability of recalling a distinct item will be greater than the probability of recalling a common item because there are fewer distinct items in their mnemonic category. This is similar to the cue-overload hypothesis, which proposes that recall of an item is a function of the number of cues associated with the item (Watkins & Watkins, 1975). For category cued recall, results show that memory performance is inversely related to the number of category instances related to the cue, that is, the category label (Tulving & Pearlstone, 1966; Watkins & Watkins, 1975). So, given the category name—which is essentially, either the "weird items" or the "common items," recall is better for the items in the smaller (weird) category than for items in the larger (common) category.

EXPERIMENTAL FINDINGS

At the outset, two critical points warrant mention. First, the existing literature involves numerous demonstrations of distinctiveness-like phenomena. It is unknown, however, to what extent all of these demonstrations rely on similar processes. Second, the most clear-cut empirical implications follow from the encoding explanations of distinctiveness effects. Accordingly, encoding views are favored when these implications are supported, whereas retrieval views generally take the role of a default position that can be embraced when encoding implications are not supported.

One basic implication of the encoding view is that more study time should be associated with distinct than with common items. Much research uses experimenter-paced presentations, and for these experiments study time is not assessed. However, in one case the presentation rate was decreased to minimize the possibility for extra study time of distinct items (sentences describing unusual events). Even so, these sentences were recalled better than were sentences describing common events (Waddill & McDaniel, 1998).

More directly, when self-paced presentations are used, differential study time has not proved to be an entirely consistent marker of effects attributed to distinctiveness across various manipulations of distinctiveness. For bizarre and common sentences, some have found a positive relation between study time and the mnemonic advantage for bizarre sentences (Kroll & Tu, 1988, Experiment 2; Richman, 1994; Worthen & Loveland, 2001). Using simpler materials, Hunt and Elliott (1980) failed to find a processing-time difference for orthographically common and distinct words. Their results showed that people studied common words for the same amount of time as they did distinct words, but orthographically distinct items were still remembered better than common items. However, processing time in this study was relatively long (10 seconds per item) and likely reflected similar study strategies across items as opposed to actual processing time. When processing time is examined using a speeded lexical decision task, decision times are longer for orthographically distinct words than for orthographically common words (Hunt & Toth, 1990).

A complementary implication of the encoding view is that divided attention at study should reduce or eliminate distinctiveness effects because resources are not available to devote additional processing to the "distinct" items. In support of this prediction, Geraci and Rajaram (2002) found that dividing attention reduced the mnemonic effects of orthographic distinctiveness. Similarly, dividing attention at study (using a secondary task of lexical decision) eliminates the recognition advantage for low-frequency words over high-frequency words (Joordens & Hockley, 2000). Also, using a response deadline at test eliminates the low-frequency word advantage (Balota, Burgess, Cortese, & Adams, 2002). In contrast, Lamb and Hunt (1999) showed in an unpublished experiment that superior memory for isolated items was not affected by divided attention.

Similarly, instructing participants to pay particular attention to salient items does not necessarily enhance memory for these items. In one experiment, participants were explicitly instructed to pay attention to items that were presented in a case (e.g., uppercase versus lowercase letters) different from the other words in the set (Bruce & Gaines, 1976). In addition, one of the uppercase items was presented within brackets. Results showed that the bracketed uppercase item was recalled better than the other uppercase words to which participants were instructed to attend. Thus, it seems that increased attention to the isolated items per se was not associated with the level of memory performance for the isolated items.

A third implication of the encoding view is that the serial position of the "distinct" items in the list should modulate the mnemonic advantage of those items. When the isolated item is in the first study position, there is nothing distinct about it until the study list is completed, at which point it is invariably too late to go back and pay more attention to the item. Consequently, an attention explanation of the distinctiveness effect would predict that in this situation there should be no memory advantage for the unusual item. Von Restorff's (1933) original work demonstrated the opposite, however. In one of her studies, she found that even when the isolated item appeared in the first serial position of the study list, people had superior memory for the isolate. Further, subsequent work has shown that isolating an item later in the list does not augment its mnemonic advantage relative to when the item is isolated early in the list (Hunt, 1995; Kelley & Nairne, 2001; McConnell, Sherman, & Hamilton, 1994; Pillsbury & Rausch, 1943). These results counter a differential encoding view and instead favor a retrieval view (e.g., Brown, Neath, & Chater, 2002; Hunt & McDaniel, 1993).[1]

Countering the above pattern, rare words are better recalled than common words when they are well mixed in a list (e.g., rare and common words alternate—see May, Cuddy, & Norton, 1979; or words assigned to serial position randomly—see DeLosh & McDaniel, 1996), but not when rare and common words are blocked in the list (May et al., 1979). These results are somewhat consistent with the incongruity version of an encoding explanation of distinctiveness effects (Schmidt, 1991). In this approach, rare words intermixed with common words would be incongruent with a conceptual framework prompted by encountering common words in the list, thereby attracting attention. On the other hand, rare words blocked in the first half of the list would be congruent with an active conceptual framework stimulated by the list context (encounter of rare words) and would therefore not attract increased attention and elaboration. In this case, better recall of rare relative to common words would not be expected from a differential processing perspective. Not explained by the incongruity formulation, however, is the presumed equivalence for rare and common words when rare words are blocked in the second half of the list. In this case, recall of rare words should benefit from increased attention stimulated by their incongruence with the conceptual framework adopted from processing the initial block of common words. The exact pattern of data is unknown, however, because the results were not examined according to the order of presentation of the blocks. Indeed, this order factor typically has not been viewed as theoretically important, and consequently not analyzed. Later in this chapter, we present new research with bizarre and common materials and with humorous and nonhumorous materials that provides initial tests of the just-mentioned predictions from the incongruity encoding formulation.

A fourth implication of the encoding view is that distinct items should appear subjectively salient at the time of encoding. Subjective judgments of salience for isolated items have been examined using judgment of learning (JOL) ratings (Dunlosky, Hunt, & Clark, 2000). Participants studied lists that contained an isolated item either at the beginning of the list, at the end of the list, or at neither, and they were asked to judge the likelihood that they would later be able to remember each item in the list. Results showed that people gave greater JOLs when the isolate occurred later in the list than when it occurred earlier, but regardless, there was no difference in memory for the early and late isolate. Thus, subjective JOLs were not predictive of finding an isolation effect, suggesting that at the time of encoding it is not necessary to see the isolated item as distinctive for it to aid subsequent memory.

This brief review underscores the apparently inconclusive and confusing state of the literature regarding whether an encoding or a retrieval process, or both, plays a major role in the wide array of findings described as distinctiveness effects. In the remainder of the chapter we propose an interpretation of these patterns of results that attempts to unify some of the apparent discrepancies.

ENCODING—RETRIEVAL REVISITED IN TERMS OF PRIMARY AND SECONDARY DISTINCTIVENESS

In one attempt to develop an understanding of distinctiveness effects in memory, Schmidt (1991) divided these effects into several classes, with two prominent classes being primary and secondary distinctiveness (a nonmutually exclusive approach to the relational/individual item account of distinctiveness; Hunt & McDaniel, 1993; see also Hunt, Chapter 1 this volume). The term *primary distinctiveness* was applied to items that are unusual with respect to their immediate encoding context. Examples would include an item printed in red in the presence of other list items printed in black, a numeral presented in a list of words, and an item not belonging to the category represented by other list items (e.g., the word *apple* presented in a list of furniture exemplars). In Schmidt's framework, primary distinctiveness was applied to situations in which the to-be-remembered material activates an overall conceptual organization or structure, within which the "distinct" item is at odds. The idea was specifically that the cognitive structure would be active during encoding, thereby bringing into relief, at study, the salient features of the item that did not match those of the preceding items (see also Worthen, Marshall, & Cox, 1998).

This formulation is restrictive, as it would not capture the original von Restorff phenomenon, which is considered the paradigm case of primary distinctiveness. In von Restorff's designs, as noted above, the "distinct" item could be presented very near the beginning of the list, making it unlikely that a conceptual structure would have emerged at the time of encountering the "distinct" item. Accordingly, we adopt a broader notion of primary distinctiveness that does *not* rest on defining the distinct item in relation to an active conceptual structure suggested by the immediately encoded items. Rather, primary distinctiveness is defined simply as the item being rendered unusual by the context of the list.

In contrast, the term *secondary distinctiveness* was applied to situations in which the item is unusual with respect to one's general knowledge—that is, information stored in permanent memory (McDaniel & Einstein, 1986; Schmidt, 1991). For instance, the sentence, "the dog road the bicycle down the street" would be distinct because this sentence would be unusual relative to people's previous experience.

In the remainder of this chapter, we explore whether the foregoing distinction may help to synthesize the apparently discrepant findings that we have noted regarding encoding and retrieval explanations of distinctiveness, and provide a framework for understanding some new findings. To anticipate, our working hypothesis is that primary distinctiveness and secondary distinctiveness may differentially rely on encoding and retrieval processes.

PRIMARY DISTINCTIVENESS

First, we suggest that primary distinctiveness is mainly a retrieval-based phenomenon and that items with primary distinctiveness do not draw upon additional online processes at encoding. It is important to note that this claim does not imply that encoding is nonessential. We assume that, in primary distinctiveness, similar or identical encoding processes are brought to bear on both distinct and common items, with these processes producing an encoding that is similar in terms of representational parameters (for instance, same type and number of features in a vector representation), though of course the content varies (different values for the features). The key claim is that the amount of encoding or type of features encoded is not differential across distinct and common items. This idea derives from the observation that the von Restorff effect was initially obtained when the isolated item was early in the list—presumably too early for the conceptual relations of the nonisolated list items to have been discerned (see Hunt, 1995), and thereby precluding differential encoding (again, in terms of the nature of the features encoded or kind of elaboration engaged).

When seen from this perspective the results of the previously reviewed studies become more consistent. None of the findings implicating differential item processing at encoding was associated with primary distinctiveness effects. Further, directing attention at study to isolated items did not uniformly affect levels of memory performance for the isolated items (Bruce & Gaines, 1976). By contrast with secondary distinctiveness, directing attention to items using intentional learning instructions produces better recall. For example, when attention is directed to low-frequency (rare) words, there is a recall advantage for low-frequency relative to high-frequency words (in mixed lists of low- and high-frequency words). In addition, minimizing attentional differences using incidental learning instructions eliminates the recall advantage of low-frequency words (Watkins et al., 2000).[2] To the extent that the advantage of low-frequency words in mixed lists can be considered a distinctiveness effect (DeLosh & McDaniel, 1996), this would be considered a secondary distinctiveness effect.

Further, research shows that at the time of encoding, items with primary distinctiveness that are isolated early in the list do not appear subjectively more salient than nonisolated items (Dunlosky et al., 2000). When participants are asked to judge how likely they are to remember isolated and nonisolated items using judgments of learning (JOL) at the time of encoding, early isolates do not receive greater JOLs than nonisolated items and yet they are still remembered better than the nonisolated items. Thus, one could argue that items with primary distinctiveness are not salient at the time of encoding.

With primary distinctiveness (physically or categorically isolated items), suppressed memory for background items is not obtained, especially when memory is assessed with recognition (Bruce & Gaines, 1976; McLaughlin, 1968; Schmidt, 1985; van Dam, Peeck, Brinkerink, & Gorter, 1974). This pattern is consistent with the idea that this class of distinctiveness effects is mediated primarily by retrieval processes. We note that the suppression of background items does occur for these primary distinctiveness effects in recall (Jenkins & Postman, 1948; Schmidt, 1985). Because people tend to recall the isolated items first, however, suppression of background items in this case appears to be due to output interference, which is consistent with a retrieval explanation of primary distinctiveness effects (see Schmidt, Chapter 3 this volume, for more extended discussion of implications of background item suppression effects).

List-position effects have been investigated in primary distinctiveness paradigms, and list position does not modulate these distinctiveness effects. List-position effects in secondary distinctiveness have received little to no attention in the literature, but as we will see below, there is a suggestion that such effects may appear in secondary distinctiveness.

While primary distinctiveness effects do not appear to be mediated by differential item processing at encoding (they are not mediated by attention, list position, or study position; they do not cause suppression of background items; and subjective uniqueness is not necessary for the effect), there is some direct support for the idea that these effects are mediated by retrieval processes. As one example, Bruce and Gaines (1976) found that physically isolated words (e.g., words in brackets), like semantically related words, were clustered at recall, suggesting that both encouraged the re-memberer to form a mnemonic category for guiding recall.

Other support for the role of retrieval factors in primary distinctiveness comes from research showing differential effects of the type of test. The majority of isolation effects that have been reported are obtained in free recall (see Wallace, 1965, for a review). When recall performance is con-trasted directly with recognition, some researchers have shown that the memory advantage for perceptually isolated items is obtained only in re-call and not in recognition (McLaughlin, 1968; van Dam et al., 1974). In McLaughlin's experiment, participants studied a list of consonant-vowel-consonant (CVC) strings. Half of the participants studied the list including one CVC that was printed in a different size and shape in the sixth posi-tion of the nine-item list. The other half of the participants studied the same list with no isolated item. Immediately after study, all participants were given a free-recall test followed by a recognition test. Results showed that people had superior recall for the isolated item than for its control item in the same position. However, there was no recognition benefit for this item.

One could argue that the recognition test was contaminated by perfor-mance on the initial free-recall test. However, when a between-subjects de-sign is used, the same general result is obtained (van Dam et al., 1974). In this experiment, participants studied lists of 15 words (Dutch words, in this case) with either all the words printed on a green background or all but one word (which appeared in position 9 of the 15-item list on a red back-ground) appearing against a green background. Immediately after study, both groups of participants either received a free-recall test or a recogni-tion test. As in the previous study, results showed superior memory for the isolated item on the free-recall test, but not on the recognition test. Both studies conclude that retrieval processes should be invoked to explain the isolation effect. McLaughlin suggests that "vividness affects processes of search and retrieval and may not affect the strength of stored information" (1968, p. 101) and van Dam et al. suggest that "the isolation effect in this study was localizable primarily in the retrieval phase" (1974, p. 502). In fact, von Restorff (1933) herself reportedly had difficulty obtaining the ef-fects of primary distinctiveness in recognition and had to go to greater lengths to see its effects on this test compared to free recall (as cited in Hunt, 1995).

Finally, it appears that the type of cue at test has a large effect on whether memory benefits from isolation. For example, Hunt and Smith (1996) show that providing test cues that access the study context increase the effects of primary distinctiveness. In this study, participants studied cat-egorized lists and indicated either how one item in the list was different from the other items or how it was similar to the other items in the list. The difference judgment led to superior memory for the item (a kind of distinctiveness effect), and this effect was magnified when participants were given a cue at test that provided information about the study context (the particular category). This result suggests that primary distinctiveness effects are affected by retrieval cues that help to delineate the particular study episode. Moreover, in studies that do not require any reference back to the study episode (studies using implicit memory tests), the effects of primary distinctiveness can be difficult to obtain (Smith & Hunt, 2000; but see Geraci & Rajaram, 2004). Taken together, the array of findings reported in the literature strongly suggests that retrieval processes mediate primary distinctiveness effects.

Thus far we have used the concept of differential encoding processes to refer to processing that occurs at the time the individual item is encountered. Our use of differential encoding processes does not include processes subsequent to encoding of the item itself that occur during the encoding phase of the study list. In other words, for primary distinctiveness it is possible that while participants do not devote more processing to the item at the moment the item is encountered, they may engage in some additional processing during the study phase of the experiment, before the actual retrieval phase. Dunlosky et al. (2000) make a similar distinction: "The idea is that when the isolate appears in the beginning of the list, it is not initially salient but becomes salient sometime after its presentation. For instance, after studying several other items on the list, the individual may attend to the isolate (e.g., through retrieval), which then induces a surprise response via conceptual salience. We call this conceptual salience because salience here does not rely on the direct perception of the isolate but instead is triggered by conceptual processes, such as retrieving the isolate and comparing it to previously presented items from the list" (p. 652; see also Geraci & Rajaram, Chapter 10 this volume, for a similar idea). The surprise mechanism described by Dunlosky et al. awaits detailed study. However, when the conceptual salience view is tested by examining whether the isolated item receives extra rehearsal, this view is not supported (Dunlosky et al., 2000). Still, the distinction between differential item processing and differential subsequent processing (all during the encoding phase of the experiment) may be important to consider. Participants might engage in some differential processing subsequent to the presentation of the isolated item that does not engender extra rehearsal. More research is needed to explore this hypothesis.

SECONDARY DISTINCTIVENESS

In contrast to our discussion of primary distinctiveness, we suggest that secondary distinctiveness effects may involve differential online encoding processes in addition to differential retrieval processes. This makes sense because, at the moment one encounters an item with secondary distinctiveness, this item is already odd with respect to one's past experience. Indeed, a closer look at the research reviewed earlier provides some initial support for the hypothesis that secondary distinctiveness effects may engender additional processes at encoding (whereas primary distinctiveness effects do not). For example, as discussed earlier, dividing attention at study negatively affects only secondary distinctiveness. Specifically, dividing attention reduces the orthographic distinctiveness effect (Geraci & Rajaram, 2002) and the recognition advantage for low-frequency words (Joordens & Hockley, 2000), but not the isolation effect (Lamb & Hunt, 1999). Recent neuroimaging evidence on orthographic distinctiveness and word frequency effects provides converging evidence. One FMRI study found that during encoding, orthographically distinct words were associated with greater bi-lateral activity in prefrontal and visual processing regions than were orthographically common words (Kirchhoff, Schapiro, & Buckner, in press). Another FMRI study found greater frontal and anterior cingulate activation during encoding of low-frequency relative to high-frequency words (Chee, Westphul, Geh, Graham, & Seng, 2003).

The study-time evidence is more complicated, however. Study time has been fairly consistently related to the effects of secondary distinctiveness as manifested in bizarre imagery, for those conditions that typically give rise to bizarreness effects (free recall in mixed list designs with simple sentences; Kroll & Tu, 1988; Worthen & Loveland, 2001). With complex bizarre and common sentences, experimenter-varied presentation rates produce effects that may implicate a role for study time. Kline and Groninger (1991) varied the presentation rate of complex bizarre and common sentences ("The yellow and orange striped cat relentlessly chases the small, scarred, rubber ball."). In two experiments, the faster presentation rate was 11 seconds and the slower rate was 15 seconds. Both experiments found a significant interaction between presentation rate and the effect of sentence type. The bizarreness effect was completely eliminated (there was an advantage for common sentences) at the fast presentation rate, but appeared at the slower presentation rate (with an increase in recall for bizarre relative to common sentences of .20 and .10 in each experiment).

These results may support the idea that additional processing time for unusual relative to common items is a factor in the bizarreness effect. In line with this idea, Kline and Groninger (1991) note that bizarreness effects for complex sentences have not been reported when study times are 11 seconds or less (Kroll, Schepeler, & Angin, 1986; McDaniel & Einstein, 1989; see also Robinson-Riegler & McDaniel, 1994). Further, in experiments in which long presentation rates were used (e.g., 30 seconds), advantages for complex bizarre sentences have sometimes been reported (Richman, 1994). Of course, these associations between presentation rate and the bizarreness effect do not directly implicate enhanced encoding of bizarre items as the underlying mediator of the effect. Worthen, Garcia-Rivas, Green, and Vidos (2000) have suggested that increased processing time for bizarre stimuli is needed to attain comprehension levels equivalent to that achieved more quickly for common stimuli (in vector-model terminology, encoding of a similar feature vector, but of course with somewhat different values for the features).

Further, in paradigms other than those using bizarre imagery, the evidence for differential study time is not forthcoming. Waddill and McDaniel (1998) presented simple sentences describing atypical events ("The boy found a huge diamond in the apple sauce") and typical events ("The boy found a huge diamond in the jewelry store") and varied the study time for these sentences. In a normally paced condition, sentences were presented for 18 seconds each, and in the fast-paced condition sentences were presented for 5 seconds each. Waddill and McDaniel reasoned that the fast-paced condition should have precluded the opportunity for participants to further elaborate the atypical events (as suggested above for forming complex bizarre images). Thus on an encoding view, the fast-paced condition might be expected to eliminate or attenuate the secondary distinctiveness effects observed in the normally paced condition. The results showed that atypical items were recalled better under both study-time conditions, with no interaction. One could argue, however, that the presentation rate in the fast condition for these simple sentences was still generous enough to allow participants to devote additional processing to the atypical sentences. As discussed earlier, the same idea might be applied to the equivalent, but somewhat long study times for orthographically distinct and nondistinct words (Hunt & Elliott, 1980).

In light of the mixed study-time findings, other types of evidence are needed to compel the idea that secondary distinctive effects depend in part on differential encoding dynamics. For example, would items with secondary distinctiveness, such as low-frequency words, orthographically distinct words, bizarre sentences, or even bizarre pictures be associated with higher ratings of JOLs that would predict superior memory for these items? Our hypothesis would predict that for items with secondary distinctiveness but not primary distinctiveness, JOLs would predict superior memory. More experimental tests like the one just mentioned are needed to provide evidence for the psychological distinction between these two types of distinctiveness. Accordingly, we next consider some newer, unpublished work to examine the role of encoding processes in secondary distinctiveness. Before doing so, a puzzling feature of secondary distinctiveness effects that is pertinent must be mentioned.

One common experimental paradigm presents unmixed lists of unusual and typical items. This unmixed list design consistently produces no recall advantage for atypical items or sometimes a slight advantage for common items (e.g., see DeLosh & McDaniel, 1996; Einstein & McDaniel, 1987; McDaniel, DeLosh, & Merritt, 2000a, Experiments 1 and 2; McDaniel, Einstein, Delosh, May, & Brady, 1995; Hunt & Elliott, 1980; Hunt & Mitchell, 1982; Waddill & McDaniel, 1998; Worthen, Chapter 7 this volume). Because these items are unusual with respect to one's general knowledge (the definition of secondary distinctiveness), unmixed lists should not undermine the enhanced encoding that we have suggested unusual items enjoy relative to common items. It was precisely this puzzle that prompted Schmidt's (1991) incongruity view. His view provides an encoding account that directly accommodates the unmixed-list findings by suggesting that enhanced encoding for unusual items follows only when those items are processed in the context of an active conceptual framework for which the unusual items are incongruent. In an unmixed list of unusual items, the active conceptual framework is congruent with those items. Thus, in this instance, no relevant context is established to engage any additional processing at encoding.

Another approach suggested by DeLosh and McDaniel (1996; see also McDaniel et al., 2000a; Serra & Nairne, 1993) is that in unmixed lists, unusual items receive more individual-item processing than do common items, but that such processing is at the expense of serial-order information that is ordinarily encoded. For memory tests for which serial-order information can be useful (e.g., free recall; DeLosh & McDaniel, 1996), the mnemonic advantage of the unusual items is thus countered by reduced order memory of the list itself. Though this newer approach seems promising (e.g., McDaniel, DeLosh, & Merritt, 2000b), the experiments that follow are considered from the perspective of the incongruity view.

New Experiments

A clear implication from the incongruity view, as developed earlier, is that the serial position of the unusual items in a mixed list of common and unusual items should be critical in obtaining secondary distinctiveness effects (as opposed to primary distinctiveness effects). That is, it should be critical to structure the list such that some common items are presented before the unusual items, thereby providing the active conceptual framework against which the unusual items will be processed. Published research directly examining this prediction is virtually nonexistent. In a correlational procedure, Worthen et al. (1998) reported that recall of a bizarre item was positively associated with the number of common items that preceded the bizarre items. A finding reported by Hirshman et al. (1989) may also be consistent with the incongruity version of the encoding view, but their article did not evaluate the data in a manner that would inform this view. In some of their experiments, bizarre sentences (e.g., "The DOG rode the BICYCLE down the STREET") were presented in one entire block and common sentences ("The DOG chased the BICYCLE down the STREET") were presented in another block. Hirshman et al. reported significantly better recall for bizarre relative as compared to common sentences. According to the ideas just outlined, this finding should have been limited to the condition in which the bizarre block followed the common block (which occurred half of the time because presentation order was counterbalanced). For the conditions in which the bizarre-sentence block is presented first, the active conceptual framework would not be incongruent with bizarre sentences. Thus, recall of bizarre sentences should not be enhanced in a bizarre-block first-presentation order.

The present formulation prompted us to reanalyze data from an unpublished experiment completed by Courtney Dornburg and one of the authors (MAM). We conducted a conceptual replication of Hirshman et al. (1989), in which participants received one blocked list of bizarre sentences followed by a blocked list of common sentences or vice versa. Originally, we had not examined the bizarreness effect as a function of block order, simply viewing it as a counterbalancing factor. In this experiment, we also attempted to further isolate the effects of encoding processes on the bizarreness advantage using a modified recall procedure. We instructed participants to first recall one block of sentences that was presented; when they finished that recall task, participants were then instructed to recall the other block of sentences that was presented (the order of recall of the two blocks was completely counterbalanced across subjects). We did not want to require recall of both blocks concurrently because in a mixed retrieval environment that includes both common and bizarre stimuli, learners could exploit bizarre features to help reconstruct or recover items for recall (McDaniel & Einstein, 1986; McDaniel et al., 1995; Knoedler et al., 1999). This possibility would cloud our attempt to illuminate the role of encoding processes in mediating these secondary distinctiveness effects. The results were in line with the prediction outlined above. When the bizarre sentences were presented first, the proportion of target nouns recalled from bizarre ($M = .36$) and common sentences ($M = .36$) was equivalent. By contrast, when the bizarre sentences followed presentation of common sentences, recall was significantly better for bizarre ($M = .40$) than for common items ($M = .27$; $F (1, 30) = 5.94$).

Melissa Guynn, Susan Clapper, Olena Connor, and one of us (MAM) recently applied this design to examine another effect that might be classified as a secondary distinctiveness effect. Paralleling the bizarreness effect, Schmidt (1994) reported that humorous sentences were better recalled than common sentences when mixed lists were presented but not when unmixed lists were presented. Assuming that humorous sentences are not as typically encountered as nonhumorous sentences in people's reading experiences, the mnemonic advantage of humorous sentences could be viewed as a distinctiveness effect.

The findings from this study using humorous sentences paralleled those reported for the experiment with bizarre and common sentences. When the humorous sentences were presented first, the recall advantage for humorous sentences was eliminated (mean proportion recall of content words for humorous sentences = .18 and for nonhumorous sentences = .28). When the humorous sentences followed the nonhumorous sentences, the humorous sentences ($M = .31$) were recalled substantially better than the nonhumorous sentences ($M = .09$). Unfortunately, these patterns are not entirely straightforward because there are recency effects as well. The more incisive experiment to test the incongruency formulation would be to compare the recall of bizarre or humorous sentences that followed a block of common sentences with recall of bizarre or humorous sentences that followed a block of like sentences (bizarre or humorous). The more general point here is that existing experimental paradigms could be fruitfully extended to help disentangle encoding versus retrieval dynamics in distinctiveness (and bizarreness and humor) effects.

Our hypothesized distinction between primary and secondary distinctiveness also prompts one to look for dissociative effects of certain manipulations across the two kinds of distinctiveness. The clear prediction from our distinction between primary and secondary distinctiveness is that there should be such dissociative effects on these classes of distinctiveness, which would contrast with the predictions from a common process approach (e.g., Schmidt, 1991). The results of a study that we just completed are in line with this expectation. We (along with Roddy Roediger) examined the effects of primary and secondary distinctiveness for older adults. In the primary distinctiveness conditions participants studied items that were either isolated in a study list (the word *table* was presented amid categorized items such as *salmon, trout, bass, tuna*, and so on) or not isolated in the study list. Older adults studied several of these lists and were then given a surprise cued-recall test. For these adults, recall of the critical targets did not significantly vary as a function of isolation: they did not show an isolation effect.

In the secondary distinctiveness conditions, we examined memory for target items embedded in bizarre sentences such as "The DOG rode the BICYCLE down the STREET." Recall of targets embedded in bizarre sentences was compared to recall of the same items embedded in common sentences ("The DOG chased the BICYCLE down the STREET"). Contrasted with the absence of a primary distinctiveness effect, there was a significant advantage in proportion recall of target nouns for bizarre relative to common sentences for older adults. Unlike isolation, older adults can take advantage of bizarreness to aid memory.

This apparently inconsistent pattern can be understood from our notion that secondary but not primary distinctiveness effects are due in part to enhanced encoding of the distinct items. Much literature has demonstrated that conditions that stimulate additional encoding produce mnemonic benefits for older adults (e.g., keyword encoding—Brigham & Pressley, 1988; organization—Hultsch, 1969; generation—McDaniel, Ryan, & Cunningham, 1989; McFarland, Warren, & Crockard, 1985; imagery-based mnemonics—Kliegl, Smith, & Baltes, 1989; Poon, Walsh-Sweeney, & Fozard, 1980).

Similarly, the absence of a primary distinctiveness effect for older adults makes sense from the perspective that this type of effect relies heavily on retrieval processes. A prominent view of age-related deficits in memory suggests that older adults are especially impaired in using internally generated cues to guide retrieval (e.g., Craik, 1986). Thus, older adults would not benefit from primary distinctiveness because they are presumably less able to exploit the unusual feature of the isolated items to augment retrieval.

One further condition in our recent study supports our focus on retrieval dynamics in primary distinctiveness and their relation to the nonsignificant effects with older adults. We augmented encoding of the distinct features of the isolated item by requiring participants to read each word and rate the degree to which it fit into the list context. If the primary distinctiveness effect were based on encoding processes that enhanced storage of the of the isolated item (cf. Schmidt, 1991), and these encoding processes needed to be guided for older adults, then under these enhanced encoding instructions a distinctiveness effect should emerge for older adults. Again, however, there was no significant distinctiveness effect for older adults. However, the rating task was effective for older adults: recall was improved over the condition with no rating task. Yet, the effectively augmented encoding did not produce an isolation effect for the older adults. According to our view, the isolation effect depends on retrieval processes that exploit the isolated item's feature that is unusual relative to the other list items— processes that are impaired in older adults.

Retrieval Processes in Secondary Distinctiveness Effects

In the bizarreness experiment with older adults, the bizarre and common sentences were intermixed in the acquisition list. More generally, the recall advantage for bizarre items is consistently found with intermixed lists but not with unmixed lists of bizarre and common items, as is true for many secondary distinctiveness effects (see Einstein & McDaniel, 1987, and McDaniel et al., 1995, for reviews). This pattern has prompted theorists to suggest that mixed lists might produce additional processing of the bizarre or unusual items (Wollen & Margres, 1987; Worthen et al., 1998; see Schmidt, 1991, for the more general notion that secondary distinctiveness effects rely in part on encoding processes stimulated by mixed lists). The idea is that mixed lists highlight the unusual nature of bizarre items, so that these items receive a greater amount of processing such as elaboration or rehearsal (Merry, 1980; Schmidt, 1991; Wollen & Cox, 1981). In turn, the more extensive, elaborative processing produces a more memorable encoding of the bizarre items.

Recent work on the bizarreness effect suggests, however, that retrieval processes also play an integral role in secondary distinctiveness effects. As discussed earlier, retrieval views assume that in a retrieval environment that includes both common and bizarre stimuli, learners exploit bizarre features to help reconstruct or recover items for recall (cf. Knoedler et al, 1999). McDaniel et al. (2000a) reasoned that if such retrieval processes were involved in the recall advantage for bizarre stimuli, then providing or encouraging reliance on alternative retrieval strategies should eliminate or attenuate the bizarreness effect. Alternatively, if differential encoding is solely responsible for the bizarreness effect, then the more elaborated and better attended bizarre items should generally be better recalled regardless of free recall strategy.

In one experiment, McDaniel et al. (2000a, Experiment 3) examined recall of mixed lists of bizarre and common sentences when participants were either instructed to recall items in serial order or recall them freely in any order (in the serial-recall group participants were also encouraged to encode serial-order information). For both groups (serial and standard instructions) recall was scored as if it were free recall—correct output order was not considered. With standard instructions, the typical bizarreness advantage was replicated (mean proportion target nouns recalled was .57 for bizarre and .49 for common). By contrast, with serial-recall instructions, a very atypical pattern for mixed lists emerged such that the advantage for bizarre items was eliminated ($M = .55$ for bizarre items and $M = .58$ for common items). Therefore, this study demonstrates that retrieval processes are also critical for secondary distinctiveness effects.

In a parallel experiment (McDaniel et al., 2000a, Experiment 4), some of the mixed lists were constructed so that the target nouns in the sentences were categorically related. Because categorical information is used prominently in recall relative to other potential sources of information (e.g., Nairne, Riegler, & Serra, 1991), we expected that the categorically related lists would foster a spontaneous recall strategy based in part on category information. If the bizarreness effect is based solely on enhanced encoding for bizarre items (a bizarreness-rating orienting task was used for both standard and categorically related lists), then the bizarreness effect should have been obtained for both types of mixed lists (categorized and uncategorized). Instead, McDaniel et al. found that the typical bizarreness effect in the standard mixed list ($M = .51$ and $M = .43$, for bizarre and common items, respectively) was eliminated in the categorized list ($M = .58$ and $M = .60$ for bizarre and common items).

Both sets of results are entirely in line with the idea that retrieval dynamics play a prominent role in the bizarreness effect. In recall, when participants were required (serial recall) or encouraged (categorized lists) to adopt a retrieval process that did not focus on item distinctiveness, bizarre items lost their mnemonic advantage. Were the bizarreness advantage simply a function of more extensive encoding, then one would expect that the bizarreness effect would persist with both a serial-order recall strategy and a category-guided strategy, given the assumption that both relational (serial order, category) and item information (extensive encoding of the individual items) promote optimal recall (Hunt & McDaniel, 1993).

The companion expectation is that if the retrieval context augments a retrieval process that focuses on item distinctiveness, then the bizarreness effect should become more pronounced. We examined this idea in the experiment conducted with Dornburg. As described earlier, in that experiment, blocked presentation of bizarre and common items was followed by blocked recall. The pattern of results implied an encoding advantage for bizarre items (a marginally significant advantage). With another group of participants not yet mentioned, we followed the identical encoding conditions with a recall test in which all sentences were to be recalled together. In this mixed-retrieval context, retrieval processes relying on distinctive features would be productive (Knoedler et al., 1999; McDaniel et al., 2000a). If, however, differential encoding is the sole determinant of bizarreness effects (and by extension, secondary distinctiveness effects), then this retrieval context should be irrelevant to the magnitude of the bizarreness effect. Countering this prediction, in the mixed retrieval condition, bizarre items ($M = .54$) showed a 50% increase over recall of common items ($M = .35$), a notable expansion (effect size, $\eta^2 = .30$) in the advantage of bizarre ($M = .38$) over common sentences ($M = .31$) in the separate recall condition ($\eta^2 = .09$). It is noteworthy that the amplified bizarreness effect in the mixed retrieval condition was entirely a result of increased recall of bizarre items relative to that obtained in the separate retrieval condition. To the extent that the bizarreness effect reflects a secondary distinctiveness phenomena (Schmidt, 1991), the corpus of results reviewed here supports our assumption that secondary distinctiveness effects are mediated in part by retrieval processes.

Summary

For years, memory theorists have wrestled with the theoretical issue of specifying the encoding or retrieval processes, or both, that underlie the mnemonic advantage of distinctiveness. The issue has been all the more challenging because the literature appears to be confusing and contradictory with regard to this central theoretical issue. In this chapter we have revisited this literature from the perspective that two kinds of distinctiveness effects, primary and secondary, may be mediated by somewhat different processes. When examined from this perspective, the literature converges on the conclusion that primary distinctiveness effects are principally driven by retrieval processes, and not encoding processes. On the other hand, for secondary distinctiveness effects, convincing findings can be marshaled for both encoding and retrieval processes. As initial demonstrations of the fruitfulness of our framework, we presented new experiments described within this framework that further the understanding of several kinds of secondary distinctiveness effects (bizarreness and humor effects) and that directly reveal differences between primary and secondary distinctiveness patterns. We offer this framework as a means for reconciling some of the inconsistent findings in the literature and for generating new questions. Further tests of this hypothesis are needed, and we think that such research has the potential to better illuminate distinctiveness and the various processes that might mediate different kinds of distinctiveness effects.

ACKNOWLEDGMENTS

Preparation of this chapter was supported in part by NIA grant AG 17481. We are grateful to Gilles Einstein, Reed Hunt, and James Worthen for helpful comments on an earlier version of this chapter.

NOTES

1. Another, somewhat similar, implication of the encoding view is that the distinctiveness effect should depend on the proportion of distinct to common items. For isolation effects, the list structure is critical and the effect is not obtained, by definition, if the isolated item is not infrequent in the list. For other distinctiveness effects, the list structure appears to be less critical. For example, the bizarreness effect is obtained even when half of the items are bizarre and half are common (McDaniel & Einstein, 1986; McDaniel et al., 1995; Worthen & Loveland, 2001). Similarly, the orthographic distinctiveness effect occurs with this same list structure (Hunt & Elliott, 1980; Hunt & Mitchell, 1978, 1982; Hunt & Toth, 1990). Even when the list is structured such that all of the items are distinct and only one is common; the orthographic distinctiveness effect is still obtained (unpublished work cited in Hunt & Mitchell, 1982). Thus, it appears that the presence of other common items influences the distinctiveness effect.
2. See the bizarreness literature for a different pattern, however (Worthen, Chapter 7, this volume).

REFERENCES

Balota, D. A., Burgess, G. C., Cortese, M. J., & Adams, D. R. (2002). Memory for the infrequent in young, old, and early stage Alzheimer's disease: Evidence for two processes in episodic recognition performance. *Journal of Memory and Language, 46*, 199–226.

Brigham, M. C., & Pressley, M. (1988). Cognitive monitoring and strategy choice in younger and older adults. *Psychology and Aging, 3*, 249–257.

Brown, G. D. A., Neath, I., & Chater, N. (2002). A ratio model of scale-invariant memory and identification. Manuscript submitted for publication.

Bruce, D. & Gaines, M. T. (1976). Tests of an organizational hypothesis of isolation effects in free recall. *Journal of Verbal Learning and Verbal Behavior, 15*, 59–72.

Chee, M. W. L., Westphul, C., Geh, J., Graham, S., & Seng, A. W. (2003). Word frequency and subsequent memory effects studied using event-related FMRI. *NeuroImage, 20*, 1042–1051.

Craik, F. I. M. (1986). A functional account of age differences in memory. In F. Klix & H. Hagendorf (Eds.), *Human memory and cognitive capabilities: Mechanisms and performances* (pp. 409–422). North Holland: Elsevier Science Publishers.

DeLosh, E. L., & McDaniel, M. A. (1996). The role of order information in free recall: Application to the word frequency effect. *Journal of Experimental Psychology: Learning, Memory, and Cognition, 22,* 1136–1146.

Duncan, C. P. (1974). Retrieval of low-frequency words from mixed lists. *Bulletin of the Psychonomic Society, 4,* 137–138.

Dunlosky, J., Hunt, R. R., & Clark, E. (2000). Is perceptual salience needed in explanations of the isolation effect? *Journal of Experimental Psychology: Learning, Memory, and Cognition, 26,* 649–657.

Einstein, G. O., & McDaniel, M. A. (1987). Distinctiveness and the mnemonic benefits of bizarre imagery. In M. A. McDaniel & M. Pressley (Eds.), *Imagery and related mnemonic processes: Theories, individual differences and applications* (pp. 78–102). New York: Springer-Verlag.

Geraci, L., & Rajaram, S. (2002). The orthographic distinctiveness effect on direct and indirect tests of memory: delineating the awareness and processing requirements. *Journal of Memory and Language, 47,* 273–291.

Geraci, L. & Rajaram, S. (2004). The distinctiveness effect in the absence of conscious recollection: Evidence from conceptual priming. *Journal of Memory and Language, 51,* 217–230.

Geraci, L., & Rajaram, S. (2006). The distinctiveness effect in explicit and implicit memory. In R. R. Hunt & J. B. Worthen (Eds.), *Distinctiveness and memory* (pp. 211–234). New York: Oxford University Press.

Graesser, A. C., Woll, S. B., Kowalski, D. J., & Smith, D. A. (1980). Memory for typical and atypical actions in scripted activities. *Journal of Experimental Psychology: Human Learning and Memory, 6,* 503–515.

Green, R. T. (1956). Surprise as a factor in the von Restorff effect. *Journal of Experimental Psychology, 52,* 340–344.

Gregg, V. H. (1976). Word frequency, recognition and recall. In J. Brown (Ed.), *Recall and recognition* (pp. 183–216). London: Wiley.

Gregg, V. H., Montgomery, D., & Castano, D. (1980). Recall of common and uncommon words from single and mixed lists. *Journal of Verbal Learning and Verbal Behavior, 19,* 240–245.

Hirshman, E., Whelley, M. M., & Palij, M. (1989). An investigation of paradoxical memory effects. *Journal of Memory and Language, 28,* 594–609.

Hultsch, D. F. (1969). Adult age differences in the organization of free recall. *Development Psychology, 1,* 673–678.

Hunt, R. R. (1995). The subtlety of distinctiveness: What von Restorff really did. *Psychonomic Bulletin & Review, 2,* 105–112.

Hunt, R. R., & Elliott, J. M. (1980). The role of nonsemantic information in memory: Orthographic distinctiveness effects on retention. *Journal of Experimental Psychology: General, 109,* 49–74.

Hunt, R. R., & Lamb, C. A. (2001). What causes the isolation effect? *Journal of Experimental Psychology: Learning, Memory, and Cognition, 27,* 1359–1366.

Hunt, R. R. & McDaniel, M. A. (1993). The enigma of organization and distinctiveness. *Journal of Memory and Language, 32,* 421–445.

Hunt, R. R. & Mitchell, D. B. (1978). Specificity in non-semantic orienting tasks and distinctive memory traces. *Journal of Experimental Psychology: Learning, Memory, and Cognition, 4,* 121–135.

Hunt, R. R. & Mitchell, D. B. (1982). Independent effects of semantic and nonsemantic distinctiveness. *Journal of Experimental Psychology: Learning, Memory, and Cognition, 8,* 81–87.

Hunt, R. R., & Smith, R. E. (1996). Accessing the particular from the general: The power of distinctiveness in the context of organization. *Memory & Cognition, 24,* 217–225.

Hunt, R. R., & Toth, J. P. (1990). Perceptual identification, fragment completion, and free recall: Concepts and data. *Journal of Experimental Psychology: Learning, Memory, and Cognition, 16,* 282–290.

Jenkins, W. O., & Postman, L. (1948). Isolation and the spread of effect in serial learning. *American Journal of Psychology, 61,* 214–221.

Joordens, S., & Hockley, W. E. (2000). Recollection and familiarity through the looking glass: When old does not mirror new. *Journal of Experimental Psychology: Learning, Memory, and Cognition, 26,* 1534–1555.

Kelley, M. R. & Nairne, J. S. (2001). Von Restorff revisited: Isolation, generation, and memory for order. *Journal of Experimental Psychology: Learning, Memory, and Cognition, 27,* 54–66.

Kirchoff, B. A., Schapiro, M. L., & Buckner, R. L. (in press). Orthographic distinctiveness and semantic elaboration provide separate contributions to verbal memory. *Journal of Cognitive Neuroscience.*

Kliegl, R., Smith, J., & Baltes, P. B. (1989). Testing-the-limits and the study of adult age differences in cognitive plasticity of a mnemonic skill. *Developmental Psychology, 25,* 247–256.

Kline, S., & Groniger, L. D. (1991). The imagery bizarreness effect as a function of sentence complexity and presentation time. *Bulletin of the Psychonomic Society, 29,* 25–27.

Knoedler, A. J., Hellwig, K. A., & Neath, I. (1999). The shift from recency to primacy with increasing delay. *Journal of Experimental Psychology: Learning, Memory, and Cognition, 25,* 474–487.

Kroll, N. E. A., Schepeler, E. M., & Angin, K. T. (1986). Bizarre imagery: The misremembered mnemonic. *Journal of Experimental Psychology: Learning, Memory, and Cognition, 12,* 42–53.

Kroll, N. E. A. & Tu, S.-F. (1988). The bizarre mnemonic. *Psychological Research, 50,* 28–37.

Lamb, C. A., & Hunt, R. R. (1999). *Extraordinary attention is not necessary for isolation effects.* Unpublished manuscript, University of North Carolina, Greensboro.

May, R. B., Cuddy, L. J., & Norton, J. M. (1979) Temporal contrast and the word frequency effect. *Canadian Journal of Psychology, 33,* 141–147.

May, R. B., & Tryk, H. E. (1970). Word sequence, word frequency, and free recall. *Canadian Journal of Psychology, 24,* 299–304.

McConnell, A. R., Sherman, S. J., & Hamilton, D. L. (1994). Illusory correlation in the perception of groups: An extension of the distinctiveness-based account. *Journal of Personality and Social Psychology, 67,* 414–429.

McDaniel, M. A., DeLosh, E. L., & Merritt, P. S. (2000a). Order information and retrieval distinctiveness: Recall of common versus bizarre material. *Journal of Experimental Psychology: Learning, Memory, and Cognition, 26,* 1045–1056.

McDaniel, M. A., DeLosh, E. L., & Merritt, P. S. (2000b, Nov.). *Order information in free recall: A new look at word-frequency effects.* Paper presented at the 41st Annual Meeting of the Psychonomic Society, New Orleans, LA.

McDaniel, M. A., & Einstein, G. O. (1986). Bizarre imagery as an effective memory aid: The importance of distinctiveness. *Journal of Experimental Psychology: Learning, Memory, and Cognition, 12,* 54–65.

McDaniel, M. A., & Einstein, G. O. (1989). Sentence complexity eliminates the mnemonic advantage of bizarre imagery. *Bulletin of the Psychonomic Society, 27,* 117–120.

McDaniel, M. A., Einstein, G. O., Delosh, E L., May, E. P., & Brady, P. (1995). The bizareness effect: It's not surprising, it's complex. *Journal of Experimental Psychology: Learning, Memory, and Cognition, 21,* 422–435.

McDaniel, M. A., Ryan, E. B., & Cunningham, C. J. (1989). Encoding difficulty and memory enhancement for young and old readers. *Psychology and Aging, 4,* 333–338.

McFarland, C. E., Jr., Warren, L. R., & Crockard, J. (1985). Memory for self-generated stimuli in young and old adults. *Journal of Gerontology, 40,* 205–207.

McLaughlin, J. P. (1968). Recall and recognition measures of the von Restorff effect in serial learning. *Journal of Experimental Psychology, 78,* 99–102.

Merry, R. (1980). Image bizarreness in incidental learning. *Psychological Reports, 46,* 427–430.

Nairne, J. S., Riegler, G. L., & Serra, M. (1991). Dissociative effects of generation on item and order retention. *Journal of Experimental Psychology: Learning, Memory, & Cognition, 17,* 702–709.

Peynircioglu, Z. & Mungan, E. (1993). Familiarity, relative distinctiveness, and the generation effect. *Memory & Cognition, 21,* 3, 367–374.

Pillsbury, W. B., & Rausch, H. L. (1943). An extension of the Koler-Restorff inhibition phenomenon. *American Journal of Psychology, 56,* 293–298.

Poon, L. W., Walsh-Sweeney, L., & Fozard, J. L. (1980). Memory skills training for the elderly: Salient issues on the use of imagery mnemonics. In L. W. Poon, J. L. Fozard, L. S. Cermak, D. Arenberg, & L. W. Thompson (Eds.), *New directions in memory and aging* (pp. 461–484). Hillsdale, NJ: Lawrence Erlbaum Associates.

Richman, C. L. (1994). The bizarreness of effect with complex sentences: Temporal effects. *Canadian Journal of Experimental Psychology, 48,* 444–450.

Robinson-Riegler, B., & McDaniel, M. A. (1994). Further constraints on the bizarreness effect: Elaboration at encoding. *Memory & Cognition, 22,* 702–712.

Schmidt, S. R. (1985). Encoding and retrieval processes in the memory for conceptually distinctive events. *Journal of Experimental Psychology: Learning, Memory, and Cognition, 11*, 565–578.

Schmidt, S. R. (1991). Can we have a distinctive theory of memory? *Memory and Cognition, 19*, 523–542.

Schmidt, S. R. (1994). Effects of Humor on Sentence Memory. *Journal of Experimental Psychology: Learning, Memory, and Cognition, 20*, 953–967.

Serra, M., & Nairne, J. S. (1993). Design controversies and the generation effect: Support for an item-order hypothesis. *Memory & Cognition, 21*, 34–40.

Smith, R. E., & Hunt, R. R. (2000). The effects of distinctiveness require reinstatement of organization: The importance of intentional memory instructions. *Journal of Memory and Language, 43*, 431–446.

Slamecka, N. J., & Graf, P. (1978). The generation effect: Delineation of a phenomenon. *Journal of Experimental Psychology: Human Learning and Memory, 4*, 592–604.

Slamecka, N. J., & Katsaiti, L. T. (1987). The generation effect as an artifact of selective displaced rehearsal. *Journal of Memory and Language, 26*, 589–607.

Stein, B. S. (1978). Depth of processing reexamined: The effects of the precision of elaboration and test appropriateness. *Journal of Verbal Learning and Verbal Behavior, 17*, 165–174.

Tulving, E., & Pearlstone, S. (1966). Availability versus accessibility of information in memory for words. *Journal of Verbal Learning & Verbal Behavior, 5*, 381–391.

Van Dam, G., Peeck, J., Brinkerink, M., & Gorter, U. (1974). The isolation effect in free recall and recognition. *American Journal of Psychology, 87*, 497–504.

von Restorff, H. (1933). Uber die Wirkung von Bereichsblidungen im Spurenfeld. Psychologishe Forschung, 18, 299–342.

Waddill, P. J., & McDaniel, M. A. (1998). Distinctiveness effects in recall: Differential processing or privileged retrieval? *Memory and Cognition, 26*, 108–120.

Wallace, W. P. (1965) Review of the historical, empirical, and theoretical status of the von Restorff phenomenon. *Psychological Bulletin, 63*, 410–424.

Watkins, M. J., LeCompte, D. C., & Kim K. (2000). Role of study strategy in recall of mixed lists of common and rare words. *Journal of Experimental Psychology: Learning, Memory, and Cognition, 26*, 239–245.

Watkins, O. C., & Watkins, M. J. (1975). Buildup of proactive inhibition as a cue-overload effect. *Journal of Experimental Psychology: Human Learning and Memory, 104*, 442–452.

Wollen, K. A., & Cox, S. (1981). Sentence cuing and the effectiveness of bizarre imager *Journal of Experimental Psychology: Human Learning and Memory, 7*, 386–392.

Wollen, K. A., & Margres, M. G. (1987). Bizarreness and the imagery multiprocess model. In M. A. McDaniel & M. Pressley (Eds.), *Imagery and re-*

lated mnemonic processes: Theories, individual differences and applications (pp. 103–127). New York: Springer-Verlag.

Worthen, J. B., Garcia-Rivas, G., Green, C. R., & Vidos, R. A. (2000). Tests of a cognitive resource allocation of the bizarreness effect. *Journal of General Psychology, 127,* 117–144.

Worthen, J. B., & Loveland, J. M. (2001). Imagery nonvividness and the mnemonic advantage of bizarreness. *Imagination, Cognition, and Personality, 20,* 373–381.

Worthen, J. B., Marshall, P. H., & Cox, K. B. (1998). List length and the bizarreness effect: Support for a hybrid model. *Psychological Research/ Psychologische Forschung, 61,* 147–156.

5

Reducing Memory Errors:
The Distinctiveness Heuristic

Daniel L. Schacter and Amy L. Wiseman

The concept of distinctiveness has an extensive history in memory research (Hunt, 1995). Numerous studies have revealed that memory for an event benefits from a variety of manipulations that increase distinctive processing during encoding of that event, including surprising items that are incongruent with the prevailing context (e.g., Hunt & Lamb, 2001; von Restorff, 1933) and various types of encoding tasks that focus attention on the properties of an item that distinguish it from others (e.g., Hunt & Smith, 1996; Jacoby & Craik, 1979; Lockhart, Craik, & Jacoby, 1976). As documented in many chapters in this volume, students of memory have devoted a good deal of empirical and theoretical attention to understanding the basis for the beneficial effects of distinctiveness on subsequent retention.

It is perhaps less widely appreciated that distinctiveness can benefit subsequent memory in a related but different manner: by helping to avoid memory errors, such as misremembering the details of prior experiences, or falsely remembering events that did not occur. Some investigators have indeed explored the role of distinctiveness in reducing errors concerning the source of recently studied information (e.g., Dobbins, Kroll, Yonelinas, & Liu, 1998; Gruppuso, Lindsay, & Kelley, 1997; Hunt, 2003), and others have examined the role of distinctiveness in avoiding false recognition (e.g., Ghetti, 2003; Strack & Bless, 1994; Dodson & Schacter, 2002a, 2002b; Israel & Schacter, 1997; Schacter, Israel, & Racine, 1999). Nonetheless, such research is in an early stage of development compared with work examining how distinctiveness increases subsequent retention.

In the present chapter, we focus on recent research concerned with understanding how distinctiveness can help to reduce memory errors—specifically those involved in false recognition, where people claim that they have previously seen or heard a novel item or event. We will focus in particular on recent studies from our laboratory that have provided evidence for a memory monitoring mechanism that we have called the *distinctiveness heuristic* (Schacter et al., 1999). As we will document later, when people rely on a distinctiveness heuristic, they *expect* to remember distinctive details of recently studied information, which in turn leads to reduced false recognition of novel items. Thus, when we speak of a distinctiveness heuristic as a monitoring mechanism invoked at the time of retrieval, we depart somewhat from the widely used definition of distinctiveness as the processing of unusual or unique features of an item during encoding that increase the subsequent discriminability of that item (e.g., Hunt, 2003; Lockhart et al., 1976). However, as we will see later in the chapter, our notion of a distinctiveness heuristic incorporates the standard conception of distinctiveness, while emphasizing that distinctive processing during encoding can greatly influence expectations during retrieval regarding the quality of to-be-retrieved information.

To set the stage for discussion of the distinctiveness heuristic, we first review more generally the role of distinctiveness in memory errors by considering the seven "sins" of memory (Schacter, 1999, 2001), and then move on to recent studies that have begun to explore the relationship between distinctiveness and false recognition. Finally, we consider possible directions for future research in this area.

THE SEVEN SINS OF MEMORY: RELATIONS TO DISTINCTIVENESS

To initiate discussion of the role of distinctiveness in memory errors, we find it is useful to have a conceptual framework for thinking about mistaken memories. Schacter (1999, 2001) provides one such framework, which holds that memory's imperfections can be divided into seven basic categories or "sins": transience, absent-mindedness, blocking, misattribution, suggestibility, bias, and persistence. The first three sins involve different forms of forgetting—that is, "sins of omission." *Transience* refers to the nature of memories that tend to become decreasingly accessible over time. This general characteristic of memory, first documented in the laboratory by Ebbinghaus (1885/1964) over a century ago, is central to all theories of remembering and forgetting. *Absent-mindedness*, in contrast, refers to lapses of attention that result in forgetting to do things, such as the common experience of failing to recall where we placed our keys or eyeglasses moments ago (Reason & Mycielska, 1982). *Blocking* refers to the temporary inability to access information that has not faded out of memory. The best known example of blocking is the "tip of the tongue" experience, where we temporarily cannot retrieve a name or word that, nevertheless, we are certain that we know (e.g., Schwartz, 1999; Maril, Wagner, & Schacter, 2001).

The next three memory errors can be viewed as "sins of commission": cases in which memory is present, but wrong. *Misattribution* occurs when we remember some aspect of an experience but attribute the memory to an incorrect source. For example, having imagined carrying out a task, we may mistakenly come to believe that we actually did it (Johnson & Raye, 1981; Johnson, Hahstroudi, & Lindsay, 1993). *Suggestibility* refers to the implanting of memories that are produced by leading questions or suggestions. Dramatic examples of suggestibility have been documented where the use of suggestive procedures contributes to the "recovery" of vivid, even traumatic memories of events that never happened (for review, see Ceci & Bruck, 1993; Loftus & Pickrell, 1995; Schacter, 2001). The final distortion-related sin, *bias*, refers to the ways in which current knowledge and beliefs can skew memories for past experiences. Numerous studies have shown that what people know, believe, and feel in the present can influence and distort the past (Ross & Wilson, 2000). Finally, the seventh sin, *persistence*, refers to unwanted recollections of difficult or even traumatic experiences that people cannot forget, even though they wish they could. Persisting memories can, in extreme cases, permanently color how we view the present, past, and future, such as the intrusive memories sometimes experienced by war veterans or survivors of sexual assault (McNally, 2003).

How is distinctiveness related to each of the seven sins? A good deal is known about how to answer this question for a few of the sins, but next to nothing is known for most of the others. For example, considering the three forgetting-related sins of transience, absent-mindedness, and blocking, we are not aware of any research that specifically links distinctiveness and blocking. By contrast, much of the classic work on distinctive processing and memory alluded to earlier in the chapter indicates that distinctive encoding serves to decrease transience, at least in the sense that distinctive encoding typically improves performance on standard recall and recognition tests. Relatively little work has been conducted on the role of distinctiveness in absent-minded forgetting, but some relevant evidence is provided by studies of prospective memory: remembering to do things in the future. Prospective memory is highly relevant to absent-mindedness because many absent-minded errors involve forgetting to carry out future tasks, such as picking up milk at the grocery store on the way home from work, or forgetting to pass on a message to an acquaintance at a later time. To avoid absent-minded errors in such situations, it is important to have access to retrieval cues at the time that a task needs to be carried out; a distinctive retrieval cue can increase the probability of prospective remembering.

Experiments by McDaniel and Einstein (1993) using a laboratory prospective memory task demonstrate the importance of cue distinctiveness. Participants were given lists of words to learn for a later test. For the prospective memory task, some participants tried to remember to push a button whenever a specific word appeared, such as *movie*, whereas others were instructed to push the button whenever a specific nonword appeared, such as *yolif*. McDaniel and Einstein reasoned that participants have many pre-existing associations to *movie* and thus might sometimes retrieve these associations instead of remembering to press the button. By contrast, participants have no associations to *yolif*. With a more distinctive association to the prospective response, participants should not be distracted by irrelevant information and therefore should be less likely to forget to push the button in response to this cue. Consistent with these ideas, results showed that participants were much more likely to remember to press the button when cued with *yolif* than with *movie*.

Turning next to the four sins of commission, we will review research related to misattribution in the next section of the chapter. We are not aware of any studies linking suggestibility and distinctiveness (we will comment on their possible relations later in the chapter), and we are likewise unaware of any work concerning bias and distinctiveness. Persistence, the seventh sin, is typically observed following emotionally arousing or traumatic events. To the extent that such events are also usually highly distinctive, one could argue that persistence and distinctiveness are closely and perhaps inextricably linked. If so, then research that attempts to disentangle the contributions of emotional arousal and distinctiveness from persisting, intrusive memories would be highly desirable (for discussion of the relation between emotion and distinctiveness, see Chapters 8 and 3 in this volume).

MISATTRIBUTION AND DISTINCTIVENESS: RECENT RESEARCH

As noted earlier, misattribution occurs when we remember some aspects of an experience, but we misattribute the memory to an incorrect source. Misattribution therefore involves a confusion about the origins of retrieved information (Jacoby, Kelley, & Dywan, 1989; Johnson et al., 1993; Schacter, 1999), and it can take various forms. For example, we can confuse two external sources of information, such as when we recall hearing about a movie from a friend, when in fact we heard it reviewed on a radio program, or we come to believe that a tidbit of gossip is true because we mistakenly remember reading about the item in a reputable newspaper, when in fact we saw it in a tabloid. In laboratory experiments, this type of misattribution error is often studied by having two different sources (e.g., male and female) present participants with lists of words, facts, or other information, and later testing memory for both the items and the sources (e.g., Dodson & Shimamura, 2000; McIntyre & Craik, 1987; Schacter, Harbluk, & McLachlan, 1984; for review, see Johnson et al., 1993). Similar types of source misattribution errors can lead to false recognition. For example, in the repetition lag paradigm introduced by Jennings and Jacoby (1997), participants are initially exposed to a list of words, and on a subsequent recognition test they make old/new recognition judgments about previously studied words and new words that did not appear previously on the study list. Critically, the new words are repeated later in the test at various lags, and participants are specifically instructed to call these repeated items new (because they had never appeared in the study list). Jennings and Jacoby (1997) found that participants still made false alarms to repeated new words, and the effect was quite pronounced in older adults. Calling a repeated new word "old" indicates a failure of source memory: participants misattribute their familiarity with the repeated new words to having encountered them on the study list. As discussed later, our laboratory has adapted this paradigm to examine the role of distinctiveness in avoiding this type of misattribution error (Dodson & Schacter, 2002a, 2002b).

A related type of misattribution involves confusing what we only imagined or thought with what we actually perceived. For instance, an individual may confuse whether he imagined having a conversation with his friend with whether he actually participated in the conversation. These types of misattribution, referred to as *reality monitoring errors*, have been extensively studied by Johnson and colleagues, among others (e.g., Johnson & Raye, 1981; Johnson et al., 1993). Similarly, people may believe that they generated an idea on their own, when in fact they had encountered it from another source, a phenomenon known as *unconscious plagiarism* or *cryptomnesia* (e.g., Marsh, Landau, & Hicks, 1997).

Source misattribution errors play an important role in recent laboratory demonstrations of robust false-recognition effects. One paradigm that has been widely used to examine false recognition was originally developed by Deese (1959), and later refined and extended by Roediger and McDermott (1995). In the Deese/Roediger–McDermott (DRM) paradigm, participants hear lists of words (e.g., *candy, sour, sugar*) that are all semantic associates of a nonpresented theme or lure word (e.g., *sweet*). When later given an old/new recognition test that contains studied words (e.g., *candy*), new unrelated words (e.g., *point*), and new related lure words (e.g., *sweet*), participants frequently and confidently claim that they previously studied the related lures. This striking false-recognition effect has been replicated and extended in a variety of experimental conditions and subject populations (cf., Brainerd & Reyna, 1998; Budson, Sullivan, et al., 2002; Ghetti, Qin, & Goodman, 2002; Norman & Schacter, 1997; Payne, Elie, Blackwell, & Neuschatz, 1996; Schacter, Verfaellie, & Pradere, 1996; Smith & Hunt, 1998; Tun, Wingfield, Rosen, & Blanchard, 1998).

One account of these findings is that when an item is studied, such as the word *candy*, participants implicitly think of the related lure word *sweet*. When *sweet* is later presented on the recognition test, participants misattribute their own prior implicit associative response to having studied the word. A related hypothesis is that when numerous associatively related words are studied, participants may later respond on the basis of general similarities between the related items, which have been termed *gist information* (e.g., Brainerd, Reyna, & Kneer, 1995). Inherent in this latter approach to understanding false recognition in the DRM paradigm is the idea that when provided lists of semantic associates, participants do not focus on, and hence later fail to recollect, distinctive characteristics of specific studied items.

Although the foregoing hypotheses are difficult to disentangle in the DRM paradigm, Koutstaal and Schacter (1997) presented evidence that false recognition can be based on gist information. They used a paradigm in which participants studied categorized pictures and were later tested on studied pictures and related lures from studied categories (along with unrelated lures). For example, after studying varying numbers of shoes, cars, or teddy bears, participants made old/new recognition decisions about the pictures they actually saw and nonstudied shoes, cars, or teddy bears. Koutstaal and Schacter reasoned that participants are not likely to specifically generate the related lures during study, in the same sense that they might generate *sweet* in the DRM paradigm. Nonetheless, participants still showed significant false recognition of related lures (i.e., nonstudied pictures from studied categories). The effect was especially pronounced in older adults who, according to Koutstaal and Schacter's analysis, are more likely than younger adults to respond on the basis of gist information.

The overall pattern of results from the foregoing studies suggests that misattribution errors can arise in situations where people initially focus on similarities that are shared among a group of items while at the same time not noticing the distinctive features that differentiate the items from one another (cf., Hunt & McDaniel, 1993). If so, then it should be possible to reduce such false-recognition effects by creating conditions that encourage participants to focus on the distinctive properties of individual items. This line of reasoning initially led us to examine the role of distinctive processing in reducing the misattribution errors observed during gist-based false recognition. We then extended our approach to false recognition involving source-memory confusions but not gist-based errors. We review these two lines of research in the next sections of the chapter.

Distinctiveness and Gist-Based Misattribution

If false recognition in the DRM paradigm is at least partly attributable to responding on the basis of gist information, then encouraging participants to focus on distinctive information should result in attenuated false-recognition effects. To evaluate this hypothesis, Israel and Schacter (1997) examined whether false recognition of semantic associates is reduced when participants encode DRM lists along with detailed pictures corresponding to each item. Israel and Schacter reasoned that presenting items as pictures should increase encoding of distinctive, specific details about studied words that should, in turn, make them easier to discriminate from nonstudied semantic associates. Israel and Schacter generated pictures of words from 21 of the DRM lists (a number of the lists were not amenable to pictorial representation). In an initial study with college students, they compared a word-encoding condition (participants both heard and saw lists of DRM semantic associates; a "hear only" word-encoding condition was also used, which did not differ from the hear + see word-encoding condition) with a picture-encoding condition (participants heard the same lists of semantic associates and also saw line drawings corresponding to each word). Following study-list presentation, previously studied words, related lures, and unrelated lures were tested on an old/new recognition task, with test items presented as pictures or as words. Israel and Schacter found that, consistent with predictions, false recognition of semantic associates was significantly reduced after pictorial encoding compared to word encoding.

Schacter et al., (1999) extended this paradigm to older adults. In an initial experiment, separate groups of younger and older adults were assigned either to a word-encoding condition (hear a study word and see the word) or a picture-encoding condition (hear a study word and see a corresponding picture). Recognition was tested either with pictures or words. Results demonstrated that older adults, just like younger adults, showed significant reductions of false recognition after picture encoding compared to word encoding (Schacter et al., 1999). Indeed, whereas false recognition was significantly higher in older than in younger adults after word encoding, there were no age differences in corrected false-recognition scores (i.e., false recognition to related lures—false recognition to unrelated lures) following picture encoding.

Schacter et al. (1999; see also, Israel & Schacter, 1997) hypothesized that reduced false recognition after picture encoding compared to word encoding depends on a shift in responding based on participants' metamemorial assessments of the kinds of information they feel they *should* remember. Having encountered pictures with each of the presented words, participants in the picture-encoding condition may have employed a general rule of thumb whereby they demanded access to distinctive pictorial information in order to support a positive recognition decision. Because access to pictorial information is diagnostic of having studied an item previously, failure to gain access to such distinctive information when tested with related lures would yield a negative recognition decision (see Strack & Bless, 1994; Rotello, 1999; and Ghetti, 2003, for discussion of a similar heuristic process). Thus, Schacter et al. (1999) hypothesized that suppression relies on a general expectation that a test item should elicit a distinctive recollection if, indeed, it had been presented previously. Participants in the word-encoding condition, by contrast, did not expect to retrieve distinctive representations of previously studied items, and hence, are much less likely to demand access to detailed recollections. We referred to the hypothesized rule of thumb in the picture-encoding condition as the *distinctiveness heuristic*. We suggested that when using a distinctiveness heuristic, participants are especially attuned to whether they recollect distinctive details about an item, and they use criteria such as "If I do not remember seeing a picture of an item, it is probably new."

However, an alternative account of the data from the aforementioned experiments by Israel and Schacter (1997) and Schacter et al. (1999) is that suppression following picture encoding depends on, and requires access to, *list-specific distinctive information* about studied items. By this view, metamemorial assessments and heuristic processes of the kind we posited are not necessary for obtaining false-recognition suppression after picture encoding. For instance, when presented with the related lure item *bread* on the recognition test, participants in the picture-encoding condition may have recalled seeing pictures of such presented associates as *milk, butter, flour,* or *dough*. Because they could remember pictures of these specific words from the study list, but failed to recall a corresponding picture for *bread*, participants may have used their recollections of particular list items to avoid false recognition responses. The idea that access to such list-specific information is a critical mechanism of false-memory suppression following picture encoding is consistent with the widely accepted idea that distinctive encoding produces differentiated and easily accessible episodic representations (cf., Hunt & McDaniel, 1993; McClelland & Chappell, 1998; Rotello, 1999).

In an attempt to distinguish between these two theoretical perspectives, Schacter et al. (1999) conducted a follow-up experiment in which a critical feature of the encoding conditions from the first experiment was altered. Picture versus word encoding had been manipulated on a between-groups basis in the first experiment, so that recollection of pictorial details was diagnostic of having studied an item. In the second experiment, picture versus word encoding was manipulated on a within-groups basis. Having studied some lists with pictures and others with words only, participants' recollection of pictorial information is no longer diagnostic of having studied a target. Under these conditions, reliance on a distinctiveness heuristic alone would not produce differential suppression of false recognition for lists studied with pictures compared to those studied with words alone—access to list-specific information would be necessary to achieve lower levels of false recognition following picture than following word encoding. Thus, if the distinctiveness heuristic is the critical mechanism underlying false memory suppression, then manipulating picture vs. word encoding on a within-subjects basis should eliminate the suppression effect. If, on the other hand, false-recognition suppression following picture encoding is based on increased access to list-specific representations for items encoded as pictures compared to items encoded as words, then reduced false recognition after picture encoding compared to word encoding should still be observed in a within-subjects design.

In the experiment, participants studied seven DRM lists as words (auditory word plus visual word presentation) and seven as pictures (auditory word plus picture presentation). On the subsequent recognition test, half of the participants were presented studied items, related lures, and unrelated lures as pictures, and half were presented the same items as words. There was no evidence for reduction of false recognition after picture encoding compared to word encoding in younger or older adults in either the word or picture test condition. These results suggest that false-recognition suppression after picture encoding depends on invoking the distinctiveness heuristic: when access to pictorial information is no longer diagnostic of having studied an item and access to list-specific information is required, the distinctiveness heuristic is rendered ineffective.

Whereas the foregoing experiments are consistent with the idea that a distinctiveness heuristic plays an important role in the reduction of false recognition, it is possible that the observed effects are specific to pictorial materials. In an attempt to extend the generality of the distinctiveness heuristic account, Dodson and Schacter (2001) drew on findings from a study by Foley, Johnson, and Raye (1983). In this experiment, participants heard words or said words during the study phase of the experiment. During a later source-memory test, participants exhibited a bias when responding to new words that were falsely judged as old: they were more likely to respond that these new words had been heard rather than said. Thus, participants appeared to be using a kind of distinctiveness heuristic, reasoning that "I would have remembered the word if I had said it." The absence of memory for the distinctive "say" information suggested to the participants that the word must have been heard.

To examine whether saying target words aloud during the study phase would produce reduction of robust false recognition, Dodson and Schacter presented DRM lists of semantic associates to two groups of college students. All participants saw the target words on a computer screen. One group also heard the words, whereas the other group also said the words. On a recognition test immediately following study-list presentation, participants made old/new judgments about studied words, related lures, and unrelated lures that were presented visually. Although saying words aloud had no effect on hit rates or unrelated lure false alarm rates, there was significantly less false recognition of related lures after "say" encoding than after "hear" encoding. In a follow-up experiment, Dodson and Schacter manipulated say vs. hear encoding on a within-subjects basis. Under these conditions, there were no differences in false recognition of related lures after the two kinds of encoding. The account of these results was identical to that of Schacter et al. (1999): when say vs. hear encoding is manipulated within subjects, the distinctive "say" information is no longer diagnostic of prior study, and access to list-specific information is required to show decreased false recognition of related lures that are associated with said than heard lists. The overall pattern of results thus suggests that saying words aloud at study, just like studying pictures, provides a basis for invoking the distinctiveness heuristic.

Although the theoretical claim advanced by Schacter et al. (1999) and Dodson and Schacter (2001) is that the distinctiveness heuristic is a strategic process that operates during retrieval, an important limitation of the evidence reviewed above is that these studies manipulated only encoding conditions. To provide a strong test of the distinctiveness heuristic hypothesis, it is necessary to show that use of the distinctiveness heuristic is sensitive to changes in retrieval conditions. Schacter, Cendan, Dodson, and Clifford (2001) tested a prediction that follows from this account: differences in false-recognition rates between picture and word encoding should be attenuated in a retrieval condition that does not encourage reliance on a distinctiveness heuristic. Schacter et al. (2001) used DRM lists that were studied as either words or pictures, as in the experiments discussed earlier. In addition, however, they contrasted performance on a standard old/new recognition condition with a "meaning recognition" test (Brainerd & Reyna, 1998) in which participants are instructed to ignore whether an item is old or new and accept all items consistent in meaning with list themes. Thus, the proportion of related lure words endorsed under the meaning-recognition instructions provides an index of memory for the semantic theme or gist of study lists, unopposed by counterveiling influences of item-specific recollection that can operate on old/new recognition tests. Schacter et al. (2001) observed an interaction between encoding and retrieval conditions that supports the distinctiveness heuristic account: "old" responses to related lures were significantly lower after picture than after word encoding on the standard recognition test, but not on the meaning recognition test. Although people appear to possess metamemorial knowledge about the aspects of past events that are likely to be remembered, using this knowledge depends on the specific goal of retrieval.

Because the evidence summarized thus far for the operation of the distinctiveness heuristic stems entirely from the DRM false-recognition paradigm, the generality of the distinctiveness heuristic is unknown. Moreover, the evidence reviewed thus far is ambiguous concerning an important point regarding the conditions necessary to "turn on" the distinctiveness heuristic. As noted earlier, Schacter et al. (1999) reported reduced false recognition after picture rather than word encoding in a between-subjects design but observed no evidence of reduced false recognition for picture lists compared to word lists in a within-subjects design where some lists were studied as pictures and others were studied as words. Dodson and Schacter (2001) reported a similar pattern in the "say" vs. "hear" version of the DRM paradigm. We argued that this finding indicates that the distinctiveness heuristic is used only when distinctive information is diagnostic of prior study. However, in the within-subjects DRM paradigm, to exhibit lower false recognition of picture lists compared to word lists, participants would have to remember, when presented with a related lure word, the form in which the relevant list of associates was originally presented (e.g., as pictures or as words). If participants fail to remember the form of list presentation, they would not be able to apply the distinctiveness heuristic selectively to the distinctive items (i.e., pictures or "say" items), even if they do attempt to invoke the heuristic under nondiagnostic conditions. Indeed, there is some evidence suggesting that subjects in the within-subjects picture vs. word conditions of the Schacter et al. (1999) experiment were attempting to apply the distinctiveness heuristic, but could not do so selectively. When pictures vs. words was manipulated within subjects, false recognition to *both* words and pictures was lower than in the word-only condition of the initial experiment, where pictures versus words was manipulated between subjects. Schacter et al. (2001) confirmed this finding in a single experiment: when participants studied all or half of the lists as pictures, they were generally less likely to falsely recognize related lure items than were participants who studied all of the items as words. However, just as in Schacter et al. (1999), in the mixed picture-word condition (i.e., within subjects), there were no differences in false recognition for lures related to word or picture lists. These findings suggest that participants were attempting to use the distinctiveness heuristic in the mixed picture-word condition, but were unable to apply it selectively to pictures, perhaps because they were unable to remember whether individual lists were presented as pictures or as words. Therefore, failure to remember the form of list presentation, rather than the diagnosticity of prior study, could account for the observed results.

In the next section, we consider a related line of experiments that has attempted to address the questions concerning the role of diagnosticity in the distinctiveness heuristic, and to evaluate the generality of the heuristic outside of the DRM paradigm considered thus far. We attempted to accomplish these goals by using an experimental paradigm in which source-based, but not gist-based, misattribution errors contribute to false recognition.

Extending the Distinctiveness Heuristic: The Repetition Lag Paradigm

To address issues of diagnosticity and generality, Dodson and Schacter (2002a, 2002b) examined the operation of the distinctiveness heuristic with the repetition lag paradigm discussed earlier (Jennings & Jacoby, 1997). To review, in this paradigm, participants study a list of unrelated words and then make old/new recognition judgments about previously studied words and new words. In addition, new words on the recognition test are repeated after varying lags. Even though participants are specifically instructed to say "old" only to words from the study list, and not to new words that are repeated, after sufficiently long lags, participants make false alarms to some repeated new words, misattributing their familiarity with the repeated new words to prior appearance in the study list. Dodson and Schacter (2002a) reasoned that studying target items as pictures, rather than words, would allow participants to invoke a distinctiveness heuristic on the recognition test and thus avoid making false alarms to repeated new words, because they would expect to remember viewing pictures in order to call test items old. Results confirmed this prediction in both younger adults (Dodson & Schacter, 2002b) and older adults (Dodson & Schacter, 2002a). Reduced false recognition following picture study was especially pronounced for older adults, who showed considerably higher false-recognition rates in the word-encoding condition than did younger adults. Dodson and Schacter argued that reduced false recognition in this paradigm in the picture study condition is attributable to the use of a distinctiveness heuristic. Because misattribution errors likely have a different basis in the repetition lag procedure than in the DRM procedure, these findings suggest that the distinctiveness heuristic has some generality.

Dodson and Schacter further used the repetition lag paradigm to evaluate the role of diagnosticity in "turning on" the distinctiveness heuristic by examining false recognition following conditions in which only 50% of the study items were pictures, and hence were no longer diagnostic of prior study. The repetition lag paradigm provides a more direct test of the role of diagnostic information in eliciting the distinctiveness heuristic than does the DRM paradigm because the repetition lag procedure is not confounded by the memory-for-mode-of-list presentation issue that, as discussed above, confounds interpretation of results from the DRM procedure. Results revealed that suppression of false recognition after studying 50% pictures was just as large as after studying 100% pictures in both younger (Dodson & Schacter, 2002b) and older (Dodson & Schacter, 2002a) adults. Indeed, Dodson and Schacter (2002b) found that false recognition suppression was just as strong after subjects studied as few as 25% pictures.

The foregoing results indicate that distinctive information need not be perfectly diagnostic to turn on the distinctiveness heuristic. Therefore, it also seems reasonable to conclude that Schacter et al.'s (1999) original finding that, in a within-subjects design, false recognition after picture study was no lower than after word study likely reflects the memory-for-mode-of-list-presentation issues discussed earlier that are specific to the DRM paradigm. However, since the diagnosticity interpretation of this finding was initially cited as support for the idea that suppression of false recognition after picture encoding reflects the operation of a distinctiveness heuristic, the newer results from Dodson and Schacter indicate that other evidence is needed to buttress this claim. Dodson and Schacter (2002b) provided such evidence by manipulating participants' *expectations* about the usefulness of previously encoded distinctive information—specifically, about whether the recognition test in the repetition lag would contain items studied as pictures. If the effects of picture study on subsequent false recognition reflect the operation of a distinctiveness heuristic that itself reflects participants' expectations about the characteristics of what they should remember, then picture study should influence false recognition only when they expect that such information will be relevant to the recognition test.

Dodson and Schacter compared two different test conditions that were identical except for instructions: participants in both conditions studied a mixture of pictures and words, but they were tested only on the items studied as words. When participants were informed that they would not be tested on the picture study items, they did not engage the distinctiveness heuristic, and consequently, falsely recognized many of the repeated new words. But when they were (incorrectly) informed that the test was based on all studied items, participants used the heuristic and rejected the repeated new words. These results indicate that the distinctiveness heuristic is under metacognitive control such that it can be turned on or off depending on participants' expectations about its usefulness.

MISATTRIBUTION AND DISTINCTIVENESS: FUTURE DIRECTIONS

The research reviewed in the present chapter represents a beginning attempt to delineate the relationship between distinctiveness and a particular type of memory "sin," misattribution, that is closely associated with the phenomenon of false recognition. We have focused in particular on recent studies indicating that people sometimes invoke the distinctiveness heuristic to successfully reduce or suppress false-recognition effects that occur following the study of semantic associates, as in the DRM paradigm, and repeated new words on a recognition test, as in the repetition lag procedure. It is clear, however, that this line of work is in an early stage of development. We conclude by noting several promising directions for future research.

First, we have emphasized that the distinctiveness heuristic critically involves participants' *expectations* regarding the distinctive properties of to-be-remembered information, and thus can be considered a type of metacognitive strategy. Others have also stressed the role of metacognitive expectations in coming to decide that an event did not happen (Ghetti, 2003; Strack & Bless, 1994; cf., Rotello, 1999). Thus, it seems clear that future work on the distinctiveness heuristic will need to link it more closely to research on the role of expectations in memory (e.g., Whittlesea & Williams, 2001), as well as more generally with work on metacognition (e.g., Reder, 1996; Shimamura, 2000). Second, in a related vein, a variety of heuristics have been proposed in connection with the evaluation and use of memory contents, including the availability heuristic (Tversky & Kahneman, 1973), fluency heuristic (Jacoby & Dallas, 1981; Whittlesea & Leboe, 2003), accessibility heuristic (Koriat & Levy-Sadot, 2001), and cue familiarity heuristic (Koriat & Levy-Sadot, 2001). How is the distinctiveness heuristic similar to the other heuristics, and how does it differ? To what extent do the various heuristics depend on shared underlying memory or judgment processes? We are not aware of any research that has specifically compared the distinctiveness heuristic with other memory heuristics, but the issue seems worth pursuing.

Third, while much of the work reviewed earlier concerning the distinctiveness heuristic involves college students, our laboratory and others are beginning to extend this research to other subject populations. We already noted studies indicating that older adults exhibit an intact ability to use the distinctiveness heuristic in both the DRM (Schacter et al., 1999) and repetition lag (Dodson & Schacter, 2002a) paradigms. Further evidence that the distinctiveness heuristic is robust across subject populations comes from a study using the repetition lag paradigm in schizophrenic patients. Though patients showed increased susceptibility to false recognition in the standard word-encoding condition, they showed a normal reduction in false recognition after picture encoding, suggesting an intact ability to use the distinctiveness heuristic (Weiss, Dodson, Goff, Schacter, & Heckers, 2002). In contrast, an initial study involving patients with Alzheimer's disease suggests that such patients are unable to use the distinctiveness heuristic to reduce false recognition in the DRM paradigm (Budson, Sitarski, Daffner, & Schacter, 2002). Further research is needed to determine the reliability and generality of each of these sets of findings (for work concerning the development of related memory-monitoring processes in young children, see Ghetti, 2003; Ghetti et al., 2002).

Fourth, it would be desirable to examine the role of the distinctiveness heuristic in a closely related memory "sin": suggestibility. Research concerning suggested false memories has grown during the past decade, as a variety of researchers have shown that leading questions and suggestions can influence a significant proportion of subjects to "remember" entire autobiographical experiences that never happened—typically events that supposedly occurred in early childhood (e.g., Hyman, Husband, & Billings, 1995; Loftus & Pickrell, 1995; Porter, Yuille, & Lehman, 1999). Interestingly, some of the events that are falsely remembered in such studies are complex, salient, and seemingly distinctive, such as spilling punch on the bride at a wedding (Hyman et al., 1995), being lost in a shopping mall (Loftus & Pickrell, 1995), or suffering a vicious animal attack (Porter et al., 1999).

Based on the studies considered earlier and our ideas about the distinctiveness heuristic, it may seem surprising that people exhibit false memories for these kinds of events. They should expect to remember vivid, distinctive details of such events—details that are presumably not available—and, hence, they should be able to avoid creating false memories in response to suggestions. Importantly, however, it seems reasonable to propose that people likely do not expect to recall experiences from childhood with vividness or clarity, in the same way that they should expect to recall vivid details for distinctive recent events. It should be extremely difficult to suggest false memories of salient experiences that supposedly occurred in recent days or months, such as having been attacked by a vicious animal, because people will invoke the distinctiveness heuristic, expecting to remember the recent events in vivid detail. By contrast, we are far less likely to expect to recall vivid details from childhood experience, and thus may be more vulnerable to interpreting ambiguous images or vague feelings of familiarity as evidence of memory for a past experience. Although we know of no research that has specifically examined this issue, it may merit further empirical and theoretical attention.

Finally, nothing is known about the neural basis of the distinctiveness heuristic. However, a number of studies using neuroimaging techniques such as positron emission tomography (PET), functional magnetic resonance imaging (fMRI), and event-related potentials (ERPS) have compared brain activity during true and false recognition, documenting both similarities and differences between the two (e.g., Cabeza, Rao, Wagner, Mayer, & Schacter, 2001; Johnson et al., 1997; Schacter, Reiman, et al., 1996; Schacter, Buckner, Koutstaal, Dale, & Rosen, 1997). Further, several recent studies have used neuroimaging, including both fMRI and event-related ERPs, to dissect component processes of retrieval, such as those involved in successful recovery of encoded information versus those involved in monitoring of retrieved contents (e.g., Dobbins, Foley, Schacter, & Wagner, 2002; Rugg, Herron, & Morcom, 2002; Wheeler & Buckner, 2003). These lines of research provide some of the foundation necessary for neuroimaging and ERP analyses of the distinctiveness heuristic. With the further development of carefully controlled paradigms for examining the role of the distinctiveness heuristic in reducing false recognition, and the increasing adaptability of imaging techniques such as fMRI for delineating subtle aspects of memory retrieval, studies examining the neural basis of distinctiveness effects on misattribution errors represent an attractive frontier for future study.

ACKNOWLEDGMENTS

Supported by NIA grant AG08441 and NIMH grant MH60941. We thank Chris Moore for help with preparation of this chapter. Portions of the chapter were presented at the 49th Annual Meeting of the Southwestern Psychological Association, New Orleans, LA, April 2003.

REFERENCES

Brainerd, C. J., & Reyna, V. F. (1998). When things that were never experienced are easier to "remember" than things that were. *Psychological Science, 9*, 484–489.

Brainerd, C. J., Reyna, V. F., & Kneer, R. (1995). False-recognition reversal: When similarity is distinctive. *Journal of Memory and Language, 34*, 157–185.

Budson, A. E., Sitarski, J., Daffner, K. R., & Schacter, D. L. (2002). False recognition of pictures versus words in Alzheimer's disease: The distinctiveness heuristic. *Neuropsychology, 16*, 163–173.

Budson, A. D., Sullivan, A. L., Mayer, E., Daffner, K. R., Black, P. M., & Schacter, D. L. (2002). Suppression of false recognition in Alzheimer's disease and in patients with frontal lobe lesions. *Brain, 125*, 2750–2765.

Cabeza, R., Rao, S., Wagner, A. D., Mayer, A., & Schacter, D. L. (2001). Can medial temporal lobe regions distinguish true from false? An event-related fMRI study of veridical and illusory recognition memory. *Proceedings of the National Academy of Sciences (USA), 98*, 4805–4810.

Ceci, S. J., & Bruck, M. (1993). Suggestibility of the child witness: A historical review and synthesis. *Psychological Bulletin, 113*, 403–439.

Deese, J. (1959). On the prediction of occurrence of particular verbal intrusions in immediate recall. *Journal of Experimental Psychology, 58*, 17–22.

Dobbins, I. G., Foley, H., Schacter, D. L., & Wagner, A. D. (2002). Executive control during episodic retrieval: Multiple prefrontal processes subserve source memory. *Neuron, 35*, 989–996.

Dobbins, I. G., Kroll, N. E. A., Yonelinas, A. P., & Liu, Q. (1998). Distinctiveness in recognition and free recall: The role of recollection in the rejection of the familiar. *Journal of Memory and Language, 38*, 381–400.

Dodson, C. S., & Schacter, D. L. (2001). "If I had said it I would have remembered it": Reducing false memories with a distinctiveness heuristic. *Psychonomic Bulletin & Review, 8*, 155–161.

Dodson, C. S., & Schacter, D. L. (2002a). When false recognition meets metacognition: The distinctiveness heuristic. *Journal of Memory and Language, 46*, 782–803.

Dodson, C. S., & Schacter, D. L. (2002b). Aging and strategic retrieval processes: Reducing false memories with a distinctiveness heuristic. *Psychology and Aging, 17*, 405–415.

Dodson, C. S., & Shimamura, A. P. (2000). Differential effects of cue dependency on item and source memory. *Journal of Experimental Psychology: Learning, Memory and Cognition, 26*, 1023–1044.

Ebbinghaus, H. (1885/1964). *Memory: A contribution to experimental psychology*. New York: Dover.

Foley, M. A., Johnson, M. K., & Raye, C. L. (1983). Age-related changes in confusion between memories for thoughts and memories for speech. *Child Development, 54*, 51–60.

Gallo, D. A., & Roediger, H. L., III. (2002). Variability among word lists in evoking memory illusions: Evidence for associative activation and monitoring. *Journal of Memory and Language, 47*, 469–497.

Ghetti, S. (2003). Memory for nonoccurrences: The role of metacognition. *Journal of Memory & Language, 48*, 722–739.

Ghetti, S., Qin, J., & Goodman, G. (2002). False memories in children and adults: age, distinctiveness, and subjective experience. *Developmental Psychology, 38*, 705–718.

Goldmann, R. E., Sullivan, A. L., Droller, D. J., Rugg, M. D., Curran, T., Holcomb, P. J., Schacter, D. L., Daffner, K. R., & Budson, A. E. (2003). Late frontal brain potentials distinguish true and false recognition. *NeuroReport, 14*, 1717–1720.

Gruppuso, V., Lindsay, D. S., & Kelley, C. M. (1997). The process-dissociation procedure and similarity: Defining and estimating recollection and familiarity in recognition memory. *Journal of Experimental Psychology: Learning, Memory and Cognition, 23*, 259–278.

Hunt, R. R. (1995). The subtlety of distinctiveness: What von Restorff really did. *Psychonomic Bulletin & Review, 2*, 105–112.

Hunt, R. R. (2003). Two contributions of distinctive processing to accurate memory. *Journal of Memory & Language, 48*, 811–825.

Hunt, R. R., & Lamb, C. A. (2001). What causes the isolation effect? *Journal of Experimental Psychology: Learning, Memory and Cognition, 27*, 1359–1366.

Hunt, R. R., & McDaniel, M. A. (1993). The enigma of organization and distinctiveness. *Journal of Memory and Language, 32*, 421–445.

Hunt, R. R., & Smith, R. E. (1996). Accessing the particular from the general: The power of distinctiveness in the context of organization. *Memory and Cognition, 24*, 217–225.

Hyman, I. E., Husband, T. H., & Billings, F. J. (1995). False memories of childhood experiences. *Applied Cognitive Psychology, 9*, 181–197.

Israel, L., & Schacter, D. L. (1997). Pictorial encoding reduces false recognition of semantic associates. *Psychonomic Bulletin and Review, 4,* 577–581.

Jacoby, L. L., & Craik, F. I. M. (1979). Effects of elaboration of processing at encoding and retrieval: Trace distinctiveness and recover of initial context. In L. S. Cermak and F. I. M. Craik (Eds.), Levels of processing in human memory (pp. 1–22). Hillsdale, NJ: Lawrence Erlbaum Associates.

Jacoby, L. L., & Dallas, M. (1981). On the relationship between autobiographical memory and perceptual learning. *Journal of Experimental Psychology: General, 110,* 306–340.

Jacoby, L. L., Kelley, C. M., & Dywan, J. (1989). Memory attributions. In H. L. Roediger, III & F. I. M. Craik (Eds.), *Varieties of memory and consciousness: Essays in honour of Endel Tulving* (pp. 391–422). Hillsdale, NJ: Lawrence Erlbaum Associates.

Jennings, J. M., & Jacoby, L. L. (1997). An opposition procedure for detecting age-related deficits in recollection: Telling effects of repetition. *Psychology and Aging, 12,* 352–361.

Johnson, M. K., Hashtroudi, S., & Lindsay, D. S. (1993). Source monitoring. *Psychological Bulletin, 114,* 3–28.

Johnson, M. K., Nolde, S. F., Mather, M., Kounios, J., Schacter, D. L., & Curran, T. (1997). The similarity of brain activity associated with true and false recognition memory depends on test format. *Psychological Science, 8,* 250–257.

Johnson, M. K., & Raye, C. L. (1981). Reality monitoring. *Psychological Review, 88,* 67–85.

Koriat, A., &, Levy-Sadot, R. (2001). The combined contributions of the cue-familiarity and accessibility heuristics to feelings of knowing. *Journal of Experimental Psychology: Learning, Memory and Cognition, 27,* 34–53.

Koutstaal, W., & Schacter, D. L. (1997). Gist-based false recognition of pictures in older and younger adults. *Journal of Memory and Language, 37,* 555–583.

Lockhart, R. S., Craik, F. I. M., &, & Jacoby, L. L. (1976). Depth of processing, recognition, and recall: Some aspects of a general memory system. In J. Brown (Ed.), *Recall and Recognition* (pp. 75–102). London: Wiley.

Loftus, E. F., & Pickrell, J. E. (1995). The formation of false memories. *Psychiatric Annals, 25,* 720–725.

Maril, A., Wagner, A. D., & Schacter, D. L. (2001). On the tip of the tongue: An event-related fMRI study of retrieval failure and cognitive conflict. *Neuron, 31,* 653–660.

Marsh, R. L., Landau, J. D., & Hicks, J. L. (1997). Contributions of inadequate source monitoring to unconscious plagiarism during idea generation. *Journal of Experimental Psychology: Learning Memory and Cognition, 23,* 886–897.

McClelland, J. L., & Chappell, M. (1998). Familiarity breeds differentiation: A subjective-likelihood approach to the effects of experience in recognition memory. *Psychological Review, 105,* 724–760.

McDaniel, M. A., & Einstein, G. O. (1993). The importance of cue familiarity and cue distinctiveness in prospective memory. *Memory, 1,* 23–41.

McIntyre, J. S., & Craik, F. I. M. (1987). Age differences in memory for item and source information. *Canadian Journal of Psychology, 41,* 175–192.

McNally, R. J. (2003). *Remembering trauma.* Cambridge, MA: Belknap Press/Harvard University Press.

Norman, K. A., & Schacter, D. L. (1997). False recognition in young and older adults: Exploring the characteristics of illusory memories. *Memory and Cognition, 25,* 838–848.

Payne, D. G., Elie, C. J., Blackwell, J. M., & Neuschatz, J. S. (1996). Memory illusions: Recalling, recognizing, and recollecting events that never occurred. *Journal of Memory and Language, 35,* 261–285.

Porter, S., Yuille, J. C., & Lehman, D. R. (1999). The nature of real, implanted, and fabricated memories for emotional childhood events: Implications for the recovered memory debate. *Law and Human Behavior, 23,* 517–537.

Reason, J., & Mycielska, K. (1982). Absent-*minded?: The psychology of mental lapses and everyday errors.* Englewood Cliffs, NJ: Prentice-Hall.

Reder, L. M. (Ed.).(1996). *Implicit memory and metacognition.* Hillsdale, NJ: Lawrence Erlbaum Associates.

Roediger III, H. L., & McDermott, K. B. (1995). Creating false memories: Remembering words not presented in lists. *Journal of Experimental Psychology: Learning, Memory, and Cognition, 21,* 803–814.

Ross, M., & Wilson, A. E. (2000). Constructing and appraising past selves. In D. L. Schacter & E. Scarry (Eds.), *Memory, brain, and belief.* Cambridge, MA: Harvard University Press.

Rotello, C. M. (1999). Metacognition and memory for nonoccurrence. *Memory, 7,* 43–63.

Rugg, M. D., Herron, J. E., & Morcom, A. M. (2002). Electrophysiological studies of retrieval processing (pp. 154–165). In L. R. Squire & D. L. Schacter (Eds.), *Neuropsychology of memory.* New York: Guilford.

Schacter, D. L. (1999). The seven sins of memory: Insights from psychology and cognitive neuroscience. *American Psychologist, 54*(3), 182–203.

Schacter, D. L. (2001). *The seven sins of memory: How the mind forgets and remembers.* Boston: Houghton Mifflin.

Schacter, D. L., Buckner, R. L., Koutstaal, W., Dale, A. M., & Rosen, B. R. (1997). Late onset of anterior prefrontal activity during true and false recognition: An event-related fMRI study. *NeuroImage, 6,* 259–269.

Schacter, D. L., Cendan, D. L., Dodson, C. S., & Clifford, E. R. (2001). Retrieval conditions and false recognition: Testing the distinctiveness heuristic. *Psychonomic Bulletin and Review, 8,* 827–833.

Schacter, D. L., Harbluk, J. L., & McLachlan, D. R. (1984). Retrieval without recollection: An experimental analysis of source amnesia. *Journal of Verbal Learning and Verbal Behavior, 23,* 593–611.

Schacter, D. L., Israel, L., & Racine, C. A. (1999). Suppressing false recognition in younger and older adults: The distinctiveness heuristic. *Journal of Memory & Language, 40,* 1–24.

Schacter, D. L., Reiman, E., Curran, T., Yun, L. S., Bandy, D., McDermott, K. B., & Roediger, H. L., III. (1996). Neuroanatomical correlates of veridical and illusory recognition memory: Evidence from positron emission to-mography. *Neuron, 17*, 267–274.

Schacter, D. L., Verfaellie, M., & Pradere, D. (1996). The neuropsychology of memory illusions: False recall and recognition in amnesic patients. *Journal of Memory and Language, 35*, 319–334.

Schwartz, B. L. (1999). Sparkling at the end of the tongue: The etiology of tip-of-the-tongue phenomenology. *Psychonomic Bulletin & Review, 6*, 379–393.

Shimamura, A. P. (2000). Toward a cognitive neuroscience of metacognition. *Consciousness & Cognition, 9*, 313–323.

Smith, R. E., & Hunt, R. R. (1998). Presentation modality affects false memory. *Psychonomic Bulletin and Review, 5*, 710–715.

Strack, F., & Bless, H. (1994). Memory for nonoccurrences: Metacognitive and presuppositional strategies. *Journal of Memory and Language, 33*, 203–217.

Tun, P. A., Wingfield, A., Rosen, M. J., & Blanchard, L. (1998). Response latencies for false memories: Gist-based processes in normal aging. *Psychology & Aging, 13*, 230–241.

Tversky, A., & Kahneman, D. (1973). Availability: A heuristic for judging frequency and probability. *Cognitive Psychology, 5*, 207–232.

von Restorff, H. (1933). Analyse von Vorgangen in Spurenfeld. I. Über die Wirkung von Bereichsbildung im Spurenfeld. *Psychologische Forschung, 18*, 299–342.

Weiss, A. P., Dodson, C. S., Goff, D. C., Schacter, D. L., & Heckers, S. (2002). Intact suppression of increased false recognition in schizophrenia. *American Journal of Psychiatry, 159*, 1506–1513.

Wheeler, M. E., & Buckner, R. L. (2003). Functional dissociation among components of remembering: control, perceived oldness, and content. *Journal of Neuroscience, 23*, 3869–3880.

Whittlesea, B. W. A., &, & Leboe, J. P. (2003). Two fluency heuristics (and how to tell them apart). *Journal of Memory & Language, 49*, 62–79.

Whittlesea, B. W., & Williams, L. D. (2001). The discrepancy-attribution hypothesis: II. Expectation, uncertainty, surprise, and feelings of familiarity. *Journal of Experimental Psychology: Learning, Memory and Cognition, 27*, 14–33.

6

Assessing Distinctiveness: Measures of Item-Specific and Relational Processing

Daniel J. Burns

Much of my research over the last few years has focused on developing and refining techniques for measuring distinctive processing. Of course, before one measures something one must know what is being measured. Unfortunately, researchers are not in complete agreement on the matter of defining distinctiveness. Traditional definitions of distinctiveness point to the processing of nonoverlapping attributes or features (e.g., Nelson, 1979). Presumably, encoding of unique or item-specific attributes facilitates retention by increasing the discriminability of the item during retrieval. This definition essentially equates distinctiveness with the encoding of differences. More recently, however, some have come to view distinctiveness as the encoding of item-specific attributes in the context of relational cues (e.g., Hunt & McDaniel, 1993; Hunt & Smith, 1996; Smith & Hunt, 2000). This latter definition implies that the distinctive benefits of item-specific processing will emerge only when they are encoded in the context of relational cues. Hence, the former definition assumes that distinctiveness results directly from item-specific processing or difference encoding, whereas the latter view suggests that distinctiveness is the combined result of item-specific and relational processing.

The approach I have taken here is to discuss the current state of affairs regarding measures of item-specific and relational processing. Since distinctiveness can be viewed as the direct result of the encoding of item-specific cues or as the result of encoding item-specific cues in the context of relational cues, measures of both item-specific and relational processing are crucial for either approach. In the following sections, I make a conscious effort to focus on item-specific and relational processing without discussing their relative contributions to distinctiveness. I come back to the notion of distinctiveness later.

THE NEED OF ASSESSMENT TOOLS FOR INDEXING ITEM-SPECIFIC AND RELATIONAL PROCESSING

Current research on distinctiveness has been heavily influenced by the seminal work of Hunt and Einstein (1981, Einstein & Hunt, 1980). This early research was of particular consequence for demonstrating that semantic processing per se was not sufficient to produce good retention. Rather, it was the type of semantic processing performed that was critical. Hunt and Einstein pointed out that organizational theory, prominent during the 1960s, focused on the beneficial effects of relational processing, whereas the levels of processing approach, which dominated the 1970s, generally focused on the beneficial effects of item-specific processing. They argued, however, that it was the combination of relational and item-specific processing that is most beneficial to memory. One of the objectives of the early research on item-specific and relational processing was to illustrate the different functions of each type of processing at time of retrieval. Initial attempts to measure relational and item-specific processing were useful for demonstrating deficiencies in each type of processing. The typical experimental procedure was similar to that of levels of processing research, in which orienting tasks were used to focus attention on relational features, item-specific features, or both types of features. The ensuing tests of memory were often designed to assess the memorial benefits and deficiencies of each type of processing. To avoid one of the shortcomings of the levels of processing approach, researchers used various measurement tools or indices to verify their claims that different orienting tasks resulted in different types of processing.

More recently, researchers have gone beyond focusing on the memorial consequences of each type of processing. They have used the relational/item-specific processing distinction as a framework for explaining a variety of seemingly unrelated memory phenomena (for a partial list of effects see Hunt & McDaniel, 1993). The importance of assessment tools for indexing the amount of relational and item-specific processing is also extremely important in these more recent pursuits. As an example, if one were to argue that the memorial benefits of pictures compared to words are due to greater item-specific (or distinctive) processing without first providing evidence that pictures enhance item-specific processing, the explanation would be circular. We believe that pictures lead to superior memory performance because of enhanced item-specific processing. How do we know that pictures enhance item-specific processing? We know because the pictures resulted in superior memory performance.

The indices of relational and item-specific processing discussed below are critical for avoiding such circular definitions. Each index described in the following sections is theoretically based on and is derived from assumptions about the functions of item-specific and relational processing during retrieval. I discuss these functions next.

THE FUNCTIONS OF ITEM-SPECIFIC AND RELATIONAL PROCESSING DURING RETRIEVAL

Retrieval from episodic memory must necessarily be guided by retrieval cues that delineate a specific event that occurred at a particular time in a particular place. When you are asked about the meeting you attended, the event to be retrieved is a particular meeting and the time and place of occurrence of that meeting are directly stated or implied by the cue. Without such stated or implied retrieval cues you could not delineate the particular episode from other episodes.

Typically, retrieval from episodic memory not only involves accessing a particular episode but also retrieving elements (items) from the episode. For example, if you are asked who was at the meeting, the elements you consider are the individuals. To the extent that a retrieval cue specifies more than one element of the event, it can be considered a relational cue. When a cue specifies a single element, it is an item-specific cue. For example, being asked which members of your department were at the meeting would be a relational cue, whereas asking who chaired the meeting would be an item-specific cue (assuming only one person was chair).

Retrieval can be conceptualized as a series of progressively finer discriminations (e.g., Begg, Vinski, Frankovich, & Holgate, 1991; Hunt & Einstein, 1981). Relational cues function to organize the items into successively smaller categories. The combination of relational cues can be especially effective in this regard (e.g., Humphreys, Wiles, & Bain, 1993; Rubin & Wallace, 1989). Without item-specific cues, however, no single item can be delineated. It is the sole function of item-specific cues to pinpoint a specific element to be retrieved and make it stand out, both among other items in the episode and among items not in the episode. Relational and item-specific cues work together to enhance retrieval. The relational cues, by producing successively smaller categories, provide a plan for organizing retrieval. Retrieval of items from one category may be attempted before retrieval of items from a second category. Item-specific cues, on the other hand, allow for the delineation of particular elements within each category.

The retrieval-guiding function of relational cues is presumed to have several memorial consequences. First, the items in an episode will tend to be clustered together by category during free recall (e.g., Einstein & Hunt, 1980). Second, the categories will be brought to mind during retrieval, resulting in items being recalled from the various categories (e.g., Burns & Brown, 2000; Cohen, 1963, 1966; Hunt & Seta, 1984). Third, to the extent that the retrieval plan is useful, it is likely to guide retrieval across repeated retrieval attempts (Burns, 1993; Hunt & McDaniel, 1993; Klein, Loftus, Kihlstrom & Aseron, 1989). The use of item-specific cues during retrieval is also presumed to have several memorial consequences. It allows individual items from within categories to be retrieved, resulting in more items from each category being recalled (e.g., Hunt & Seta, 1984; Tulving

& Pearlstone, 1966). It also makes discrimination easier between a particular item and other items not present in the episode, which is particularly beneficial for tests of recognition memory (e.g., Einstein & Hunt, 1980). Finally, since each item-specific cue specifies only one particular item (and each item may have several item-specific cues), it is often the case that not all of the item-specific cues will be exhausted during a single retrieval attempt. Those remaining item-specific cues, however, may be used on later retrieval attempts (e.g., Klein et al., 1989).

The expected memorial consequences of relational and item-specific processing have provided researchers with several methods for verifying hypothesized processing differences. In the next two sections I will discuss the measures of relational and item-specific processing, respectively. I will focus on the advantages and disadvantages of each measure, pointing out the experimental situations in which each measure is likely to be useful and/or accurate and when it is likely to be inappropriate. For convenience, I list the indices in Table 6.1 and point out the appropriateness of each index in various experimental situations. Keep in mind, however, that the measures of relational and item-specific processing are indirect measures: They are not perfect indicators of the underlying processes they are intended to measure. Rather, they are indices that are correlated with the underlying mechanisms. Therefore, the best measures to use will likely depend on the specific experimental situation. In Shuell's (1975) words, when selecting among the alternative measures, "the best strategy to follow is to realize that there is no such thing as the best measure" (p. 723).

Measures of Relational Processing

Mandler (1970, 1972) argued that organizational (relational) processing can take several forms, including serial-order processing, categorical processing, and the processing of shared features that are not categorical in nature. Although, in long-term memory research study of serial-order processing recently has enjoyed a resurgence of interest (e.g., Burns; 1996; Engelkamp & Dehn, 2000; Nairne, Riegler, & Serra, 1991; Mulligan, 2000), my discussion of measures of relational processing will focus only on the latter two types. For those readers interested, Greene, Thapar, and Westerman (1998) offer an excellent discussion of the measures of order processing.

Categorical Clustering

The most frequently used measures of relational processing are the categorical clustering measures, such as the adjusted ratio of clustering (ARC) and the modified ratio of repetition (MRR). Categorical clustering measures all compute the tendency for categorically related words to be recalled together. Although there is some disagreement concerning the best formula for determining the degree of clustering, categorical clustering is generally

TABLE 6.1 Experimental Situations for Which Each Measure of Relational or Item-Specific Processing is Appropriate

	Experimental Situation				
Measure	UnKnown Categories	Mixed-List Design	Single Recall Test	Single Memory Test	Comments
Relational Processing					
Category Clustering	N	N	Y	Y	Misses non-categorical relational processing.
Subjective Clustering	Y	Y	N	Y	Misses new relational processing during later trials. Insensitive to large clusters.
Category Access	N	N	Y	Y	Accuracy is dependent on all groups processing some relational information. Adjustments must be made for recall-level differences.
Item Losses	Y	N	N	N	Accuracy of measure not known with long intervals between successive tests.
Item-Specific Processing					
Recognition	Y	Y	Y	N	Accuracy is dependent on the type of distracter items given.
Items Per Category Recalled	N	N	Y	Y	Accuracy is dependent on all groups processing some relational information. Adjustments must be made for recall-level differences.
Item Gains	Y	Y	N	N	Accuracy is dependent on length of recall tests.
Cumulative Recall Analysis	Y	Y	Y	Y	A lengthy recall test must be given. Cumulative recall must be monitored.

accepted as a fairly accurate index of relational processing (e.g., Einstein & Hunt, 1980). Most of the categorical clustering measures make adjustments for differences in recall levels across conditions, although some do it more effectively than others (see Murphy, 1979).

Despite fairly wide consensus that differences in categorical clustering accurately reflect differences in relational processing, the approach is limited in a few respects. First, and perhaps most limiting, categorical clustering measures can be used only with categorized lists (or when the specific relational cues are known by the experimenter). There are many experimental situations using categorically unrelated word lists in which differences in relational processing have been inferred (e.g., Klein, Loftus, Kihlstrom, & Schell, 1994; Mulligan & Duke, 2002). For example, the self-reference effect—better memory for information encoded with reference to oneself than for information encoded semantically (e.g., Rogers, Kuiper, & Kirker, 1977)—has typically been studied by requiring participants to perform either a self-referent encoding orienting task or a semantic orienting task on a list of trait adjectives. The superior retention for the items encoded with reference to oneself relative to those encoded semantically has been hypothesized to be the result of more relational processing for the self-encoded items (e.g., Klein & Loftus, 1988). However, since the adjectives in the list are not categorically related (other than the fact that they are all traits), one cannot measure categorical clustering.

Additionally, categorical clustering only measures one type of relational processing—categorical processing—and therefore may miss the use of other types of relational cues. For example, if participants are instructed to categorize a randomly ordered list of categorically related words, they will undoubtedly produce a high level of category clustering. However, they may not have processed any more relational information than participants who formed interactive images between successive words in the list. The category clustering measure simply misses forms of relational processing other than categorical processing.

Another shortcoming of the categorical clustering measures is that most of them are not appropriate when the variables presumed to produce differences in relational processing are manipulated within subject (or within lists). This shortcoming has become more relevant in recent years because several phenomena, which are presumed to be due to differences in relational and item-specific processing, tend to be dependent on mixed-list designs (e.g., the generation, enactment, simultaneous acquisition, perceptual interference, and bizarre imagery effects). There are some techniques for measuring category clustering in mixed-list designs (e.g., Klein & Kihlstrom, 1986), but little is known about these measures and their use is limited.

Subjective Clustering

The subjective clustering measures were developed to assess clustering by relational cues when those cues are not obvious to the experimenter. The basic technique is to determine the extent to which the output order on an earlier recall test is related to the output order on a later test. This is usually accomplished in a multitrial free-recall situation, but it is important to realize that subjective organization can be used when only one presentation trial is given as long as it is followed by successive recall attempts. As with categorical clustering, there has been debate over the best formula for measuring subjective clustering. The paired frequency (PF) measure (Anderson & Watts, 1969), championed by Sternberg and Tulving (1977), appears to have become the preferred method. The PF measure is based on the number of paired words recalled in adjacent output positions on two successive tests.

In addition to the inconvenience of requiring the administration of successive recall tests, several other factors limit the use of subjective-clustering measures. Perhaps of most concern is the fact that most subjective-clustering measures are insensitive to clusters larger than two items (cf. Pellegrino & Ingram, 1979). In addition, at least in the case of multitrial free recall, the procedure may miss new relational cues encoded during the second study trial, which might alter the order of items on the second test. As an example, on the first trial a participant might relate the items *dollar* and *grass* based on their greenness and recall them in adjacent output positions. On the next learning trial, however, the item *lime* might also be encoded as being green. If the participant were to output *lime* between *dollar* and *grass*, the PF measure would not reflect this relational processing. Note that this problem, which results from additional learning on later trials, is not a concern when successive recall tests are given without additional learning trials.

Category Access

The category access (CA) measure is another technique that can be used to gauge the extent to which relational cues are used to guide retrieval. CA is usually defined as the number of categories from which at least one item has been recalled. It is generally believed that CA scores increase with increases in relational processing (e.g., Cohen, 1963, 1966; Hunt & McDaniel, 1993; Hunt & Seta, 1984). The assumption is that recall of at least one item indicates that the relational information is available. The published studies using the CA measure have consistently produced results in which variables expected to increase relational processing increased CA scores (e.g., Basden, Basden, Bryner, & Thomas, 1997; Cohen, 1963, 1966; Hunt & Seta, 1984; McDaniel, Waddill, & Einstein, 1988; Schmidt & Cherry, 1989).

Murphy (1979) pointed out, however, that CA scores are correlated with recall level: CA scores increase with increases in recall. It is possible, therefore, that observed CA differences are due to differences in recall level rather than differences in relational processing. Burns and Brown (2000) proposed an adjusted CA (ACA) measure that corrects for differences in recall level. The ACA measure was shown to be sensitive to presumed differences in relational processing even after correction for recall-level differences. Hence, although recall level is an important consideration, the ACA measure can be used when recall level differences exist. One problem with the ACA measure, however, is that it is likely to overadjust for recall differences (see Burns & Brown). This overcorrection may occasionally conceal small differences in relational processing.

Burns and Brown (2000) described another problem with the CA (or ACA) measure. They showed that CA scores do not accurately reflect differences in relational processing when one of the groups processes little or no relational information. They presented a list of 48 items, 4 from each of 12 ad hoc (or nonobvious) categories (e.g., things that can be hot, round things, and things that can fly) and required participants to perform either a relational orienting task (name the categories to which the items belong) or an item-specific orienting task (generate a word associate for each item). Analysis of clustering on the ensuing recall test revealed that the item-specific orienting task produced virtually chance-level clustering (mean ARC = .06), whereas the relational orienting task resulted in an extremely high clustering score (mean ARC = .88). Despite the fact that both the ARC scores and common sense suggested that the relational orienting task induced greater relational processing, the CA scores were actually higher for the item-specific processing group.

Burns and Brown (2000) suggested that the relationship between relational processing and CA scores is curvilinear: high levels of relational processing produce higher CA scores than low levels of relational processing. However, the highest CA scores are actually obtained when very little or no relational processing is performed. This finding suggests that the CA scores are inappropriate for comparisons in which one of the groups did not perform any relational processing. Burns and Brown suggested that the advantage for the group processing no relational information is predicted by organizational theory. According to organizational theory, items within the list are not retrieved independently. Rather, recall of a particular item is dependent on the recall of related items (see Wood, 1972, for a review). For example, Rundus (1973) assumed that recall begins with retrieval of a category name followed by recall of the category members. Moreover, the clustering data suggest that for highly organized recall, nearly all of the items from one category are recalled before accessing another category. Therefore, the CA (and ACA) scores are likely to be well below those predicted if items were retrieved independently. Since purely item-specific processing is likely to produce recall in which items are likely to be recalled more independently of each other, CA scores are likely to be higher than those for relational processing.

The CA scores, therefore, are inappropriate for comparisons in which one of the groups may not have used any relational information. Additionally, the CA measure suffers from some of the same limitations as do the category-clustering measures. First, it can only be used with categorized lists. Second, it has not been used with mixed-list designs.

Item Losses

I proposed an alternative measure of relational processing (Burns, 1993), which was derived from Klein et al.'s (1989) work on hypermnesia—the improvement in memory across repeated tests. Hypermnesic recall is dependent on the number of newly recalled items on a later test that were not recalled on an earlier test (item gains) being greater than the number of items forgotten on a later test that were remembered on an earlier test (item losses). Klein et al. demonstrated that manipulations enhancing relational processing decrease item losses.

On the basis of Klein et al.'s (1989) discovery, I suggested that item losses could be used to assess the amount of relational processing performed. Across a series of experiments, I showed that differences in relational processing consistently produced differences in item losses. Presumably, relational processing results in the encoding of a relatively small number of relational cues (e.g., category names) that provide an organized retrieval plan. These relational cues are usually exhausted by the end of the first recall period (see Klein et al., 1994), which means that the same relational cues are likely to be used again on later attempts at retrieval. Since the same organized plan is used on later tests, it is likely that the same items will be retrieved, thus resulting in few item losses.

The item-loss measure of relational processing has enjoyed considerable success (e.g., Burns & Gold, 1999; Klein et al. 1994; Mulligan, 2000, 2001, 2002). Other than the fact that it requires the administration of repeated tests, there appear to be few concerns with the measure. One difficulty is that item losses increase with longer retention intervals, regardless of the type of processing originally performed. In other words, forgetting occurs. Hence, when the repeated recall tests are not given in close temporal proximity, it can be difficult to determine whether item losses are due to a lack of an organized retrieval plan or, rather, are simply the result of normal forgetting. Of course, the forgetting of items over time might occur at different rates following relational and item-specific processing. For example, if relational information were forgotten more slowly over time relative to item-specific information, then item losses would continue to be a veridical measure of relational processing across different retention intervals. Unfortunately, until more is known about the time course of forgetting of relational and item-specific information, the item-loss measure should be interpreted with caution when lengthy retention intervals are used.

The only other concern with the item-loss measure to date is that it may not work when type of processing is manipulated within subjects in a mixed-list design. For example, Burns & Hebert (2005) found that those conditions that presumably processed more relational information produced numerically more item losses than their counterparts in a mixed-list design, although none of the conditions produced many losses.

Measures of Item-specific Processing

Recognition-Test Performance

Perhaps the most oft-used measure of item-specific processing is performance on a recognition test (e.g., Einstein & Hunt, 1980). Since the main objective in a recognition test is to discriminate previously presented items from those not presented, item-specific retrieval cues are particularly important. Moreover, presenting the item itself on the recognition test would seem, on the face of it, to be the quintessential item-specific retrieval cue. Thus, increases in recognition are presumed to reflect increases in item-specific processing. The use of a recognition test to assess the amount of item-specific processing has met with considerable success (e.g., Burns, Curti, & Lavin, 1993; Einstein & Hunt, 1980; Engelkamp & Dehn, 2000; McDaniel & Waddill, 1990; Nairne et al. 1993; Schmidt, 1985). However, the relative importance of relational and item-specific information for retention is dependent on the specific test conditions, and it is clear that even recognition test performance can be affected by relational processing under some conditions (Hunt & Seta, 1984; Mandler, 1972; Neely & Balota, 1981). To the extent that the lures on the recognition test come from different categories than the target items, relational processing would be expected to facilitate recognition. That is, participants could base their recognition decision on category membership. This point was clear to Hunt and Seta (1984), who pointed out that "accurate recognition can occur on the basis of relational information under some circumstances" (p. 462). Specifically, they suggested that as the number of distractor items sharing the relational features of the targets decreases, relational information becomes more beneficial.

There are also several variables (e.g., word frequency, presentation rate, and item repetition) that influence recognition performance that are not necessarily assumed to influence the amount of item-specific processing. Furthermore, inclusion of a recognition test can sometimes be burdensome. While it is quite easy to append a final recognition test to the end of an experimental session, this simple approach is problematic because recognition test performance may be contaminated by performance on the earlier (recall) test. For example, if one group recalled twice as many items as a second group on an earlier test, the former group would have a distinct advantage on the recognition test regardless of the type of processing performed, simply because of their superior recall performance. A more methodologically sound approach is to test separate groups that are given the recognition test *instead* of the recall test. This procedure, however, often requires the testing of twice the number of participants.

Items Recalled per Category

Once a category is accessed, item-specific cues supposedly facilitate discrimination among the category members. This allows access to the specific items within the category. Thus, item-specific processing is presumed to increase the number of items recalled per category (IPC) (see Burns & Brown, 2000; Hunt & Seta, 1984). A number of published studies have verified this relationship (e.g., Jacoby, 1973; McDaniel, Waddill, & Einstein, 1988; Sowder, 1973). However, the IPC measure suffers from the same problems as are inherent in the CA measure. First, IPC scores are correlated with recall level: IPC scores increase with increases in recall. Burns and Brown (2000) developed the adjusted IPC (AIPC) score, which corrects for recall-level differences. The AIPC scores continued to be correlated with variables thought to affect the amount of item-specific processing even after correction. Hence, the AIPC score should be used for situations in which recall-level differences exist. However, as with the ACA score, the AIPC measure overcorrects, and therefore, may be insensitive to small differences in item-specific processing.

Burns and Brown (2000) also argued that the IPC measure is inaccurate when any of the groups being compared performed little or no relational processing. In their experiment, which was described when discussing the CA measure, they showed that a group performing only item-specific processing (and little or no relational processing) actually produced lower IPC scores than a group performing only relational processing. Hence, item-specific information produces an advantage in IPC scores only when it is encoded in the context of relational information. Therefore, the IPC measure is inappropriate when one of the conditions being compared performs little or no relational processing.

Item Gains

Klein et al. (1989), in their study on hypermnesia, demonstrated that item-specific processing produces hypermnesic recall because it increases the number of new items recalled on later tests (item gains). I further explored the relationship between item-specific processing and item gains, and across several experiments, I showed that item gains tend to increase as amount of item-specific processing increases (Burns, 1993). I proposed that item gains could be used as an index of the amount of item-specific processing. The item-gain measure has since been used extensively and has proved to be quite successful (e.g., Burns & Gold, 1999; Engelkamp & Seiler, 2003; Klein et al., 1994; Mulligan, 2000, 2001, 2002; Mulligan & Duke, 2002). When proposing the item-gain measure, however, I pointed out that it is likely to be inaccurate in several experimental situations (Burns, 1993). The main problem is that the number of item gains observed is dependent on the rather arbitrary choice of recall-test length. When two groups differing in amount of item-specific processing have both processed a great deal of relational information, the item-gain measure will be more sensitive to item-specific processing differences only with short recall tests. Across two experiments, a list of categorically related items was given to participants who either rated the items for pleasantness or sorted them into categories. Two lengthy recall tests were then given and the results revealed no item-gain difference between groups. However, when shorter (2.5 minutes) recall tests were given in experiment 2, the pleasantness-rating group (item-specific processing) produced significantly more gains than the category-sorting group (relational processing).

I have also argued that regardless of the amount of item-specific processing performed, *relational* processing may produce considerable item gains when very short recall tests are given (Burns, 1993). The relational retrieval cues may not be exhausted at the end of a relatively short test. The remaining relational cues may be retrieved on a later test, allowing new items to be retrieved (see also Burns & Hebert, 2005; Burns & Schoff, 1998).

The difficulties with the item-gain measure should be correctable by giving several successive, relatively short recall tests. The brevity of the tests should ensure that any item-specific processing difference existing between groups that processed a great deal of relational information would be detected. Further, the fact that multiple recall tests are given should allow one to verify that an item-gain difference is due to item-specific processing, not relational processing. Specifically, if an item-gain difference exists both on early trials and on later trials, then it is not likely due to relational processing. The difficulty with giving several recall tests, however, is that it can become rather boring for participants, who may become less motivated on later trials.

ANALYSIS OF CUMULATIVE-RECALL CURVES: A NEW MEASURE OF ITEM-SPECIFIC AND RELATIONAL PROCESSING

Recently, Burns and Hebert (2005) proposed an alternative technique for measuring item-specific and relational processing. This new approach relies on analysis of cumulative-recall scores. Wixted and Rohrer (1994) published an excellent review of the literature on cumulative-recall curves. The research reveals that the relationship between recall duration and the cumulative number of items recalled can be reasonably well described by the exponential equation:

$$n(t) = n(\infty)(1 - e^{-\lambda t}) \tag{1}$$

where $n(t)$ is the number of items recalled at time t, $n(\infty)$ is asymptotic recall level, e is the base of the natural logarithm, and λ is the rate of approaching asymptote (e.g., Bousfield & Sedgewick, 1944; Indow & Togano, 1970; Roediger, Stellon, & Tulving, 1977). With few exceptions, the research has demonstrated an inverse relationship between asymptotic level of recall and rate of approaching asymptote (e.g., Bousfield & Sedgewick, 1944; Hermann & Chaffin, 1976; Hermann & Murray, 1979; Johnson, Johnson, & Marks, 1951; Indow & Togano, 1970; Kaplan, Carvellas, &

Metlay, 1969). In terms of Equation 1, as $n(\infty)$ increases, λ decreases. In other words, those conditions that produce good overall recall tend to result in a slower approach to asymptote. Of the few exceptions to this inverse relationship, (e.g., Rohrer & Wixted, 1994; Wixted & Rohrer, 1994), only one involves manipulation of an encoding variable. Burns and Schoff (1998) demonstrated that manipulations of item-specific and relational processing have profound effects on the shape of cumulative-recall curves. They used orienting tasks to promote the processing of item-specific information, relational information, or both types of information. Following the incidental learning phase, participants were given a lengthy recall test and the number of items each participant recalled during each minute of the recall period was recorded.

Across several experiments, Burns and Schoff (1998) found that relational processing produces very good recall early in the recall period, whereas item-specific processing tended to produce poorer initial recall, but resulted in more items being recalled during later stages of the recall period. Moreover, a different cumulative-recall pattern emerged when both item-specific and relational processing was performed. Some of Burns and Schoff's results are reproduced in Figure 6.1. The top panel of Figure 6.1 displays the results from experiment 1, in which one group categorically sorted a list of items from ad hoc categories (relational processing) and the second group both rated each item for pleasantness and also generated a word that was related to each item (item-specific processing). As can be seen, the relational-processing group produced greater initial recall, whereas the item-specific group tended to recall more items per minute during the later portion of the recall period. This resulted in equivalent estimates of asymptotic recall levels, but λ was lower for the item-specific group.

The middle panel of figure 6.1 shows the results from Burns and Schoff's (1998) experiment 4, in which one group was given the category sorting task (relational processing) while the second group was required both to sort the items into categories and to rate them for pleasantness (relational and item-specific processing). As you can see, the group processing both relational and item-specific information recalled more items per minute of recall throughout the entire recall period, resulting in a roughly equivalent rate of approach to asymptote, but a much higher estimate of asymptotic recall level.

The comparison in the bottom panel of Figure 6.1 is between a group given both the category-sorting and pleasantness-rating tasks (relational and item-specific processing) and a group given two item-specific processing tasks (pleasantness rating and word generation). The group processing both item-specific and relational information produced better initial recall, but after the first 4 minutes, the two groups recalled about the same number of items per minute. The estimates of both λ and $n(\infty)$ were higher for the relational and item-specific processing group than for the item-specific group.

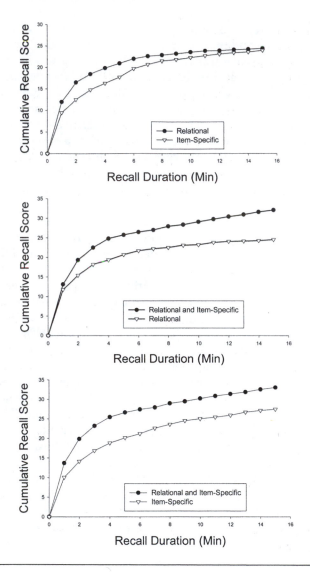

FIGURE 6.1 Mean cumulative-recall scores for various conditions tested in Burns and Schoff's (1998) experiments.

Burns and Hebert (2005) pointed out that the shapes of the cumulative-recall curves and their resulting parameter estimates could be used to assess the amount of item-specific and relational processing performed. They suggested that conditions processing primarily relational information produce cumulative-recall curves that approach asymptote very quickly relative to conditions processing primarily item-specific information. Conditions processing both item-specific and relational information produce cumulative-recall curves that demonstrate both very rapid initial recall and good recall throughout the remainder of the recall period.

Burns and Hebert (2005) also demonstrated that the cumulative-recall analysis adequately indexed item-specific and relational processing differences even in a within-subjects (or mixed-list) design. They presented two groups a list of items constructed from both obvious and ad hoc categories, requiring one of the groups to rate the words for pleasantness while the other group categorically sorted the items. Following presentation, two successive 8-minute recall tests were administered. Consistent with previous research, the obvious-category items were expected to receive relational processing regardless of the type of orienting task, whereas the items from ad hoc categories were expected to receive item-specific processing regardless of orienting task.

The resulting cumulative-recall curves, plotted across both recall periods and shown in Figure 6.2, were similar to those obtained when type of category was manipulated between subjects. The items that presumably received only item-specific processing (the ad hoc-category items rated for pleasantness) produced low initial recall levels, but their approach to asymptote was quite slow. The items presumably receiving only relational processing (the obvious-category items that were categorically sorted) produced relatively high initial levels of recall, but approached asymptote more quickly. A comparison between these two groups reveals a pattern of results quite similar to those obtained by Burns and Schoff (1998), shown in the top panel of Figure 6.1.

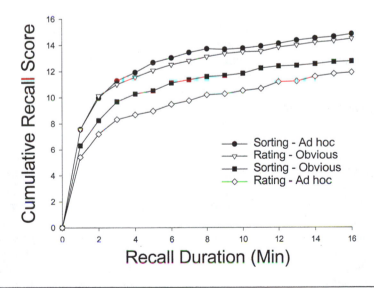

FIGURE 6.2 Mean cumulative-recall scores for each of the four conditions tested in Burns and Hebert (2005) experiment.

The two types of items that presumably received both types of processing (the obvious-category items that were rated and the ad hoc items that were sorted) produced very similar curves, and a comparison of these curves to that produced by the items receiving only item-specific processing produces a pattern of results nearly identical to that displayed in the bottom panel of Figure 6.1.

In addition to demonstrating that the cumulative-recall analysis works when type of processing is manipulated within-lists, Burns and Hebert (2005) also demonstrated that cumulative recall is sensitive to item-specific processing differences under conditions (lengthy recall tests) in which an item-gain analysis failed to detect them. Similarly, the cumulative-recall analysis detected relational processing differences under conditions in which the item-loss measure failed to detect them. Hence, the cumulative-recall analysis may prove to be a very useful approach to measuring item-specific and relational processing differences.

One potential limitation with the cumulative-recall analysis is that, to date, it has been used primarily in situations in which type of processing is manipulated by using particular orienting tasks (e.g., pleasantness rating, categorization). It is possible that other methods of inducing item-specific and relational processing might invoke additional processes that could affect the cumulative-recall curves above and beyond that of item-specific and relational processing. This possibility seems doubtful for two reasons. First, the shape of cumulative-recall curves is intricately related to the item-gain measure (see Burns, 1993; Burns & Schoff, 1998), and the item-gain measure has been applied to several experimental situations with great success (e.g., Klein et al., 1994; Mulligan, 2000). There is good reason, therefore, to believe that the cumulative-recall analysis will generalize to other experimental situations. Second, in recent research conducted by my students and me, we have applied the cumulative-recall analysis to several list-learning phenomena, including the generation effect, the self-reference effect, and the picture-superiority effect. The results are quite encouraging, with hypothesized differences in relational and item-specific processing producing cumulative-recall curves described in the foregoing analysis.

SUMMARY OF MEASURES

There are various measurement tools available for assessing the amount of relational and item-specific processing performed. Each has its advantages and limitations, some of which are summarized in Table 6.1. Concerning relational processing, the category clustering and category access measures both rely on experimenter-defined categories and neither has been shown to work well in mixed-list designs. Moreover, the CA measure should not be used when one of the comparison groups may have performed little or no relational processing. The subjective-clustering measures, although quite universal, seem to suffer from a lack of sensitivity. Specifically, they may be insensitive to large clusters. The item-loss measure seems particularly promising, but it is not clear that it can be applied to mixed-list designs.

The item-specific processing measures are also limited. Recognition test performance has been shown to be sensitive to relational processing in some circumstances and may require the testing of additional groups of participants. The IPC measure suffers from the same limitations as CA; namely, it is correlated with recall level, and it does not work when one condition has performed little or no relational processing. The accuracy of the item-gain measure is dependent on test length. Although problems with the item-gain measure can be solved by giving several successive recall tests this approach may be unrealistic in many circumstances. The cumulative-recall measure, which allows for the simultaneous assessment of item-specific and relational processing, seems to be quite promising. Moreover, it has been shown to be accurate in mixed-list designs.

There are other limitations concerning each of the measures discussed. For example, it is not clear how well the various measures assess relational and distinctive processing in situations in which the unit of analysis is something other than individual items in list-learning tasks. It is not clear, for example, whether the CA or IPC measures would reflect processing differences when sentences are the unit of analysis. Further research in this area is clearly needed.

MEASURING DISTINCTIVENESS

Heretofore, I have discussed the techniques available to assess the extent of item-specific and relational processing. Since this volume is dedicated to issues concerning distinctiveness, I now return to the question of using these measurement tools to substantiate presumed differences in distinctive processing. Whether one believes distinctiveness results from the encoding of unique properties of an item relative to other items in the encoding context (e.g., Hunt & Einstein, 1981; Nelson, 1979), or as the result of processing differences among items that are related on some dimension (e.g., Hunt & Lamb, 2001; Smith & Hunt, 2000), the measurement techniques discussed above should prove useful. To the extent that distinctiveness is considered the sole consequence of item-specific processing, the application of the tools is straightforward: The item-specific processing measures can be applied directly to assess the degree of distinctiveness. When distinctiveness is defined as the combined result of item-specific and relational processing, then the item-specific and relational processing measures can be used in conjunction: distinctiveness would be expected to influence both sets of measures and therefore, the combination of item-specific and relational processing measures could be used to index distinctiveness. For example, an increase in item gains in conjunction with a decrease in item losses would be indicative of distinctive processing, whereas an increase in item gains only or a decrease in item losses only would not be indicative of distinctive processing.

The Cumulative Recall Analysis and Recent Conceptualizations of Distinctiveness

Interestingly, the cumulative-recall analysis seems particularly valuable for researchers who have begun to define distinctiveness as the product of both item-specific and relational processing. Whereas each of the other indices discussed either one type of processing or the other, the cumulative-recall analysis can be used to assess both types of processing. Different cumulative-recall patterns should emerge as a function of whether item-specific, relational, or both types of processing (i.e., distinctive processing) are performed. Distinctive processing should produce cumulative-recall curves with a higher estimate of $n(\infty)$ than those produced by relational processing (see the middle panel of Figure 6.1) and with higher estimates of both λ and $n(\infty)$ than the curves produced by item-specific processing (see the bottom panel of Figure 6.1).

The cumulative-recall analysis may also provide insight regarding the specific mechanisms by which distinctiveness affects retrieval. The finding that the combination of relational and item-specific processing (distinctiveness) produces a pattern of cumulative recall that is unique from the pattern obtained following either relational or item-specific processing not only suggests that there are unique memorial consequences to performing both types of processing but also elucidates the nature of those memorial consequences. Distinctive processing seems to enhance retrieval by allowing item-specific cues to become aligned or associated with relational cues. The item-specific cues apparently become part of the organized retrieval plan. As part of the retrieval plan, the item-specific cues may enjoy not only quicker access but also a greater probability of access. The rapid access of the item-specific cues leads to initial recall that is greater than that produced following purely item-specific or purely relational processing. The greater probability of access leads to continued high recall throughout the remainder of the period, since the cues are less likely to become exhausted.

Regardless of the manner in which one chooses to define distinctiveness, however, it is a psychological process and not an independent variable (or property of objects). Hence, it is critical that one provides converging evidence for hypothesized differences in distinctiveness. It is hoped that the foregoing discussion will aid researchers in this endeavor.

ACKNOWLEDGMENTS

Portions of this paper were presented at the 49th meeting of the Southwestern Psychological Association, New Orleans, LA.

REFERENCES

Anderson, R. C., & Watts, G. H. (1969). Bidirectional associations in multi-trial free recall, *Psychonomic Science, 15*, 288–289.

Basden, B. H., Basden, D. R., Bryner, S., & Thomas, R. L. (1997). A comparison of group and individual remembering: Does Collaboration disrupt retrieval strategies? *Journal of Experimental Psychology: Learning, Memory, and Cognition, 23*, 1176–1189.

Begg, I., Vinski, E., Frankovich, L., & Holgate, B. (1991). Generating makes words memorable, but so does effective reading. *Memory & Cognition, 19*, 487–497.

Bousfield, W.A., & Sedgewick, C. H. W. (1944). An analysis of restricted associative responses. *Journal of General Psychology, 30*, 149–165.

Burns, D. J. (1993). Item gains and losses during hypermnesic recall: Implications for the item-specific—relational information distinction. *Journal of Experimental Psychology: Learning, Memory, and Cognition, 19*, 163–173.

Burns, D. J. (1996). The item-order distinction and the generation effect: The importance of order information in long-term memory. *American Journal of Psychology, 109*, 567–580.

Burns, D. J., & Brown, C. A. (2000). The category access measure of relational processing. *Journal of Experimental Psychology: Learning, Memory, and Cognition, 26*, 1057–1062.

Burns, D. J., Curti, E. T., & Lavin, J. C. (1993). The effect of generation on item and order retention in immediate and delayed recall. *Memory & Cognition, 21*, 846–852.

Burns, D. J., & Gold, D. E. (1999). An analysis of item gains and losses in retroactive interference. *Journal of Experimental Psychology: Learning, Memory, and Cognition, 25*, 978–985.

Burns, D. J., & Hebert, T. (2005). Using cumulative-recall curves to assess the extent of relational and item-specific processing. *Memory, 13*, 189–199.

Burns, D. J., & Schoff, K. M. (1998). Slow and steady often ties the race: The effects of item-specific and relational processing on cumulative recall. *Journal of Experimental Psychology: Learning, Memory, and Cognition, 24*, 1041–1051.

Cohen, B. H. (1963). Recall of categorized word lists. *Journal of Experimental Psychology, 65*, 368–376.

Cohen, B. H. (1966). Some or none characteristics of coding behavior. *Journal of Verbal Learning and Verbal Behavior, 5*, 182–187.

Einstein, G. O., & Hunt, R. R. (1980). Levels of processing and organization: Additive effects of individual item and relational processing. *Journal of Experimental Psychology: Human Learning and Memory, 6*, 588–598.

Engelkamp, J., & Dehn, D. M. (2000). Item and order information in subject-performed tasks and experimenter-performed tasks. *Journal of Experimental Psychology: Learning, Memory, and Cognition, 26*, 671–682.

Engelkamp, J., & Seiler, K. H. (2003) Gains and losses in action memory. *Quarterly Journal of Experimental Psychology, 56*, 829–848.

Greene, R. L., Thapar, A., & Westerman, D. L. (1998). Effects of generation on memory for order. *Journal of Memory and Language, 38*, 255–264.

Hermann, D. J., & Chaffin, R. J. S. (1976). Number of available associations and rate of association for categories in semantic memory. *Journal of General Psychology, 95*, 227–231.

Hermann, D. J., & Murray, D. J. (1979. The role of category size in continuous recall from semantic memory. *Journal of General Psychology, 101*, 205–218.

Humphreys, M. S., Wiles, J., & Bain, J. D. (1993). Memory retrieval with two cues: Think of Intersecting Sets. In D. E. Meyer & S. Kornblum (Eds.), *Attention and performance XIV: Synergies in experimental psychology, artificial intelligence, and cognitive neuroscience* (pp. 489–507). Hillsdale, NJ: Lawrence Erlbaum Associates.

Hunt, R. R., & Einstein, G. O. (1981). Relational and item-specific information in memory. *Journal of Verbal Learning and Verbal Behavior, 20*, 497–514.

Hunt, R. R., & Lamb, C. A. (2001). What causes the isolation effect? *Journal of Experimental Psychology: Learning, Memory, and Cognition, 27*, 1359–1366.

Hunt, R. R., & McDaniel, M. A. (1993). The enigma of organization and distinctiveness. *Journal of Memory and Language, 32*, 421–445.

Hunt, R. R., & Seta, C. E. (1984). Category size effects in recall: The roles of relational and individual item information. *Journal of Experimental Psychology: Learning, Memory, and Cognition, 10*, 454–464.

Hunt, R. R., & Smith, R. E. (1996). Assessing the particular from the general: The power of distinctiveness in the context of organization. *Memory & Cognition, 24*, 217–225.

Indow, T., & Togano, K. (1970). On retrieving sequence from long-term memory. *Psychological Review, 77*, 317–331.

Jacoby, L. L. (1973). Test appropriate strategies in categorized lists. *Journal of Verbal Learning and Verbal Behavior, 12*, 675–682.

Johnson, D. M., Johnson, R. C., & Mark, A. L. (1951). A mathematical analysis of verbal recall. *Journal of General Psychology, 44*, 121–128.

Kaplan, I. T., Carvellas, T., & Metlay, W. (1969). Searching for words in letter sets of varying size. *Journal of Experimental Psychology, 82*, 377–380.

Klein, S. B., & Kihlstrom, J. F. (1986). Elaboration, organization and the self-reference effect in memory. *Journal of Experimental Psychology: General, 115*, 26–38.

Klein, S. B., & Loftus, J. (1988). The nature of self-referent encoding: The contribution of elaborative and organizational processes. *Journal of Personality and Social Psychology, 55*, 5–11.

Klein, S. B., Loftus, J., Kihlstrom, J. F., & Aseron, R. (1989). Effects of item-specific and relational information on hypermnesic recall. *Journal of Experimental Psychology: Learning, Memory, and Cognition, 15*, 1192–1197.

Klein, S. B., Loftus, J., Kihlstrom, J. F., & Schell, T. (1994). Repeated testing: A technique for assessing the roles of elaborative and organizational processing in the representation of social knowledge. *Journal of Personality and Social Psychology, 66,* 830–839.

Mandler, G. (1970). Words, lists and categories: An experimental view of organized memory. In J. L. Cowan (Ed.), *Studies in thought and language* (pp. 252–271). Tucson: University of Arizona Press.

Mandler, G. (1972). Organization and recognition. In E. Tulving & W. Donaldson (Eds.), *Organization and memory* (pp. 139–166). New York: Academic Press.

McDaniel, M. A., & Waddill, P. J. (1990). Generation effects for context words: Implications for item-specific and multi-factor theories. *Journal of Memory and Language, 29,* 201–211.

McDaniel, M. A., Waddill, P. J., & Einstein, G. O. (1988). A contextual account of the generation effect: A three factor theory. *Journal of Memory and Language, 27,* 521–536.

Mulligan, N. W. (2000). Perceptual interference at encoding enhances item-specific encoding and disrupts relational encoding: Evidence from multiple recall tests. *Memory & Cognition, 28,* 539–546.

Mulligan, N. W. (2001). Generation and hypermnesia. *Journal of Experimental Psychology: Learning, Memory and Cognition, 27,* 436–450.

Mulligan, N. W. (2002). The emergence of item-specific encoding effects in between-subjects designs: Perceptual interference and multiple recall tests. *Psychonomic Bulletin and Review, 9,* 375–382.

Mulligan, N. W., & Duke, M. D. (2002). Positive and negative generation effects, hypermnesia, and total recall time, *Memory & Cognition, 30,* 1044–1053.

Murphy, M. D. (1979). Measurement and category clustering in free recall. In C. R. Puff (Ed.), *Memory organization and structure* (pp. 51–83). New York: Academic Press.

Nairne, J. S., Riegler, G. L., & Serra, M. (1991). Dissociative effects of generation on item and order retention. *Journal of Experimental Psychology: Learning, Memory and Cognition, 17,* 702–709.

Nelson, D. L. (1979). Remembering pictures and words: Appearance, significance, and name. In L. S. Cermak & F. I. M. Craik (Eds.), *Levels of processing in human memory* (pp. 45–85). Hillsdale, NJ: Lawrence Erlbaum Associates.

Neely, J. H., & Balota, D. A. (1981). Test-expectancy and semantic-organization effects in recall and recognition. *Memory & Cognition, 9,* 283–300.

Pellegrino, J. W., & Ingram, A. L. (1979). Process, Products, and Measures of Memory Organization. In C. R. Puff (Ed.), *Memory organization and structure* (pp. 21–49). New York: Academic Press.

Roediger, H. L., Stellon, C. C., & Tulving, E. (1977). Inhibition from part-list cues and rate of recall. *Journal of Experimental Psychology: Human Learning and Memory, 3,* 174–188.

Rogers, T. B., Kuiper, N. A., & Kirker, W. S. (1977). Self reference and the encoding of personal information. *Journal of Personality and Social Psychology, 35,* 677–688.

Rohrer, D. & Wixted, J. T. (1994). An analysis of latency and interresponse time in free recall. *Memory & Cognition, 22,* 511–524.

Rubin, D. C., & Wallace, W. T. (1989). Rhyme and reason: Analysis of dual retrieval cues. *Journal of Experimental Psychology: Learning, Memory, and Cognition, 15,* 689–709.

Rundus, D. (1973). Negative effects of using list items as recall cues. *Journal of Verbal Learning and Verbal Behavior, 12,* 43–50.

Schmidt, S. R. (1985). Encoding and retrieval processes in the memory for conceptually distinctive events. *Journal of Experimental Psychology: Learning, Memory, and Cognition, 11,* 565–578.

Schmidt, S. R., & Cherry, K. (1989). The negative generation effect: Delineation of a phenomenon. *Memory & Cognition, 17,* 359–369.

Shuell, T. J. (1975). On sense and nonsense in measuring organization in free recall. *Psychological Bulletin, 82,* 720–724.

Smith, R. E., & Hunt, R. R. (2000). The effects of distinctiveness require reinstatement of organization: The importance of intentional memory instructions. *Journal of Memory and Language, 43,* 431–446.

Sowder, C. (1973). Mediated unlearning. *Journal of Experimental Psychology. 100,* 50–57.

Sternberg, R. J. & Tulving, E. (1977). The measurement of subjective organization in free recall. *Psychological Bulletin, 84,* 539–556.

Tulving, E., & Pearlstone, Z. (1966). Availability versus accessibility of information in memory for words. *Journal of Verbal Learning and Verbal Behavior, 5,* 381–391.

Wixted, J. T., & Rohrer, D. (1994). Analyzing the dynamics of free recall: An integrative review of the empirical literature. *Psychonomic Bulletin & Review, 1,* 89–106.

Wood, G. (1972). Organizational processes and free recall. In E. Tulving & W. Donaldson (Eds.), *Organization of memory* (pp. 49–91). New York: Academic Press.

II

BIZARRENESS

7

Resolution of Discrepant Memory Strengths: An Explanation of the Effects of Bizarreness on Memory

James B. Worthen

Research investigating the relationship between bizarreness and memory began as an attempt to determine the effectiveness of bizarre mental imagery as a mnemonic device. Although some researchers still investigate the mnemonic effectiveness of bizarre imagery, a new wave of research has begun to address the topic of bizarreness more generally. Researchers are now exploring a wide range of bizarreness effects (including both memory-facilitating and memory-disruptive effects) that have important implications not only for those interested in education and learning but also for those interested in fields such as criminal justice, advertising, marketing, and clinical psychology. The following pages provide a review of both types of bizarreness research and a description of the major theoretical accounts that have been offered to explain the basic findings related to the influence of bizarreness on memory. The limitations of existing explanations are discussed and a comprehensive explanation of both the facilitative and disruptive effects of bizarreness is offered.

Before reviewing the literature on bizarreness and memory, it may be helpful to define the term *bizarreness*. Throughout this chapter, I will use the term to refer to an extreme form of distinctiveness whereby the stimulus is in the proportional minority relative to all previously stored knowledge. This operational definition is theoretically similar to Schmidt's (1991) definition of *secondary distinctiveness* and Berlyne's (1960) definition of *absolute novelty*. Schmidt and Berlyne each recognized that stimuli can be distinct relative to either a specified and immediate context or relative to all prior experience and knowledge. Schmidt describes the former type of distinctiveness as *primary distinctiveness* and the latter as *secondary* distinctiveness, whereas, in terms of novelty, Berlyne described the former case as *relative novelty* and the latter as *absolute novelty*. I will make the argument later that, as an extreme form of distinctiveness, bizarreness induces an exaggerated form of item-specific processing (see Hunt, Chapter 1 this volume, for a discussion) at the expense of intraitem-relational processing.

BIZARRENESS AS A MNEMONIC

The most traditional research in the area of bizarreness and memory is that which examines the use of bizarre elaboration as a mnemonic. Thought to have been used to enhance memory by Greek poets dating back to 500 BC (Yarmey, 1984), bizarre imagery was advanced in popular literature (e.g., Lorayne, 1972; Lorayne & Lucas, 1974; Roth, 1961; Yates, 1966) as an important mnemonic technique. Despite the claims made in the popular literature, early empirical research investigating the mnemonic advantage of bizarre imagery produced a litany of inconsistent results and controversial interpretations.[1] In fact, solid conclusions regarding the pattern of results from early bizarre imagery research were not reached until the mid-1980s, when McDaniel and Einstein (1986) published an influential article that elucidated important boundary conditions that serve to constrain the mnemonic effectiveness of bizarre imagery in free recall. Although recent research has questioned the role of imagery in obtaining a mnemonic advantage of bizarreness, a variety of bizarre elaborative techniques continue to be tested. For purposes of this discussion, any study that employs the use of bizarre and common contexts as a vehicle to facilitate memory for individual target items will be referred to as research investigating bizarreness as a mnemonic. Research that addresses memory for entire bizarre events will be addressed separately.

Typical Methodology

Research in the mnemonic tradition typically manipulates the context in which target stimuli (usually words) are embedded in order to induce bizarre and common elaboration.[2] Most commonly, elaboration is induced by embedding target word triplets in common and bizarre sentences. For example, a mnemonic researcher may present participants with a bizarre sentence such as "The GRAPES burned the ARTIST with the CANDLE" in an effort to enhance memory for the target constituents *grapes, artist*, and *candle*. After the presentation of the stimuli, participants are engaged in a short distractor task followed by instructions to recall the target words from each stimulus sentence. Recall is typically scored in terms of the proportion of stimulus arrays accessed, the number constituents recalled per accessed array, and the total number of constituents recalled. Using the example from above, a sentence would be considered accessed if at least one target word from the sentence was recalled. The number of target words recovered per sentence accessed would be measured by noting how many target words were recovered from each accessed sentence. The proportion of target words recalled would be computed by dividing the number of total number of target words recalled by the total number of target words presented.

Boundary Conditions

Mental imagery

Despite the fact that the phrase "bizarre imagery effect" is often used to refer to the bizarre recall advantage, recent research suggests that it is elaboration, not imagery per se, that produces a bizarreness advantage. Weir and Richman (1996) demonstrated a bizarre recall advantage for noun pairs regardless of whether elaboration involved image generation, sentence generation, or a combination of sentence and image generation. Similarly, Worthen (1997) found a mnemonic advantage of bizarreness regardless of whether images accompanying word pairs were generated by the learner or provided by the experimenter. Additionally, greater recall was found for bizarre than for common word pairs under conditions designed to encourage semantic processing and minimize imaginal processing. These findings are consistent with research (i.e., Anderson & Buyer, 1994; Zoller, Workman, & Kroll, 1989) that has failed to find a significant positive relationship between imaging ability and the bizarre recall advantage. As such, it appears that the phrase "bizarre imagery effect" connotes a higher degree of constraint than is warranted and thus has been aptly replaced in the literature with more general terms such as "bizarre context effect" and "bizarreness effect." In keeping with the recent literature, the latter term will be used throughout the remainder of this paper.

List composition

It has been firmly established that the mnemonic advantage of bizarreness occurs in lists containing both bizarre and common items (within-groups designs), but not in pure lists (between-groups designs;[3] McDaniel & Einstein, 1986). However, more recent research has further illuminated the role of list composition as it relates to the bizarre-recall advantage. Several researchers have failed to obtain a bizarre-recall advantage (Hirshman, Whelley, & Palij, 1989, Experiment1; Kroll & Tu, 1988, Experiment 5; Worthen, Marshall, & Cox, 1998) and, under some conditions, found a commonness advantage (Worthen, 1997, Experiment 2; Worthen & Marshall, 1996) in mixed lists containing a disproportionate number of bizarre items. Conversely, the magnitude of the bizarreness advantage has been shown to increase as the ratio of bizarre to common items decreases within lists (Sharpe & Markham, 1992; Worthen, 1997; Worthen & Marshall, 1996).

Stimulus complexity

A good deal of research suggests that the bizarreness effect is constrained by the complexity of stimulus materials. For example, several studies (Kroll, Shepeler, & Angin, 1986, Experiment 1; McDaniel & Einstein, 1989; Richman, Dunn, Kahl, Sadler, & Simmons, 1990; Robinson-Riegler & Mc-Daniel, 1994) that used verbally complex[4] stimuli have failed to obtain significant bizarreness effects while testing free recall in mixed lists. Robinson-Riegler and McDaniel (1994) suggest that the failure to find the effect with complex stimuli is the result of the learner's using complexity rather than bizarreness as a retrieval cue. That is, the authors suggest that cues associated with the complexity of stimuli may be stronger than cues associated with bizarreness. Although bizarreness would cue only some of the learned material, complexity would cue both common and bizarre items and thus increase memory for both item types. Robinson-Riegler and McDaniel supported these arguments by demonstrating greater overall recall for target words embedded in complex relative to simple sentences despite the failure to obtain a significant bizarreness effect.

Findings from other research suggest that the failure to find bizarreness effects using complex stimuli may be related processing time. Specifically, both Kline and Groninger (1991) and Richman (1994) demonstrated a positive relationship between processing time and the magnitude of the bizarreness effect. Thus, it appears that when the allotted processing time is sufficient to comprehend verbally complex bizarre and common information, the bizarreness effect emerges. Based on such findings, it may be the case that complexity merely makes bizarre stimuli more difficult to fully comprehend. However, given that Robinson-Riegler and McDaniel (1994) failed to find bizarreness effects using both self-paced processing and stimulus presentations equal to or longer than those that have produced an effect with complex stimuli, further research is needed before firm conclusions regarding stimulus complexity and processing time can be drawn.

Stimulus plausibility

Research has also addressed the way in which bizarre elaboration is defined and the influence of that definition on memory. The first systematic studies examining the operations used to create bizarre mnemonics were conducted by Marshall, Nau, and Chandler (1979, 1980). Most relevant are the findings of the 1980 study, which indicated that, in terms of single operations, giving human or living features to nonhuman animals or objects led to the most successful recall. In keeping with this finding, Cornoldi, Cavedon, De Beni, & Pra Baldi (1988) found that bizarre elaboration depicting implausible scenarios was more effective than both common elaboration and bizarre elaboration depicting plausible scenarios. Similarly, Worthen and Marshall (1996) found stronger bizarreness effects for bizarre stimuli that contained 74% anthropomorphic scenes relative to bizarre stimuli that depicted only 24% anthropomorphic scenes when using predominantly common and 50/50 lists. However, the bizarreness effect was reversed (a commonness effect was found) when anthropomorphic bizarre stimuli were used in predominantly bizarre lists (see also Worthen, 1997, Experiment 2).

Imai and Richman (1991) provided results that indicate a relationship between plausibility and processing time with regard to the mnemonic effectiveness of bizarre stimuli. Specifically, these authors found plausible bizarre elaboration to be more effective than both common elaboration and implausible bizarre elaboration when stimulus duration was brief (7 seconds), but implausible bizarre elaboration to be most effective with a longer) stimulus duration (35 seconds). This finding is quite similar to the findings regarding the relationship between stimulus complexity and processing time (e.g., Kline & Groninger, 1991; Richman, 1994) and may indicate that implausibility makes experimenter-generated bizarre stimuli more difficult to comprehend. In keeping with these arguments, Worthen, Garcia-Rivas, Green, & Vidos (2000) demonstrated that even simple bizarre materials require more processing time than common materials and that isolated bizarre stimuli (bizarre items in predominantly common lists) require more cognitive effort for comprehension. As such, it seems safe to conclude that sufficient processing time is necessary for any type of bizarre mnemonic to be successful.

Lang (1995) provides evidence that suggests that the level of association among target components of stimuli also influences the magnitude of the bizarreness effect. Specifically, Lang varied the degree of association between target words embedded in common and in bizarre sentences. Her results indicated significant bizarreness effects with highly associated stimuli, but a significant commonness effect with weakly related stimuli. Clearly, the level of association of to-be-remembered target items must be considered when using bizarreness as a mnemonic. In terms of future work, it would be interesting to investigate the relation between level of association and processing time. That is, it may be the case that, like implausible items, weakly associated items are more difficult to comprehend than strongly associated stimuli and thus require more processing time.

Intention to learn

A relatively small amount of research investigating bizarreness as a mnemonic has addressed intention to learn and those results have been somewhat mixed. Although several studies (Merry & Graham, 1978; Hirshman et al., 1989; Tess, Hutchinson, Treloar, & Jenkins, 1999; Webber & Marshall, 1978) have demonstrated significant bizarreness effects under intentional learning conditions, a recent study (Burns, 1996) has failed to demonstrate the bizarre advantage under intentional learning conditions. Based on his results and those that preceded, Burns offered the conservative conclusion that, in the very least, intentional learning reduces the magnitude of the bizarreness effect. Although Burns' (1996) results are incongruent with previous research in the area of bizarreness mnemonics and with much of the research investigating memory for whole bizarre verbal stimuli (e.g., Engelkamp, Zimmer, Mohr, & Sellen, 1994; Mohr, Engelkamp, & Zimmer, 1989; Worthen & Roark, 2002), further research may be needed in this area.

Type of memory tested

As noted by other researchers (Einstein & McDaniel, 1987), bizarreness effects are most frequently obtained when free recall is tested and typically do not occur when cued recall is tested after short retention intervals (5 minutes or less). However, a systematic exception can be found in the literature. A bizarreness advantage can be obtained in cued recall when cues other than parts of target stimuli are used. For example, the use of a word from a target sentence to cue other words within the same target sentence generally fails to produce a bizarreness advantage. However, two studies (Nicolas & Marchal, 1996, 1998) that used moderate associates of target stimuli as cues have demonstrated facilitative effects of bizarreness in cued recall. The different outcomes resulting from the two methods of testing cued recall may be related to differences in the strength of intra-item relations for bizarre and common stimuli. Given that research suggests that bizarre stimuli have weaker intra-item relations than common stimuli (e.g., Worthen & Loveland, 2003; Worthen & Wood, 2001a, 2001b), the inability to obtain a bizarreness advantage in cued recall may be limited to cued-recall tests that are dependent on strong intra-item relations for success. Clearly, a test that uses parts of target stimuli as cues would be more dependent on intra-item relations than a test that uses associated stimuli as cues.

Despite the findings regarding cued recall after short retention intervals, a growing body of literature suggests that bizarreness effects can be found when cued recall is tested after a substantial delay (i.e., a week or longer). Importantly, this effect has been demonstrated using both parts of target stimuli as cues (Iaccino, Dvorak, & Coler, 1989; Iaccino & Spirek, 1988; Ironsmith & Lutz, 1996, Experiment 4; Marshall et al., 1980; O'Brien & Wolford, 1982; Webber & Marshall, 1978) and associates as cues (Nicolas & Marchal, 1996, 1998).

Interestingly, only two studies investigating bizarreness as a mnemonic (Emmerich & Ackerman, 1979; McDaniel & Einstein, 1986, Experiment 4) have tested recognition memory and both failed to produce a significant bizarreness effect. However, experiments examining recognition memory for bizarre action events (to be discussed later in this chapter) have found a bizarreness advantage under certain conditions. Clearly, additional research investigating the relationship between bizarre elaboration and recognition memory is needed.

Effectiveness and Accuracy

Based on previous research, it appears that bizarre elaboration can be more effective than common elaboration when free recall is tested. Although less consistently demonstrated, it may also be the case that bizarre elaboration leads to greater cued recall than does common elaboration when memory is tested after a substantial delay. Regardless of whether memory is tested with free or cued recall, the relative advantage of bizarre elaboration appears to fluctuate with list composition. Bizarre elaboration is likely to be most effective when common elaboration is also used or when exposure to common information intervenes between encoding and testing.

Mnemonic costs and gains

Despite the consistency of the bizarre-recall advantage under the boundary conditions outlined above, it must be noted that the inclusion of bizarre elaboration does not necessarily enhance total recall of a list. Several researchers (e.g., Einstein & McDaniel, 1987; Kroll & Tu, 1988; Lang, 1995) have noted that the recall advantage associated with bizarre elaboration is usually gained at the expense of common-item recall. That is, although information encoded with bizarre elaboration is recalled better than is information encoded with common elaboration, the overall proportion of items recalled in a mixed list typically does not exceed that of an unmixed list. This pattern of results suggests that, although the inclusion of bizarre elaboration at learning allows one to select which list items are most likely to be recalled, it does not increase the overall amount of information retained.

Although a trade-off between common and bizarre recall is the typical pattern of results found in bizarreness research, it should be noted that, under some very limited conditions, the inclusion of bizarre items has occasionally been found to increase overall memory for a list. First, Iaccino and colleagues have demonstrated an overall recall advantage for mixed lists relative to pure bizarre or pure common lists when cued recall was tested after a one-week delay (Iaccino et al., 1989; Iaccino & Sowa, 1989). Unfortunately, a subsequent study (Iaccino, 1996) failed to demonstrate the overall list facilitation after a 5-day delay and instead found a mixed-list advantage when cued recall was tested immediately and after a 3-day delay. Second, in tests of free recall, overall memory for list items has occasionally been found to be greater in predominantly common lists (e.g., 75% common) than in predominantly bizarre lists (Worthen et al., 1998) and lists containing equal numbers of common and bizarre items (Sharpe & Markham, 1992, Experiment 2; Worthen, 1997, Experiment 1; Worthen & Marshall, 1996, Experiment 1). However, in each of the studies referenced to support an overall recall advantage for predominantly common lists relative to lists containing equal numbers of common and bizarre items, the cited authors reported an additional experiment in which the overall recall advantage was not found. Thus, the evidence of an overall memory advantage associated with the use of bizarre elaboration in mixed lists is rather weak.

Even when considering all of the boundary conditions of the bizarreness effect, the trade-off between recall of common and bizarre items may be the most important limitation in using bizarre elaboration as mnemonic in an educational setting. Essentially, the trade-off renders the bizarre mnemonic advantage a curious phenomenon rather than a versatile tool for learning. However, the bizarre-common trade-off may actually be used to the advantage of those working in fields such as advertising and marketing. In advertising, for example, one could present or induce bizarre elaboration among consumers in order to make one's product more memorable than the product of a competitor. Even those with minimal exposure to television can draw the conclusion that this notion has not at all been ignored by the advertising industry as television commercials are replete with savvy frogs, talking lizards, culinary elves, and cuddly dough figures that are used to make a product or a product name most memorable to the consumer.

Accuracy and detail of bizarre memories

Another important issue concerning the effectiveness of bizarre elaboration as a mnemonic is the amount of target-stimulus detail recovered. As mentioned previously, research in the mnemonic tradition typically manipulates the context in which target stimuli are embedded in order to induce bizarre and common elaboration. As such, the goal is not necessarily to increase memory for the entire stimulus array (e.g., an entire bizarre sentence), but to increase memory for the target constituents (words) without concern about whether contextual details are accurately remembered. In fact, using the typical procedures and scoring methods, bizarre elaboration would be considered successful if the learner remembered the target constituents even if the exact manner in which those constituents were associated was forgotten or remembered incorrectly.

Perhaps most revealing regarding the effectiveness of bizarre elaboration is the typical finding of a bizarre advantage in the sentence access measure (one or more target words recalled), but not in the items-per-access measure of recall. In fact, several researchers (Burns, 1996; Kroll & Tu, 1988, Experiments 4 and 5; McDaniel & Einstein, 1986, Experiment 2; Worthen et al., 2000, Experiments 1 and 4) have demonstrated higher items-per-access scores with common elaborations than with bizarre elaborations. These findings indicate that bizarre elaboration does not lead to the recovery of more detail than does common elaboration and, to the contrary, the reverse may be true. Thus, even if one were to ignore to the bizarre-common trade-off discussed earlier, the lack of detail (and possibly accuracy) of memories resulting from bizarre elaboration suggest that the mnemonic advantages of bizarre elaboration are extremely limited.

MEMORY FOR ENTIRE BIZARRE EVENTS

Partly in response to the limitations (both in scope and utility) of traditional bizarre mnemonic research, researchers have begun to take a more general approach to memory for bizarre stimuli. Unlike bizarre mnemonic research that addresses bizarre elaboration as a method of enhancing memory for target constituents of elaborated stimuli, the event-based approach examines memory for the entire stimulus array. This approach views bizarreness not as a vehicle with which to present target components of learning but as a characteristic of an experience that influences information processing. Thus, the event-based approach to memory for bizarre stimuli seeks to uncover both the facilitative and the disruptive effects of bizarreness on memory for all aspects of a bizarre experience.

The feature that most clearly distinguishes the event-based approach from traditional bizarre mnemonic research is its level of analysis. The event-based approach emphasizes memory for whole events whereas the mnemonic approach ignores all aspects of a memory except for specific target components. This emphasis on memory for entire stimulus arrays allows researchers to gather more detail about the accuracy of recovered memories than could be achieved by using the traditional methods. When testing free recall, for example, participants are encouraged to recall stimuli in as much detail as possible and label whether their partially recovered memories were derived from common or bizarre memories (Worthen & Roark, 2002). As such, researchers are able to investigate issues previously ignored by bizarreness researchers, such as recall clustering (Roark & Worthen, 1999) and memory distortion (Worthen & Loveland, 2003; Worthen & Roark, 2002). Similarly, recognition memory, which has been generally ignored by traditional bizarreness researchers, is routinely tested by those taking a more general approach to bizarreness research. The inclusion of tests of recognition memory have allowed researchers to investigate not only the accuracy of recognition judgments but also issues such as memory discrimination and response bias (e.g., Michelon, Snyder, Buckner, McAvoy, & Zacks, 2003; Mohr, Engelkamp, & Zimmer, 1989; Worthen & Eller, 2002; Worthen & Wood, 2001a, 2001b).

An issue that is potentially salient with the event-based approach to bizarreness research is stimulus plausibility. From the traditional bizarre mnemonic perspective, bizarre elaboration is merely a vehicle in which to embed target stimuli. Thus, the plausibility of stimuli is not a concern to mnemonic researchers above and beyond its influence on the effectiveness of elaboration. However, because those researching the event-based approach to bizarreness are interested in entire stimulus arrays, one might argue that investigations of memory for implausible bizarre stimuli are too artificial to be extended in any meaningful way to real-world situations. This issue has been raised with regard even to traditional bizarreness research (Yarmey, 1984) and has roots in the classic debate over the relative importance of internal versus external validity (e.g., Henshel, 1980; Mook, 1982). As can easily happen in any area of basic research, the means of bizarreness research is often mistaken for its ends. That is, although event-based bizarreness researchers may use simple bizarre phrases or pictures in order to examine the influence of bizarreness on memory, one should not conclude that the purpose of the research is to determine the best way to remember such sentences and pictures if they were to be encountered in the real world. On the contrary, event-based bizarreness researchers are interested in the cognitive principles that are involved in processing any experience that is subjectively bizarre. Toward this end, implausible sentences and pictures are used as stimuli in order to consistently induce the experience of bizarreness. Although the perception of bizarreness is personal and idiosyncratic, the rigorous norming of stimuli allows researchers to be confident that their materials will be considered bizarre by most normal populations. Furthermore, it is assumed that the cognitive processes induced by experimental stimuli are similar to those induced during more subjective (or naturally occurring) bizarre experiences.

Another characteristic of event-based bizarreness research that distinguishes it from the traditional approach is the wide variety of domains examined from the event-based perspective. Whereas traditional bizarreness research is conducted mainly by those interested in verbal learning, event-based researchers have investigated memory for common and bizarre dream reports (Cipolli, Bolzani, Cornoldi, De Beni, & Fagioli, 1993; Worthen, Eisenstein, Budwey, & Varnado-Sullivan, 2005), hand-drawn pictures (Schmidt & Williams, 2004; Worthen & Eller, 2002), self-performed acts (e.g., Engelkamp, Zimmer, Mohr, & Sellen, 1994; Knopf, 1991; Mohr et al., 1989), other-performed acts (Worthen & Loveland, 2003; Worthen & Wood, 2001b), imagined acts (e.g., Thomas & Loftus, 2002; Worthen & Wood, 2001a), and script-based narratives (Davidson, Larson, Luo, & Burden, 2000; Davidson, Malmstrom, Burden, & Luo, 2000). Recent research has also investigated such topics as frequency encoding for common and bizarre stimuli (Kroll, Jaeger, & Dornfest, 1992; Marchal & Nicolas, 2000; Worthen, Hutchens, Nicodemus, & Baker, 2002) and mental imagery vividness (Baddeley & Andrade, 2000). The variety of stimulus domains tested allows event-based bizarreness research to have much more versatile applications than its traditional counterpart. Since it is no longer limited in application to education, marketing, and advertising, the general scope of event-based bizarreness research allows implications to be drawn in areas such as criminal justice and clinical psychology. For example, research examining memory distortion and response bias for performed acts may have important implications regarding the accuracy of eyewitness and self-defense testimony in the legal system. Similarly, research examining false recognition and response bias for imagined acts may have implications regarding the effectiveness of certain types of therapies (e.g., regression therapy, role playing, and imaginal desensitization).

Recent Findings

Free recall

Similar to research in the bizarre mnemonic tradition, event-based bizarreness research has found the most consistent bizarreness advantage when free recall is tested. A free-recall advantage for bizarre relative to common items has been found for several types of stimuli, including narratives (Davidson, Malmstrom, et al., 2000; Davidson, Larson et al., 2000), dream reports (Cipolli et al., 1993; Worthen et al., 2005), and sentences (Worthen & Roark, 2002). However, in a study examining memory for hand-drawn pictures, Schmidt and Williams (2004) found no free-recall advantage associated with bizarreness.

The bizarre free-recall advantage has been demonstrated less consistently in the area of memory for action events. Mohr et al. (1989) found a bizarre free-recall advantage for verbally-described acts, but not for self-performed acts. A similar study by Knopf (1991), however, failed to produce a bizarre recall advantage for either type of stimuli. Worthen and Loveland (2003), on the other hand, demonstrated a consistent free-recall advantage for objects associated with bizarre other-performed acts but mixed results regarding objects associated with self-performed acts. It is also important to note that Worthen and Loveland demonstrated facilitative effects of bizarreness only when recall was scored very leniently (e.g., using an access measure). Also, the authors found higher levels of memory distortion for bizarre than for common stimuli of both types. Specifically regarding memory distortion, objects associated with bizarre actions were more likely to be incorporated into a false memory than were objects associated with common actions (cf. Worthen & Roark, 2002).

Cued recall

Although it was routinely tested during the early days of bizarreness mnemonic research, cued recall has not often been tested by event-based researchers. To the extent that is has been tested, event-based research suggests that bizarreness does not lead to a cued-recall advantage (Engelkamp et al., 1994) and may result in higher levels of false memory than commonness. Regarding false memory, Worthen and Loveland (2003) tested memory for objects associated with self-performed and other-performed acts using verbs as cues for target nouns. Their results indicated more misplacement of bizarre than common target nouns at recall.

Recognition

Most of the studies investigating recognition memory for common and bizarre stimuli have used action events as stimuli. The typical findings of such research include a bizarre correct recognition advantage for verbally described acts but no difference between common and bizarre self-performed acts (Engelkamp, Zimmer, & Biegelmann, 1993; Engelkamp et al., 1994; Heil et al., 1999; Knopf, 1991; Mohr et al., 1989). Similarly, Worthen and Wood (2001a) found a bizarre correct-recognition advantage for imagined acts but not for self-performed acts. Furthermore, a bizarre recognition advantage was not found in either condition when self-performed and other-performed acts were directly compared (Worthen & Wood, 2001b).

Two studies (Michelon et al., 2003, and Worthen & Eller, 2002) have tested recognition memory for bizarre and common hand-drawn pictures, and the results were mixed. Worthen and Eller (2002) found no bizarreness advantage when recognition memory was tested after a 48-hour delay. However, Michelon et al. (2003) found a significant bizarreness advantage when testing recognition memory after a 2-week delay. Although differences in retention interval may explain the differing results of these studies, other stark differences in methodology preclude confident acceptance of this possibility. Thus, further research is needed to assess the influence of delayed testing on recognition memory for bizarre and common pictures.

Perhaps the most interesting findings regarding recognition memory for common and bizarre information are those related to false recognition and response bias. First, two studies (Engelkamp et al., 1993,1994) that have used completely novel items as lures have found more false recognition for common than for bizarre verbally described acts, but no difference between stimulus types for self-performed acts. Also using completely novel items as lures, Thomas & Loftus (2002) found equivalent levels of false recognition for common and bizarre acts in both a performance and an imaginal condition. However, research that has used transformed target stimuli as lures has indicated that bizarre memories are more susceptible to memory distortion than are common memories. For example, Worthen and Wood (2001a) demonstrated that participants were more likely to confuse the objects associated with separate, previously performed or imagined bizarre acts than they were to confuse the objects associated with separate, previously performed or imagined common acts. Similarly, Worthen and Wood (2001b) found that objects associated with bizarre acts were more likely to be falsely recognized in an incorrect context (bizarre or common) than were objects associated with common acts. Importantly, these false recognition results were obtained for both self-performed and other-performed acts.

Evidence in support of the notion that bizarreness disrupts information processing is also provided by studies that have examined response bias. Specifically, several studies (Michelon et al., 2003; Mohr et al., 1989; Worthen & Wood, 2001a, 2001b) have found that participants use a more liberal decision-making criterion when making judgments about bizarre memories than when making judgments about common memories.

Memory for frequency

Three studies (Kroll et al., 1992; Marchal & Nicolas, 2000; Worthen et al., 2002) have examined memory for frequency of bizarre and common stimuli. Kroll et al. concluded that memory for frequency of bizarre stimuli was more accurate than memory for frequency of common stimuli. In keeping with this general conclusion, Marchal and Nicolas demonstrated that common items were overestimated relative to bizarre items under some encoding conditions but not others. However, it must be noted that neither the Kroll et al. study nor the Marchal and Nicolas study directly compared judged frequencies and actual frequencies. Moreover, both studies used equal numbers of bizarre and common stimulus items that appeared only once each. Thus, very gross measures of bizarre and common frequency were obtained.

Using lists that varied actual frequency of stimuli, Worthen et al. (2002) compared judged and actual frequencies made by intentional and unintentional processors after a 2-minute or a 48-hour retention interval. Although bizarreness was not a significant factor after the 2-minute retention interval, bizarre frequency judgments were found to be less accurate (owing to overestimation) than were common frequency judgments after a 48-hour delay. Moreover, the delayed-testing results of Worthen et al. are consistent with previous research that has examined frequency judgments for atypical (Williams & Durso, 1986) and novel stimuli (Wiggs, 1993).

The Emerging Picture and Theoretical Explanations

Taking into consideration research from both the traditional and the event-based approaches to memory for bizarre information, it appears that bizarreness both facilitates and disrupts memory. Bizarreness enhances memory most consistently when either verbal or imaginal stimuli are used and either free recall or recognition memory is tested. Moreover, the facilitative effects of bizarreness are most pronounced when memory is scored leniently. Regardless of whether the conditions of memory facilitation are met, it appears that stimulus bizarreness negatively affects the accuracy of memory reports and memory judgments. Thus, a comprehensive explanation of the influence of bizarreness on memory must address both the memory-facilitating and memory-disrupting aspects of bizarreness. Although several theories have been offered in explanation of the facilitative effects of bizarreness, the disruptive effects of bizarreness have only recently begun to be addressed. Regardless, each of the major theoretical explanations described below is discussed in light of recent research.

Encoding-Based Explanations

Cognitive resource allocation

The most parsimonious and intuitively appealing explanations of the bizarre-recall advantage are those that suggest that the facilitative effects of bizarreness are the result of additional cognitive resources (e.g., attention, mental effort) allocated to the processing of bizarre relative to common items (e.g., Cox & Wollen, 1981; Wollen & Cox, 1981; Wollen & Margres, 1987). Although this type of explanation is supported by many basic findings of bizarreness research (e.g., processing and image times are longer for bizarre than for common items, the bizarreness advantage is typically found in mixed lists, and the recall of bizarre items is associated with the reduction of recall for common items), empirical research (Hirshman et al., 1989, Experiment 4; Worthen et al., 2000) has failed to support the notion that differences in cognitive resource allocation are significantly related to the bizarre-recall advantage. In order to test the hypothesis that the bizarre-recall advantage is the result of the bizarre items' attracting attentional resources away from common items, Hirshman et al. compared lists of alternating bizarre and common items to lists of bizarre and common items that were blocked by item type. According to the cognitive-resource-allocation account, the facilitative effects of bizarreness should be strongest in alternating lists because bizarre items would attract cognitive resources away from common items in alternating, but not blocked, lists. However, Hirshman et al. found no reduction in the magnitude of the bizarre-recall advantage for blocked relative to alternating lists. Worthen et al. examined response latencies to a secondary task as a measure of cognitive resource allocation during comprehension (Experiments 1 and 2) and imaging (Experiments 3 and 4) of bizarre and common stimuli. Contrary to the predictions of the cognitive-resource-allocation explanation, the authors found no compelling evidence to support the notion that cognitive-resource-allocation differences account for the facilitative effects of bizarreness.

Ironically, and despite the fact that it was offered to address the memory facilitating effects of bizarreness, the cognitive-resource-allocation explanation may be more suited to explain the disruptive effects of bizarreness. As has been noted in earlier work (e.g., Worthen et al., 2000), bizarreness may make a stimulus more difficult to comprehend. Thus, additional cognitive resources may be necessary to make sense of bizarre stimuli, but not sufficient to lead to an advantage in memory. Moreover, it seems likely that insufficient processing time would be related to increased bizarre memory distortion and response bias.

Expectation violation

Other encoding-based explanations specify expectation-violation and/or surprise as the crucial factors underlying the facilitative effects of bizarreness. In its original form (Hirshman et al., 1989), the expectation-violation explanation suggests that bizarre stimuli induce a surprise or orienting response that increases associations between target stimuli and general contextual cues. Although some support exists for this type of explanation (see Hirshman et al., 1989; Michelon et al., 2003; Worthen et al., 1998), other research (Davidson, Larson, et al., 2000; McDaniel et al., 1995; Worthen, Starns, Loveland, & Eisenstein, in press) that has directly tested the relationship between expectancy and recall has failed to support the notion that the facilitative effects of bizarreness are the result of an expectation-violating mechanism. Specifically, McDaniel et al. found no reduction in the magnitude of the bizarre-recall advantage under conditions designed to minimize the surprise of bizarre stimuli (Experiment 2) and no increase in the bizarreness advantage under conditions designed to maximize surprise (Experiment 3). Similarly, both Davidson, Larson, et al. and Worthen et al. (in press) failed to find a positive relationship between expectation-violation and recall for bizarre and common items. In fact, Worthen et al. (in press) provided evidence suggesting that surprise was significantly related to memory disruption rather than correct recall. This finding is consistent with previous research (e.g., Detterman, 1975; Detterman & Ellis, 1972; Ellis, Detterman, Runcie, McCarver, & Craig, 1971; Schmidt, 2002) that has demonstrated memory disruption after exposure to intensely distinctive and surprising stimuli.

Order encoding

An encoding account of the facilitative effects of bizarreness that has acknowledged some disruptive influence of bizarreness has been offered by McDaniel and colleagues (DeLosh & McDaniel, 1996; McDaniel, Einstein, DeLosh, May, & Brady, 1995). Based on the assumption that the encoding of serial-order information is a crucial factor in free recall (cf. Serra & Nairne, 1993; Toglia & Kimble, 1976), McDaniel et al. suggest that the bizarre-recall advantage found in mixed lists is the result of a disruption in the encoding of common-item order information induced by the presence of bizarre items within the list. Specifically, it is suggested that, although common items benefit from greater order encoding than do bizarre items in unmixed lists, the inclusion of both item types in a mixed list eliminates this common-item advantage. Thus, in a mixed list, common and bizarre items do not differ in terms of relational encoding, but the bizarre items benefit from more extensive item-specific encoding (cf. Wollen & Margres, 1987). Although this explanation has the attraction of providing a straightforward explanation of list composition effects and of addressing at least a minor disruptive effect of bizarreness, research has failed to fully support the order-encoding account of bizarreness effects. Specifically, McDaniel, De Losh, & Merritt (2000) and McDaniel et al. (1995) have provided support for the notion that bizarreness disrupts order encoding for common items in mixed lists, but has failed to demonstrate that this disruption is related to the recall differences found in mixed lists.

Retrieval-Based Explanations

On might argue that the general class of encoding-based accounts are unlikely to explain the facilitative effects of bizarreness on memory because those effects are most robust in free recall and least robust when cued recall is tested. The basis for this argument is that free recall is thought to be more dependent on retrieval factors than is cued recall because the burden of generating a learned item is minimized by provided cues in the latter type of recall (Riefer & Rouder, 1992; Tulving & Pearlstone, 1966). However, it should also be noted that cued recall is also more dependent on intra-item relations than is free recall when parts of target stimuli are used as cues. Given that research (e.g., Worthen & Loveland, 2003; Worthen & Wood, 2001a, 2001b) has demonstrated that bizarre stimuli have weaker intra-item relations than do common stimuli, it is possible that the failure to find a consistent bizarreness advantage in cued recall is related to poor encoding of intra-item relations in addition to the role played by retrieval factors (cf. Lang, 1995). Regardless, there has been an increasing tendency for researchers attempting to explain the facilitative effects of bizarreness to shift emphasis to retrieval and away from encoding in accounting for the bizarreness advantage.

Initial evidence in favor of a retrieval explanation of bizarreness effects was provided by Riefer and colleagues (Riefer & LaMay, 1998; Riefer & Rouder, 1992). Using multinomial analyses of cued and free-recall data, Riefer and colleagues determined that bizarre information is retrieved better than common information (Riefer & Rouder), but that common information is stored better than bizarre information (Riefer & LaMay). Although these results are generally consistent with both the facilitative and the disruptive effects of bizarreness, subsequent retrieval-based accounts have focused primarily on facilitative effects.

The differential-retrieval-process account (McDaniel et al., 2000) of bizarreness effects acknowledges the disruption of order encoding, but unlike the order-encoding account, it suggests that the facilitative effects of bizarreness are the result of better retrieval of bizarre than of common items. Specifically, the differential-retrieval-process view states that the bizarre-recall advantage emerges as a result of the distinctiveness of bizarre items relative to other items (e.g., common items) at retrieval. Thus, according to this account, the distinctiveness of bizarre items is used as the dominant retrieval cue at recall (cf. Nicolas & Marchal, 1998). This explanation of the facilitative effects of bizarreness is supported by two experiments (McDaniel et al., 2000, Experiments 3 and 4), which demonstrated an elimination of the bizarre-recall advantage in mixed lists when the use of retrieval cues other than distinctiveness was encouraged at recall. However, other research (Worthen et al., in press) using similar retrieval manipulations have failed to provide strong support for a pure-retrieval explanation.

The differential-retrieval-process account provides a simple explanation of the facilitative effects of bizarreness and at least some acknowledgment of a disruptive influence of bizarreness at encoding. However, as originally offered, the differential-retrieval-process account does not address the more salient disruptive effects of bizarreness, such as increased memory distortion and response bias. Also, any pure-retrieval account must somehow reconcile findings of a bizarreness advantage in tests of recognition memory. Given that tests of recognition are thought to be less dependent on retrieval than is free recall (Hanley & Morris, 1987; Hogan & Kintsch, 1971), it is unlikely that a pure-retrieval explanation will account for the entire pattern of results related to bizarreness and memory.

Resolution of Discrepant Memory Strengths

As mentioned earlier, a comprehensive account of the effects of bizarreness on memory must explain both the facilitative and the disruptive effects of bizarreness across a variety of empirical domains. Although the task of accounting for the facilitative and disruptive effects of bizarreness may seem daunting, it can be done with reference to item-specific and relational forms of processing (see Hunt, Chapter 1 this volume). *Item-specific processing* refers to the encoding of features unique to a particular stimulus item. *Relational processing* typically refers to the encoding of similarities between stimulus items. However, consonant with Hunt's (Chapter 1 this volume) discussion of event-based and item-based processing, relational processing can be further broken down in terms of similarities among components within a stimulus event (intra-item relations) and similarities between stimulus events (inter-item relations). The present account of the effects of bizarreness on memory is based on the notion that bizarreness induces an exaggerated form of item-specific processing that compromises intra-item relational processing. According to this account, the exaggerated form of item-specific processing induced by bizarreness leads to better memory for the phenomenological experience of bizarreness than for details of the bizarre event. To resolve the discrepancy between the strong memory for the experience of bizarreness and the relatively weaker memory for the details of the bizarre event, processors adopt a more liberal decision-making strategy with regard to bizarre than common memories at retrieval.

The resolution of discrepant memory strengths (RODMS) account of the effects of bizarreness has several advantages. First, this explanation accounts for both the facilitative and the disruptive effects of bizarreness. The tendency to find a bizarreness advantage in lenient measures (e.g., access), but not strict measures (e.g., items per sentence), of recall can be explained by poor binding of the elements of bizarre stimuli as a result of compromised intra-item relational processing. In essence, the exaggerated form of item-specific processing induced by bizarreness leads to the storage of only fragments of bizarre stimuli. However, those bizarre memory fragments are remembered better than common memories owing to a liberal response bias in favor of bizarre items. Thus, in keeping with the conclusions of Riefer & LaMay (1998) and Riefer & Rouder (1992), the RODMS account suggests that the details of bizarre stimuli are encoded poorly, but the resulting bizarre representation is easily and readily retrieved (or accepted in the case of recognition).

The RODMS account also explains why bizarreness leads to facilitative and disruptive effects for some stimulus domains, but only disruptive effects for others. Specifically, this account hypothesizes that bizarreness will be most disruptive for stimuli that typically induce item-specific processing even without bizarreness (e.g., pictures, performed acts). On the other hand, stimuli that do not naturally induce a high degree of item-specific processing (e.g., simple verbal materials) are more likely to incur the benefits of bizarreness. The pattern of previous results indicating consistent facilitative effects of bizarreness with verbal stimuli, but not with performed acts or hand-drawn pictures, is consistent with these hypotheses.

The findings from previous research investigating cued recall can also be explained by the RODMS account. As noted earlier, previous research has consistently failed to demonstrate a facilitative effect of bizarreness in cued recall when recall is cued with parts of target stimuli. However, if associates of target stimuli are used as cues, the bizarreness advantage is obtained. This pattern of results is consistent with the notion that intra-item relational processing is compromised by bizarreness. Specifically, a test that uses parts of target stimuli as cues is more dependent on intra-item relations than is a test that uses associates as cues. As such, cued recall for items whose intra-item relations are not encoded well would be at a disadvantage when parts of target stimuli are used as cues. However, weak intra-item relations would not be exploited by associate cues. Moreover, previous research demonstrating a reversal of the bizarreness advantage (a commonness advantage) when parts of target stimuli are used as cues (e.g., McDaniel & Einstein, 1986; McDaniel et al., 2000) provides additional support for the RODMS account.

Unlike recent explanations of the bizarreness advantage, the RODMS account suggests that the facilitative effects of bizarreness are the result of both encoding and retrieval factors. Put simply, it is suggested that the bizarreness advantage is the result of differential encoding for bizarre items and, subsequently, a more liberal decision-making criterion for those items at retrieval. However, the differential encoding described here is different from that described in the previous literature. Previous accounts of differential encoding (e.g., Wollen & Margres, 1987; Worthen et al., 2000) refer to a greater amount of encoding of bizarre stimuli. In contrast, the present formulation of differential encoding refers to a different type of encoding induced by bizarre stimuli. Thus, although the RODMS account suggests that encoding plays a significant role in determining the bizarreness advantage, it is unfazed by research indicating no relationship between the amount of elaboration and the bizarreness advantage.

CONCLUSIONS

Research across a variety of empirical domains suggests that bizarreness can enhance memory under certain conditions, but that bizarreness is also related to memory distortion and biased memory-based judgments. Although several explanations have been offered to account for the facilitative effects of bizarreness, few explanations have addressed both the facilitative and the disruptive effects of bizarreness. The explanation offered here (the RODMS account) suggests that bizarreness induces an exaggerated form of item-specific processing at the expense of intra-item relational processing. The differential processing induced by bizarreness ultimately leads to a more liberal decision-making criterion for bizarre relative to common items during retrieval and/or recognition. Unlike its predecessors, the RODMS account explains both the facilitative and the disruptive effects of bizarreness. Moreover, RODMS accounts for the failure to obtain a bizarreness advantage using some stimulus materials, but not others, and explains why the bizarreness advantage is typically not found using traditional cued-recall procedures.

ACKNOWLEDGMENTS

Portions of this paper were presented at the 49th Annual Meeting of the Southwestern Psychological Association, New Orleans, LA. Thanks are extended to Dan Burns, Susan Coats, Matt Rossano, and Reed Hunt who provided comments helpful in the preparation and/or revision of this chapter. This chapter is dedicated to the memory of Jason C. Reck.

NOTES

1. Those interested in early bizarreness research are referred to excellent reviews by Einstein and McDaniel (1987) and Wollen and Margres (1987).
2. See McDaniel and Einstein (1986) for a popular procedure used to induce bizarre and common elaboration of target stimuli.
3. The bizarre imagery effect can be obtained when imagery type is manipulated between groups if common intervening material is introduced as a distractor prior to recall (see Einstein, McDaniel, & Lackey, 1989).
4. In this case, verbally complex refers to simple sentences with heavily modified nouns. For example, a bizarre complex sentence used by Kroll et al. (1986) was "The large reddish *cockroach*, waving its feelers, carries off the dirty *stove*."

REFERENCES

Anderson, D. C., & Buyer, L. S. (1994). Is imagery a functional component of the "bizarre imagery" phenomenon? *American Journal of Psychology, 107,* 207–222.

Baddeley, A. D., & Andrade, J. (2000). Working memory and the vividness of imagery. *Journal of Experimental Psychology: General, 129,* 126–145.

Berlyne, D. E. (1960). *Conflict, arousal, and curiosity.* New York: McGraw-Hill.

Burns, D. J. (1996). The bizarre imagery effect and intention to learn. *Psychonomic Bulletin & Review, 3,* 254–257.

Cipolli, C., Bolzani, R., Cornoldi, C., De Beni, R., & Fagioli, I. (1993). Bizarreness effect in dream recall. *Sleep, 16,* 163–170.

Cornoldi, C., Cavedon, A., De Beni, R., & Pra Baldi, A., (1988). The influence of the nature of material and of mental operations on the occurrence of the bizarreness effect. *Quarterly Journal of Experimental Psychology, 40,* 73–85.

Cox, S. D., & Wollen, K. A. (1981). Bizarreness and recall. *Bulletin of the Psychonomic Society, 18,* 244–245.

Davidson, D., Larson, S. L., Luo, Z., & Burden, M. J. (2000). Interruption and bizarreness effects in the recall of script-based text. *Memory, 8,* 217–234.

Davidson, D., Malmstrom, T., Burden, M. J., & Luo, Z. (2000). Younger and older adults' recall of typical and atypical actions from script-based text: Evidence for interruption and bizarre-imagery effects. *Experimental Aging Research, 26,* 409–430.

DeLosh, E. L., & McDaniel, M.A. (1996). The role of order information in free recall: Application to the word-frequency effect. *Journal of Experimental Psychology: Learning, Memory, and Cognition, 22,* 1136–1146.

Detterman, D. K. (1975). The von Restorff effect and induced amnesia: Production by manipulation of sound intensity. *Journal of Experimental Psychology: Human, Learning, and Memory, 1,* 614–628.

Detterman, D. K., & Ellis, N. R., (1972). Determinants of induced amnesia in short-term memory. *Journal of Experimental Psychology, 95,* 308–316.

Einstein, G. O., & McDaniel, M. A. (1987). Distinctiveness and the mnemonic benefits of bizarre imagery. In M.A. McDaniel & M. Pressley (Eds.), *Imagery and related mnemonic processes: Theories, individual differences and applications* (pp.78–102). New York: Springer-Verlag.

Einstein, G. O., McDaniel, M. A., & Lackey, S. (1989). Bizarre imagery, interference, and distinctiveness. *Journal of Experimental Psychology: Learning, Memory, and Cognition, 15,* 137–146.

Ellis, N. R., Detterman, D. K., Runcie, D., McCarver, R. B., & Craig, E. M. (1971). Amnesic effects in short-term memory. *Journal of Experimental Psychology, 89,* 357–361.

Emmerich, H. J., & Ackerman, B. P. (1979). A test of bizarre interaction as a factor in children's memory. *Journal of Genetic Psychology, 134,* 225–232.

Engelkamp, J., Zimmer, H. D., & Biegelmann, U. E. (1993). Bizarreness effects in verbal tasks and subject-performed tasks. *European Journal of Cognitive Psychology, 5,* 393–415.

Engelkamp, J., Zimmer, H. D., Mohr, G., & Sellen, O. (1994). Memory of self-performed tasks: Self-performing during recognition. *Memory & Cognition, 22,* 34–39.

Hanley, J., & Morris, P. (1987). The effects of amount of processing on recall and recognition. *Quarterly Journal of Experimental Psychology: Human Experimental Psychology, 39,* 431–439.

Heil, M., Rolke, B., Engelkamp, J., Rosler, F., Ozcan, M., & Hennighausen, E. (1999). Event-related brain potentials during recognition of ordinary and bizarre action phrases following verbal and subject-performed encoding conditions. *European Journal of Cognitive Psychology, 11,* 261–280.

Henshel, R. L. (1980). The purposes of laboratory experimentation and the virtues of deliberate artificiality. *Journal of Experimental Social Psychology, 16,* 466–478.

Hirshman, E., Whelley, M. M., & Palij, M. (1989). An investigation of paradoxical memory effects. *Journal of Memory and Language, 28,* 594–609.

Hogan, R. M., & Kintsch, W. (1971). Differential effects of study and test trials on long-term recognition and recall. *Journal of Verbal Learning and Verbal Behavior, 10,* 562–567.

Iaccino, J. F. (1996). A further examination of the bizarre imagery mnemonic: Its effectiveness with mixed context and delayed testing. *Perceptual and Motor Skills, 83,* 881–882.

Iaccino, J. F., Dvorak, E., & Coler, M. (1989). Effects of bizarre imagery on the long-term retention of paired associates embedded within variable contexts. *Bulletin of the Psychonomic Society, 27,* 114–116.

Iaccino, J. F., & Sowa, S. J. (1989). Bizarre imagery in paired-associate learning: An effective mnemonic aid with mixed context, delayed testing, and self-paced conditions. *Perceptual and Motor Skills, 68,* 307–316.

Iaccino, J. F., & Spirek, P. (1988). Long-term retention of plausible vs. Bizarre paired associates as a function of cued recall. *Perceptual and Motor Skills, 67,* 531–537.

Imai, S., & Richman, C. L. (1991). Is the bizarreness effect a special case of sentence reorganization? *Bulletin of the Psychonomic Society, 29,* 429–432.

Ironsmith, M., & Lutz, J. (1996). The effects of bizarreness and self-generation on mnemonic imagery. *Journal of Mental Imagery, 20,* 113–126.

Kline, S., & Groninger, L. D. (1991). The imagery bizarreness effect as a function of sentence complexity and presentation time. *Bulletin of the Psychonomic Society, 29,* 25–27.

Knopf, M. (1991). Having shaved a kiwi fruit: Memory for unfamiliar subject-performed actions. *Psychological Research/Psychologische Forschung, 50,* 203–211.

Kroll, N. E. A., Jaeger, G., & Dornfest, R. (1992). Metamemory for the bizarre. *Journal of Mental Imagery, 16,* 173–190.

Kroll, N. E. A., Schepeler, E. M., & Angin, K. T. (1986). Bizarre imagery: The misremembered mnemonic. *Journal of Experimental Psychology: Learning, Memory, and Cognition, 12,* 42–53.

Kroll, N. E. A., & Tu, S. F. (1988). The bizarre mnemonic. *Psychological Research/Psychologische Forschung, 50,* 28–37.

Lang, V.A. (1995). Relative association, interactiveness, and the bizarre imagery effect. *American Journal of Psychology, 108,* 13–35.

Lorayne, H. (1972). *Good memory—good student: A guide to remembering what you learn.* Nashville, TN: Nelson.

Lorayne, H., & Lucas, J. (1974). *The memory book.* New York: Ballantine.

Marchal, A., & Nicolas, S. (2000). Is the picture bizarreness effect a generation effect? *Psychological Reports, 87,* 331–340.

Marshall, P. H., Nau, K., & Chandler, C. K. (1979). A structural analysis of common and bizarre visual mediators. *Bulletin of the Psychonomic Society, 14,* 103–105.

Marshall, P. H., Nau, K., & Chandler, C. K. (1980). A functional analysis of common and bizarre visual mediators. *Bulletin of the Psychonomic Society, 15,* 375–377.

McDaniel, M. A., DeLosh, E. L., & Merritt, P. S. (2000). Order information and retrieval distinctiveness: Recall of common versus bizarre material. *Journal of Experimental Psychology: Learning, Memory, and Cognition, 26,* 1045–1056.

McDaniel, M. A., & Einstein, G. O. (1986). Bizarreness as an effective memory aid: The importance of distinctiveness. *Journal of Experimental Psychology: Learning, Memory, and Cognition, 12,* 54–65.

McDaniel, M. A., & Einstein, G. O. (1989). Sentence complexity eliminates the mnemonic advantage of bizarre imagery. *Bulletin of the Psychonomic Society, 27,* 117–120.

McDaniel, M. A., Einstein, G. O., DeLosh, E. L., May, C. P., & Brady, P. (1995). The bizarreness effect: It's not surprising, it's complex. *Journal of Experimental Psychology: Learning, Memory, and Cognition, 21,* 422–435.

Merry, R., & Graham, N. C. (1978). Image bizarreness in children's recall of sentences. *British Journal of Psychology, 69,* 315–321.

Michelon, P., Snyder, A. Z., Buckner, R. L., MacAvoy, M., & Zacks, J. M. (2003). Neural correlates of incongruity: An fMRI study. *NeuroImage, 19,* 1612–1626.

Mohr, G., Engelkamp, J., & Zimmer, H. D. (1989). Recall and recognition of self-performed acts. *Psychological Research/Psychologische Forschung, 51,* 181–187.

Mook, D. G. (1982). In defense of external invalidity. *American Psychologist, 38,* 379–387.

Nicolas, S., & Marchal, A. (1996). Picture bizarreness effect and word association. *Cahiers de Psychologie Cognitive, 15,* 629–643.

Nicolas, S., & Marchal, A. (1998). Implicit memory, explicit memory and the picture bizarreness effect. *Acta Psychologica, 99,* 43–58.

O'Brien, E. J., & Wolford, C. R. (1982). Effect of delay in testing on retention of plausible versus bizarre mental images. *Journal of Experimental Psychology: Learning, Memory, and Cognition, 8,* 148–152.

Richman, C. L. (1994). The bizarreness effect with complex sentences: Temporal effects. *Canadian Journal of Experimental Psychology, 48,* 444–450.

Richman, C. L., Dunn, J., Kahl, G., Sadler, L., & Simmons, K. (1990). The bizarre sentence effect as a function of list length and complexity. *Bulletin of the Psychonomic Society, 28,* 185–187.

Riefer, D. M., & LaMay, M. L. (1998). Memory for common and bizarre stimuli: A storage and retrieval analysis. *Psychonomic Bulletin & Review, 5,* 312–317.

Riefer, D. M., & Rouder, J. N. (1992). A multinomial modeling analysis of the mnemonic benefits of bizarre imagery. *Memory & Cognition, 20,* 601–611.

Roark, B., & Worthen, J. B. (1999, April). Toward an associative storage and retrieval model of bizarreness effects in memory. In J. B. Worthen (Chair),

Memory for unusual events. Symposium conducted at the 45th Annual Meeting of the Southwestern Psychological Association, Albuquerque, NM.

Robinson-Riegler, B., & McDaniel, M. A. (1994). Further constraints on the bizarreness effect: Elaboration at encoding. *Memory & Cognition, 22,* 702–712.

Roth, D. M. (1961). *Roth memory course*. Hackensack, NJ: Wehman.

Schmidt, S. R. (1991). Can we have a distinctive theory of memory? *Memory & Cognition, 19,* 523–542.

Schmidt, S. R. (2002). Outstanding memories: The positive and negative effects of nudes on memory. *Journal of Experimental Psychology: Learning, Memory, & Cognition, 28,* 353–361.

Schmidt, S. R., & Williams, A. R. (2001). Memory for humorous cartoons. *Memory & Cognition, 29,* 305–311.

Serra, M., & Nairne, J. S. (1993). Design controversies and the generation effect: Support for an item-order hypothesis. *Memory & Cognition, 21,* 34–40.

Sharpe, L., & Markham, R. (1992). The effect of the distinctiveness of bizarre imagery on immediate and delayed recall. *Journal of Mental Imagery, 16,* 211–220.

Tess, D. E., Hutchinson, R. L., Treloar, J. H., & Jenkins, C. M. (1999). Bizarre imagery and distinctiveness: Implications for the classroom. *Journal of Mental Imagery, 23,* 153–170.

Thomas, A. K., & Loftus, E. F. (2002). Creating bizarre false memories through imagination. *Memory & Cognition, 30,* 423–431.

Toglia, M. P., & Kimble, G. A. (1976). Recall and use of serial position information. *Journal of Experimental Psychology: Human Learning and Memory, 2,* 431–445.

Tulving, E., & Pearlstone, Z. (1966). Availability versus accessibility of information in memory for words. *Journal of Verbal Learning and Verbal Behavior, 5,* 381–391.

Webber, S. M., & Marshall, P. H. (1978). Bizarreness effects in imagery as a function of processing level and delay. *Journal of Mental Imagery, 2,* 291–300.

Weir, D., & Richman, C. L. (1996). Subject-generated bizarreness: Imagery or semantic processing. *American Journal of Psychology, 109,* 173–185.

Wiggs, C. L. (1993). Aging and memory for frequency of occurrence of novel, visual stimuli: direct and indirect measures. *Psychology and Aging, 8,* 400–410.

Williams, K. W., & Durso, F. T. (1986). Judging category frequency: Automaticity or availability. *Journal of Experimental Psychology: Learning, Memory, and Cognition, 12,* 387–396.

Wollen, K. A., & Cox, S. (1981). Sentence cuing and the effectiveness of bizarre imagery. *Journal of Experimental Psychology: Human Learning and Memory, 7,* 386–392.

Wollen, K. A., & Margres, M. G. (1987). Bizarreness and the imagery multiprocess model. In M. A. McDaniel & M. Pressley (Eds.), *Imagery and related mnemonic processes: Theories, individual differences and applications* (pp.103–127). New York: Springer-Verlag.

Worthen, J. B. (1997). Resiliency of bizarreness effects under varying conditions of verbal and imaginal elaboration and list composition. *Journal of Mental Imagery, 21,* 167–194.

Worthen, J. B., Eisenstein, S. A., Budwey, S. C., & Varnado-Sullivan, P. (2005). Tests of structural hypotheses in free recall for bizarre and dream reports: Implications for sleep research. *Imagination, Cognition, and Personality, 24,* 315–330.

Worthen, J. B., & Eller, L. S. (2002). Test of competing of competing explanations of the bizarre response bias in recognition memory. *Journal of General Psychology, 129,* 36–48.

Worthen, J. B., Garcia-Rivas, G., Green, C. R., & Vidos, R. A. (2000). Tests of a cognitive-resource-allocation account of the bizarreness effect. *Journal of General Psychology, 127,* 117–144.

Worthen, J. B., Hutchens, S. A., Nicodemus, P. D., & Baker, J. D. (2002). Memory for frequency of bizarre and common stimuli: Limitations of the automaticity hypothesis. *Journal of General Psychology, 129,* 212–225.

Worthen, J. B., & Loveland, J. M. (2003). Disruptive effects of bizarreness in free and cued recall for self-performed and other-performed acts: The costs of item-specific processing. In F. Columbus (Ed.), *Advances in psychology research, 24* (pp. 3–17). Hauppage, NY: Nova Science Publishers.

Worthen, J. B., & Marshall, P. H. (1996). Intralist and extralist distinctiveness and the bizarreness effect: The importance of contrast. *American Journal of Psychology, 109,* 239–263.

Worthen, J. B., Marshall, P. H., & Cox, K. B. (1998). List length and the bizarreness effect: Support for a hybrid model. *Psychological Research/ Psychologische Forschung, 61,* 147–156.

Worthen, J. B., & Roark, B. (2002). Free recall accuracy for common and bizarre verbal information. *American Journal of Psychology, 115,* 377–394.

Worthen, J. B., Starns, J. J., Loveland, J. M., & Eisenstein, S. A. (in press). Influence of orienting task on memory for bizarre and common stimuli: Evidence against a surprise-based explanation. In S. P. Shohov (Ed.), *Advances in cognitive psychology.* Hauppage, NY: Nova Science Publishers.

Worthen, J. B., & Wood, V. V. (2001a). Memory discrimination for self-performed and imagined acts: Bizarreness effects in false recognition. *Quarterly Journal of Experimental Psychology: Human Experimental Psychology, 53A,* 49–67.

Worthen, J. B., & Wood, V. V. (2001b). A disruptive effect of bizarreness on memory for relational and contextual details of self-performed and other-performed acts. *American Journal of Psychology, 114,* 535–546.

Yarmey, A. D. (1984). Bizarreness effects in mental imagery. In A. A. Sheikh (Ed.), *International Review of Mental Imagery, 1* (57–76). New York: Human Sciences Press.

Yates, F. A. (1966). *The art of memory.* London: Routledge & Kegan Paul.

Zoller, C. L., Workman, J. S., & Kroll, N. E. A. (1989). The bizarre mnemonic: The effect of retention interval and mode of presentation. *Bulletin of the Psychonomic Society, 27,* 215–218.

8

Memory for Bizarre and Other Unusual Events: Evidence from Script Research

Denise Davidson

Numerous studies have examined the extent to which adults remember both common and less common, or unusual, events. Often these studies have presented uncommon events that are "bizarre," by presenting bizarre sentences within a list format (e.g., Einstein & McDaniel, 1987; McDaniel & Einstein, 1986; McDaniel, Einstein, DeLosh, May & Brady, 1995; Worthen & Wood, 2001a; 2001b). Although research on the mnemonic effectiveness of bizarreness has produced disparate results, generally, bizarre sentences such as "The dog rode a bicycle down the street" are better recalled than more common sentences, particularly when both are presented within a mixed-list format. Although it is believed that the mnemonic advantage of bizarreness occurs in lists containing both bizarre and common sentences, recent research has provided more detailed information about the roles list composition and stimulus context play in the bizarreness effect (see Worthen, Chapter 7 this volume). In my research, bizarreness effects have been examined within the context of script-based stories, although the motivation for my studies was not to examine bizarreness effects per se, but individuals' memory for a range of unusual events. In addition, my work has included individuals across the life span, for reasons that will be discussed shortly. The purpose of the present chapter is to review this work, examining children's, younger adults', and older adults' memory for unusual events, including bizarre events. In this chapter, the empirical findings of my research are presented first, and then possible explanations of these findings are discussed in terms of text-processing research.

Overview of Chapter

Initially, the goal of my research was to examine individuals' memory for typical and atypical actions from story texts. These stories consisted of scripted events, such as dining at a restaurant or getting up in the morning. Typical actions were scripted actions, or actions that typically occurred for the event, such as ordering food at a restaurant. Atypical actions were actions that did not typically occur, such as the waiter's bringing the wrong food order. In our initial studies, these atypical actions either interrupted the script or were irrelevant to the script, although both could plausibly occur in the story. Later, however, the plausibility of these actions was varied, so that memory for implausible, or bizarre, script-interruptive and script-irrelevant actions was examined. Thus, we were able to examine the effects of bizarreness within story texts. Although our findings were not always compatible with the findings of list research, in most cases they were. Both compatible and incompatible findings are presented in this chapter, in addition to some thoughts about the role of encoding and other factors underlying bizarreness effects. This chapter begins with a review of our work with children, and then presents our findings with college-age adults and older adults.

Research with Children

The first studies we conducted examined children's memory for typical and atypical, or unusual, actions from stories. Script-based stories were written that consisted of events that were thought to have a prototypical sequence of actions that usually took place. For example, a story was created about going to a grocery store, with typical or scripted actions including "going up and down the aisle with a shopping cart" or "putting food in the shopping cart." Less typical actions were also included in these stories, such as "A boy was looking at the vegetables," or, in its "bizarre" form, "A zebra was looking at the vegetables." The main goal of these early studies was to examine how well children remembered typical or script actions from stories. At the time of these initial studies, little was known about how children, particularly young children, remember the prototypical sequences of events that often take place in real life. Even less was known about the extent to which script knowledge might influence children's memory for these events. As described in more detail below, in the course of studying these aspects of development, it became clear that children not only remembered typical or scripted events, but they also had a propensity for remembering unusual, or atypical, events. Eventually, this finding led to my work with adults, both college students and the elderly, who too showed a memory advantage for atypical events.

At the time we began this work with children, a handful of studies had examined adults' memory for typical and atypical actions in script-based text (e.g., Bower, Black & Turner, 1979; Graesser, Woll, Kowalski, & Smith, 1980; Smith & Graesser, 1981). Subsequently, these studies provided the framework for studying children's memory for typical and atypical events. Specifically, most of these early studies with adults found that scripted actions were better recalled than atypical actions as the retention interval increased (e.g., Bower et al., 1979; Graesser et al., 1980; Smith & Graesser, 1981). This finding was not surprising, as it was compatible with the predictions of various schema models that existed at the time.

Although specific predictions from these models are dependent upon the length of retention interval and type of retrieval task, in general, it is believed that on recognition tasks, individuals' memory for scripted actions appearing in the stories would be confused with scripted actions not appearing in the story. Recognition data from adult studies supported this assumption, as the false-alarm rates for script actions not present in the stories was often quite high (e.g., Graesser, Gordon & Sawyer, 1979; Davidson, 1994; Maki, 1990; Smith & Graesser, 1981). For recall, atypical actions were usually better recalled at short delays, but at approximately 48 hours after testing, and again at 1-week and 3-week intervals, recall memory was better for typical actions [e.g., Smith & Graesser, 1981]. According to Smith and Graesser (1981), this pattern of findings was consistent with the assumption that, "as the retention interval increases, the tagged atypical actions in the (memory) trace become less accessible because retrieval becomes more dependent upon the generic schema (p. 557)." However, at the time these adult studies were conducted, little was known about the extent to which children would recognize or recall typical and atypical actions from text.

Children's Recall of Typical (Script) and Atypical (Script-Irrelevant, Script-Interruptive) Text

Analogous to the early adult studies of Bower et al. (1979) and Graesser and his colleagues (e.g., Graesser et al., 1979, 1980; Smith & Graesser, 1981), in the first set of studies we presented to children stories that contained scripted and nonscripted actions. As described above, the scripted actions included actions that typically occurred for scripted events, such as shopping at a grocery store. Similar to adult studies, atypical actions were also included in these stories. In the first of these studies, atypical actions included script-irrelevant and script-interruptive actions. Script-irrelevant actions were those actions that could plausibly occur for a particular scripted event, such as putting dog treats in a shopping cart, but did not always occur for the event. Script-interruptive actions were those actions that disrupted the script in some way, such as not being able to go down an aisle because people were blocking it with their shopping carts. Although script-interruptive actions could plausibly occur for the event, they were not seen as scripted actions because they did not always occur.

Presenting these actions to children through script-based stories revealed that script-interruptive actions were better recalled than both script and script-irrelevant actions at an immediate *and* a 24-hour delay (e.g., Davidson & Jergovic, 1996; Hudson, 1988). A recall advantage for script-interruptive atypical actions at a 24-hour delay was a bit surprising, given the predictions of schema models. Of interest was why interruptive actions were better recalled by children at both delays.

It was possible that script-interruptive actions were better recalled at both delays because these actions were perceived as more important, and subsequently stored more efficiently, than other actions. For example, it was argued that script interruptions were more causally connected to antecedent and subsequent actions than script-irrelevant actions because the interruptions caused situations or problems that had to be remedied in order for the events of the story to proceed (Davidson & Jergovic, 1996). In fact, it was often these interruptions or problems that provided a point to the story, or at the very least, made the story more interesting (Davidson & Jergovic, 1996). Additionally, this assumption was consistent with text-processing research that suggested that any type of coherence break in text may lead the reader to think about the information more and, subsequently, better recall it (Graesser, Singer, & Trabasso, 1994).

Unfortunately, however, a limitation existed in these studies. As with the early adult studies, the script-irrelevant actions used in the stories were relatively pallid and mundane. Of interest in a second set of studies was how well children would recall script-irrelevant actions that were more "vivid" (Davidson & Jergovic, 1996). This was examined by presenting children with stories that consisted of script actions (e.g., "At the theatre, they gave their tickets to the usher") and script-irrelevant actions that were written in either a pallid form (e.g., "At the theatre, Sam noticed that the carpet was red") or a more vivid form (e.g., "At the theatre, Sam noticed that the carpet was red and incredibly dirty and stained").

As shown, vividness was manipulated by the increased use of modifiers in each sentence. This was somewhat different from Bower et al.'s (1979,) conception of vividness, who stated that vivid irrelevant actions were those actions that would have, if experienced, a "vivid impact" (p. 210) on the reader (e.g., "The waitress was stark naked"). However, children were not asked to imagine story actions, nor was a test conducted to determine if children could visualize vivid actions better than their pallid counterparts. Such a test would be difficult to administer to children, particularly because they may not understand what it means to "imagine" a sentence and its actions. However, a sample of college students rated the vivid forms as having "more of an impact" on them and easier to visualize. Specifically, this group rated the vividness of a sentence by selecting a number from 1 ("not very clear image") to 5 ("very clear image"), similar to that used by Einstein, McDaniel, & Lackey (1989). The results of increasing the vividness of the script-irrelevant actions on children's memory are shown in Figure 8.1.

As shown, children did indeed recall vivid script-irrelevant actions better than their pallid counterparts. Interestingly, children also remembered these vivid, atypical actions better than scripted actions at both an immediate and a 24-hour delay. However, a causal-connection hypothesis used to explain a recall advantage for script-interruptive actions could not justify these findings because the script-irrelevant actions were not well connected to other story items. Thus, it became clear that script-irrelevant ac-

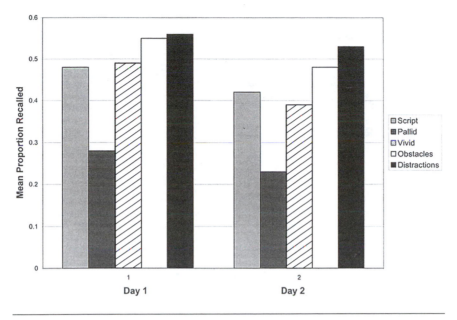

FIGURE 8.1 Children's mean proportion of script, script-irrelevant (pallid and vivid), script-interruptive actions recalled, collapsed over age groups.

tions were well recalled for other reasons, including the possibility that the vividness of the action increased the distinctiveness of the action in some way and subsequently, memory for the action.

On a general level, in script-based stories, script actions form a homogenous background whereby atypical actions may stand out from the script actions, particularly if they are vivid. At the very least, it has been suggested that vivid irrelevant actions should lead to a von Restorff, or isolation, effect (Bower et al., 1979). The von Restorff effect refers to the phenomenon whereby isolating an item against a homogenous background facilitates the learning and retention of the isolated item (see Hunt, 1995; Wallace, 1965; for discussions). According to Schmidt (1991), the distinctiveness hypothesis is a direct descendent of the von Restorff effect, which was studied extensively in the 1950s and 1960s and was discussed in detail by Wallace (1965). In fact, primary distinctiveness includes all three types of the von Restorff phenomenon in Wallace's (1965) classification and discussion of the effect.

However, it should be noted that the issue may not be why some items are better remembered, but why some items are not so well remembered. According to Hunt and Lamb (2001), memory in the isolation paradigm reflects poor memory for the nonisolated items, the reasons for which are explored in their work on the isolation effect (see also Hunt, 1995; Hunt, Chapter 1 this volume; Hunt & McDaniel, 1993). Although controversy exists as to how to frame the issue—should one consider why certain items are better remembered or why other items are not so well remembered?—it is clear that children remembered some items, or actions, from the stories better than others. Of interest, however, was whether atypical actions could be varied in other ways so as to make them more memorable. Answers to this question would shed light on processes underlying the memory advantage for atypical items.

Children's Recall of Bizarre (Script-Irrelevant) Text

At the time we were conducting this work with children, considerable research was available on bizarreness effects in adult memory (e.g., Cox & Wollen, 1981; Einstein & McDaniel, 1987; McDaniel & Einstein, 1986; McDaniel et al., 1995). A common finding was the bizarre-imagery effect. The *bizarre-imagery effect* refers to the finding that bizarre sentences are generally better recalled than more plausible, common sentences, at least when both are presented using a list format (e.g., Einstein & McDaniel, 1987; McDaniel & Einstein, 1986). In fact, later studies have revealed that the reader does not even have to imagine the sentences to receive the memory advantage (e.g., Weir & Richman, 1996; Worthen, 1997), leading to its dubbing as the "bizarreness effect." Of interest was whether bizarreness effects would also be found with children. An easy way to determine this was to present bizarre items in stories for children to recall.

Specifically, it was possible to alter the script-irrelevant actions so that some of them were bizarre. This was done in several of our studies (e.g., Davidson & Hoe, 1993) by altering the plausibility of the script-irrelevant action presented in the stories. Three types of script-irrelevant actions were presented in the stories read to children: plausible script-irrelevant actions (e.g., "At the theatre, a girl was eating a piece of pizza"); plausible within the sentence, but not within the context of the story actions (e.g., "At the theatre, a cat was eating cat food"); and implausible, script-irrelevant actions that were bizarre (e.g., "At the theatre, a cat was eating a pickle"), which were implausible both within the context of the story and the context of the sentence. It should be noted that these implausible sentences resulted in bizarre sentences, or bizarre happenings, to the extent that the subject, object, or context of the action in the sentence resulted in actions that were implausible or unusual. Importantly, the implausible, bizarre sentences used in our stories were similar to bizarre sentences used to examine the bizarre-imagery effect with adults. In fact, the bizarre sentences in the stories were often made bizarre by giving human or living features to nonhuman animals or objects. This is in line with Worthen and Marshall (1996), who found stronger bizarreness effects for bizarre stimuli that contained predominately anthropomorphic scenes provided the bizarre stimuli were presented with predominately common or 50/50 mixed lists.

The results of presenting bizarre actions in the stories are shown in Figure 8.2. As shown, a recall advantage was found for bizarre (implausible) sentences, as children in an immediate and delayed (24 hours) recall con-

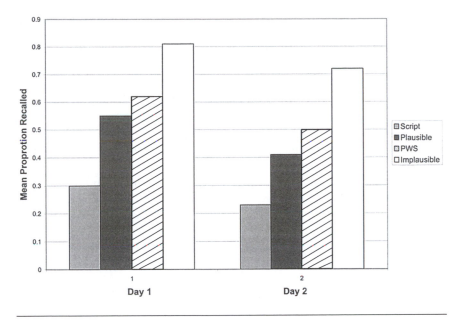

FIGURE 8.2 Children's mean proportion of script and script-irrelevant (plausible, plausible within sentence, implausible) actions recalled, collapsed over age groups.

dition recalled bizarre, implausible information better than the other sentences in the stories (Davidson & Hoe, 1993).

Adult research on bizarreness effects provided us with other interesting aspects of bizarreness to explore with children. For example, Worthen and his colleagues (e.g., Worthen & Wood, 2001a, 2001b) have found that bizarreness can disrupt memory for the general context in which the actions occurred, at least when using a list format (Worthen & Wood, 2001b). In addition, distortions in the recall of bizarre sentences can occur. However, in re-examining our data, no evidence was found that children remembered less information from stories that included bizarre sentences, nor were bizarre sentences more prone to distortions. However, because children's recall was generally poor in our studies, these effects may not have been obtained.

Additional limitations exist when working with children, particularly when trying to create stories that enable one to examine both bizarreness and interruption effects. For example, in separate studies (e.g., Davidson & Hoe, 1993; Davidson & Jergovic, 1996), interruption effects (i.e., better memory for script-interruptive actions by children in immediate and 24-hour recall conditions) and bizarreness effects (i.e., better memory for bizarre, script-irrelevant actions by children in immediate and 24-hour recall conditions) were found. However, given the limits of children's memory, we were not able to assess children's memory for bizarre, script-irrelevant actions and script-interruptive actions in the same study. The limits of children's memory also made it difficult to assess their free recall of stories beyond 24 hours. In fact, it may have been these limits that led to floor effects when testing children at longer delays.

A more basic problem involved the development of children's script knowledge. Although children were more likely to remember atypical actions than script actions, it was possible that children's memory for atypical actions was better than their memory for scripted actions because children's knowledge of scripts was not well developed. This may have been particularly true for our particular sample of children who were young—between kindergarten and third grade.

The question became, How well developed is young children's script knowledge? Past research provided an answer, as studies showed children as young as 4 or 5 years of age have at least some rudimentary knowledge of scripts or scripted events. Furthermore, this knowledge appeared to develop quickly in childhood (e.g., Fivush, 1984; Nelson, 1986). In our studies, older children were found to have more well-developed script knowledge than younger children, although this did not lead to better memory for scripted actions than atypical actions by older children (Davidson & Hoe, 1993; Davidson & Jergovic, 1996). Thus, children's limited memory for scripted actions does not appear to have been due to their limited knowledge of scripted events. Of course, one way around these problems was to examine bizarreness and interruption effects with adults. An upcoming section of this chapter reports the results of these adult studies.

Although limitations existed in our research with children, and sometimes made it difficult to compare bizarreness effects found with children to those found with adults, explanations for bizarreness effects found with adults provided some clues as to why children remembered similar actions from stories. It has been suggested that bizarreness effects may be accounted for, in part, by a distinctiveness explanation (e.g., Einstein et al., 1989; McDaniel & Einstein, 1986). Distinctiveness can be defined in a relative manner, whereby the distinctiveness of a sentence is determined by its relation to other sentences. Implausible bizarre sentences are thought to orient attention and produce more distinct encodings in the context of other more plausible sentences, subsequently leading to their better recall. At the very least, bizarre actions may lead to a von Restorff, or isolation, effect (although see Hirshman, Whelley & Palij, 1989, or Hunt and Lamb, 2001, for additional views). In script-based stories, script actions may form a homogenous background whereby less common, bizarre actions may stand out from this background. Such isolation of bizarre items may lead to their enhanced recall.

This explanation is also compatible with the schema confirmation-deployment model of Farrar & Goodman (1992). According to Farrar and Goodman (1992), if a schema for an event exists and is functioning as a coherent mental unit, then actions consistent with the schema should be absorbed by the schema (schema confirmation). In contrast, actions that can be isolated from the script (e.g., bizarre, script-irrelevant actions) should not only be better attended but may also lead to separate memory (schema deployment) for the schema-discrepant information. This in turn should lead to better memory for the isolated item, an assumption consistent with Worthen, Garcia-Rivas, Green, & Vidos (2000), who demonstrated that even simple bizarre materials require more processing time than common materials. Additional research we conducted with college-age and elderly adults enabled us to further assess these assumptions.

RESEARCH WITH COLLEGE-AGE ADULTS

In our initial studies, college students were asked to read and recall several script-based stories, the first of which consisted of script actions, script-irrelevant actions, and script-interruptive actions. Similar to our research with children, three types of script-irrelevant actions were present in the stories: plausible script-irrelevant actions (or actions that could plausibly occur within the context of the sentence and story); plausible within the sentence, but not within the story actions (or actions that were plausible within the sentence context but not within the context of the story); and implausible script-irrelevant actions. These implausible actions resulted in bizarre actions very similar to those used to study bizarreness effects using a list format (e.g., Einstein & McDaniel, 1987; McDaniel & Einstein, 1986; Worthen & Wood, 2001a).

Three types of script-interruptive actions were also present in the stories: obstacles, errors, and distractions. Although the reader is referred to Schank and Abelson (1977) for a detailed discussion of these types of actions, they can be described as follows. Obstacles result when an enabling condition for an imminent action is missing or when the flow of actions is blocked in some way (e.g., "At the movies, tall people were blocking the view of the screen"). Errors are incorrect actions, or actions that lead to inappropriate outcomes (e.g., "At the movies, they got in the wrong line to buy tickets"). Distractions are usually mishaps or accidents (e.g., "At the movies he tripped and his popcorn spilled"). Consistent with previous research (Davidson, 1994), it was predicted that all three types of script-interruptive actions would be well recalled. The primary advantage to using these three types of interruptive actions was that it provided a means to thoroughly examine the interruptive effect (i.e., better memory for interruptive actions), particularly when bizarre actions were also in the stories. That is, it was not known whether interruptive actions would be better recalled than bizarre actions.

In addition to providing a means of studying bizarreness and interruption effects in the same study, our work with adults allowed examination of bizarreness effects beyond the list format commonly used in most studies with adults. Aspects of bizarreness effects could also be studied outside the list format, such as whether the presence of bizarre sentences in stories resulted in less recall of central information or memory distortions—effects that have been found when using list formats (e.g., Worthen & Wood, 2001a, 2001b). Other interference effects could be assessed. For example, Einstein and his colleagues have found that the bizarreness effect can be diminished when subjects are asked to imagine other bizarre sentences on an intervening task or when the number of bizarre sentences is increased (Einstein et al., 1989).

Perhaps more important, this initial study provided a means for assessing an expectation-violation explanation for bizarreness (and interruption) effects. Bizarre, script-irrelevant actions and script-interruptive actions may be well recalled from script-based stories because they may stand out from, or are distinct from, the scripted context. Thus, the question becomes, What is it about these atypical actions that lead them to be distinct and subsequently better remembered? As Hunt and Lamb (2001) and others note (e.g., Schmidt, 1991), although distinctiveness itself cannot be used as an explanation for the effects of distinctiveness, it does not preclude one from examining why distinctiveness may lead to better memory.

One possibility is that interruption and bizarreness effects are due to a violation of expectancy. That is, readers may not expect these actions, in part because they do not typically occur for the script-based event. Subsequently, this violation of expectancy may result in more distinct encodings, and better memory, of these actions. For example, Hirshman et al. (1989) suggest that bizarreness effects may be subsumed under the larger class of expectation-violation effects. Surprise responses to bizarre sentences increase the association of bizarre sentences to the general contextual cues, which in turn aid free recall (see also Green, 1956; Schmidt, 1991). Thus, it may be the unexpected nature of the bizarre action that leads to it being better recalled. This possibility was explored in several studies we conducted (Davidson, Malmstrom, Burden, & Luo, 2000).

In these studies, a sample of college students were asked to rate the typicality, or "scriptedness," of the script, the script-irrelevant and script-interruptive actions in our stories, and the expectancy of the actions. For the latter, college students were asked to rate how expected each action (sentence) was as they read each story. As shown in Figure 8.3, these students judged these actions along the same lines as we did in terms of scripted and nonscripted actions. They also judged these actions as varying in expectedness. As shown in figure 8.3, script and script-interruptive actions were rated more expected than the implausible script-irrelevant actions. This finding suggested that the less expected bizarre actions in the stories would be better recalled than the other actions, at least following an expectation-violation hypothesis.

In order to examine this possibility, an additional group of college students was asked to read and recall stories with these script, script-irrelevant (plausible; plausible within the sentence, but not within the story; and implausible), and script-interruptive actions (obstacles, errors, and distractions) in them. Subjects recalled these stories at one of three delays, either 1 hour after reading them, 48 hours after reading them or 168 hours

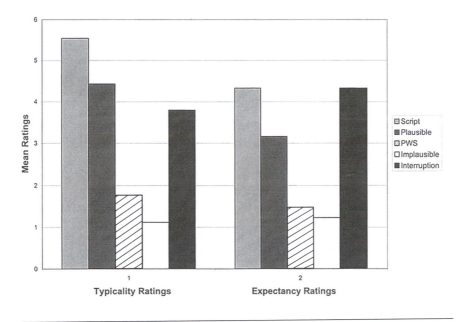

FIGURE 8.3 Mean typicality (6 = very typical) and expectancy ratings (5 = very expected) by adults.

(one week) after reading them (Davidson, Larson, Luo, & Burden, 2000). As shown in Figure 8.4, implausible (bizarre) script-irrelevant actions and script-interruptive actions were better recalled than the more plausible script-irrelevant actions and scripted actions, suggesting that both bizarreness and interruption effects were present. Importantly, this was true across all three delays. No significant differences were found in the recall of script-interruptive actions—errors, obstacles, and distractions—that were better recalled than all other actions at the immediate and 48-hour delays. At the 1-week delay, bizarre actions were better recalled than all other actions, including interruptive actions. Thus, both bizarreness and interruption effects were found in our work, consistent with our results with children.

Of interest, however, was why memory advantages for bizarre and interruptive actions were found. The data did not support the expectation-violation hypothesis to the extent that script-interruptive actions were rated more expected than bizarre actions but were generally better recalled (1-hour, 48-hour delays) or almost as well recalled (1 week). Thus, expectancy in and of itself could not explain these results. Additional studies were conducted to determine the factors that might lead to these effects. Unfortunately, one problem with the initial studies, and the interpretation of them, was that students' recall was poor, particularly at the 1-week delay. One reason for such poor memory may have been the number of items in each story. To overcome this limitation, a second study was conducted.

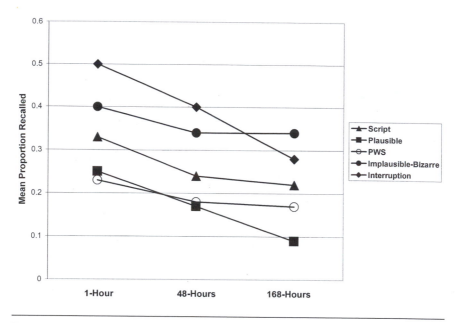

FIGURE 8.4 Mean recall proportions for script, script-irrelevant, and script-inter-ruptive actions by adults. From Davidson, Larson et al., 2000. (Copyright 2000 by Psychology Press. Reprinted with permission.)

This time the script-based stories consisted of only three types of actions: scripted actions, implausible (bizarre) script-irrelevant actions, and script-interruptive actions. The more plausible, script-irrelevant actions were re-moved from the stories. The results of this study are shown in Figure 8.5.

Once again, bizarre script-irrelevant and script-interruptive actions were better recalled than scripted actions across all three—1-hour, 48-hour, and 168-hour—delays. Note, however, that bizarre actions were not better re-called than script-interruptive actions at any of the delays, providing fur-ther support for an interruption effect and the need to further examine it. However, before this examination was done, a third study was conducted to determine whether script-interruptive actions that were bizarre would be better recalled than more plausible script-interruptive actions (David-son, Larson, et al., 2000). That is, would bizarreness add anything to the recall of interruptive items?

In order to examine this, two types of script-interruptive actions were presented in stories to college students. Plausible script-interruptive actions were similar to those used in previous studies. Implausible or bizarre ver-sions of these actions were also presented. To illustrate, the script-inter-ruptive action, "At the movies they got into the wrong ticket line" was changed to "At the movies a horse told them that they got into the wrong ticket line." In most cases (70%), the sentence was made bizarre by giving human or living features to nonhuman animals or objects, in line with list

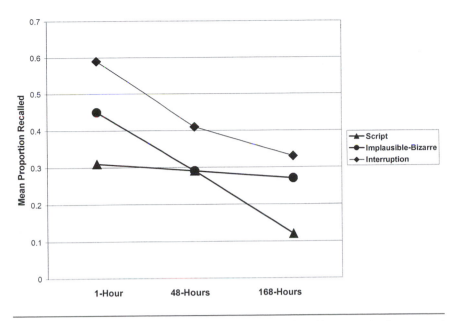

FIGURE 8.5 Mean recall proportions for script, implausible script-irrelevant, and script-interruptive actions by adults. From Davidson, Larson, et al., 2000. (Copyright 2000 by Psychology Press. Reprinted with permission.)

research that had found stronger bizarreness effects for this type of stimuli (Worthen & Marshall, 1996). The result of this manipulation is shown in Figure 8.6. Although interruption effects were found once again, bizarreness did not add to these effects. In fact, bizarre script-interruptive actions were not as well recalled as their more plausible counterparts. This suggested that while bizarreness effects may be found in script-based stories, interruption effects may supercede these effects and should be explored further. In particular, the reasons underlying interruption effects should be examined.

RESEARCH WITH OLDER (70+) ADULTS

However, before exploring explanations for interruption and bizarreness effects, it should be noted that both effects have been found with older (70+) adults (Davidson, Malmstrom, Burden, & Luo, 2000). The importance of these findings is that they run counter to previous studies that have shown that older adults tend to rely more on their schematic knowledge to aid their deteriorating memory. As basic information-processing skills become less efficient, older adults increase their reliance on script knowledge to remember (e.g., Hess, 1990). For example, in a story about dining at a restaurant (Hess & Tate, 1992), older adults were

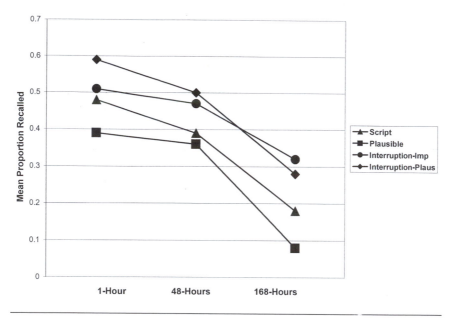

FIGURE 8.6 Mean recall proportions for script, plausible script-interruptive and implausible script-interruptive actions by adults From Davidson, Larson, et al., 2000. (Copyright 2000 by Psychology Press. Reprinted with permission.)

less likely than younger adults to recall story actions that were low in both typicality and relevance (e.g., "Jack put a pen in his pocket"), whereas fewer age effects were found for actions that were high in both typicality and relevance (e.g., "Jack asked the waiter for the check") and for actions that were low in typicality but high in relevance (e.g., "The waiter was impolite to Jack"). Note that the latter finding may have been due to the fact that items low in typicality, but high in relevance, were interruptive of the script.

Based on these findings, we predicted that script items, and possibly script-interruptive items, would be well recalled by older adults in our research. In contrast, bizarre script-irrelevant actions were not predicted to be well recalled by the older adults, not only because they were not related to the script in any way but also because previous research had found less evidence for bizarreness effects in older adults. For example, older adults resisted using bizarre imagery in learning paired words (Poon & Walsh-Sweeny, 1981). Nevertheless, both bizarreness and interruption effects were found in our research with older adults (see Fig. 8.7), suggesting that the same mechanisms that led to their appearance in young adults are operating in older adults. This provided further evidence for the need to explore these effects and their causes.

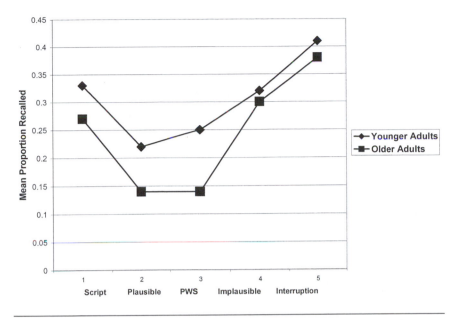

FIGURE 8.7 Mean recall proportions for script, script-irrelevant, and script-interruptive actions by younger and older adults. Note that implausible actions were bizarre actions. From Davidson, Malstrom, et al., 2000. (Copyright 2000 by Taylor & Francis. Reprinted with permission.)

EXPLANATIONS FOR INTERRUPTION AND BIZARRENESS EFFECTS IN TEXT

In general, text-processing models examine both the role of causal connections between story items and the role of causal inferences made by readers when reading these items to explain memory advantages found for specific text. The roles of other factors, such as the role of emotion in remembering, are also examined.

Text Processing Models: The Role of Causal Inference

A serendipitous finding in one of our studies suggested a reason for interruption effects, and possibly, bizarreness effects, too (Davidson, 1994). Although we consistently found interruption effects in numerous studies, in one study no effect occurred. The failure was found for the script-interruptive "errors" used in several stories (Davidson, 1994). As noted previously, we often used three types of script-interruptive actions in our stories—errors, obstacles, and distractions (mishaps)—and found that while they each interrupted the story in a different way, they usually did not interrupt the text to significantly different degrees. The exception was adults' poor recall of script-interruptive errors at a 1-week delay. These results are shown in Figure 8.8. One possibility was that obstacles and distractions were seen as less typical than errors. However, typicality could not account for the enhanced recall of obstacles and distractions because no significant differences were found in the typicality ratings of errors, obstacles, and distractions. Interruptive actions were also rated as equally vivid, and equally expected—ruling out these factors.

Another possibility, however, was the number of connections between story actions, as numerous studies have shown that actions with more connections are better recalled than actions with fewer connections (e.g., Trabasso & van den Broek, 1985; van den Broek, 1988). In examining the number of connections between story statements, trained raters judged that errors had fewer connections than the other interruptions. However, the number of connections alone could not have accounted for the recall differences because script actions, for example, had the most connections but were not better recalled than the interruptive actions.

Although the number of connections alone may not have accounted for the recall differences, the type of connection between story statements may have influenced recall. An examination of the interruptive actions used in this experiment revealed that errors were corrected significantly more often in the text than were obstacles or distractions. To illustrate, the error

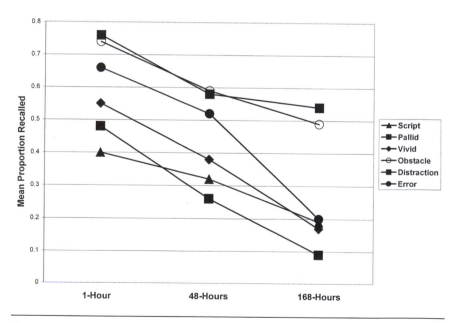

FIGURE 8.8 Mean recall proportions for script, script-irrelevant (pallid, vivid), and script-interruptive (errors, obstacles, distractions) actions by adults. From Davidson, 1994. (Copyright 1994 by Elsevier. Reprinted with permission.)

"At the movies they got into the wrong ticket line" was corrected in the next statement participants read with, "but then they got into the right line." Thus, in a second study the same errors were presented, although this time they were presented in their uncorrected form. The results of this study are shown in Figure 8.9. As shown, errors were now as well recalled as the other interruptions.

Uncorrected interruptions may be better recalled by subjects because interruptions not explicitly corrected in the text are corrected by the reader. That is, because of the continual flow of events in the story, the reader has to assume that somehow the interruption was corrected, or at least was temporary. It may be this extra inference on the part of the reader that contributes to the enhanced recall. Because interruptive actions are generally perceived as important to story comprehension (e.g., Dopkins, Klin & Meyers, 1993; Grice, 1975; McKoon & Ratcliff, 1992), an uncorrected interruption may have provided an even more compelling or noteworthy disruption in the story because readers tried to make sense out of the action and its possible consequences. These results are compatible with causal network theories of text processing (e.g., Trabasso & van den Broek, 1985; van den Broek, 1988). According to causal theories, interruptions play an important role in text processing, not only because they lead to coherence breaks but also because they generally demand explanation or inferences about why they happened and what may have occurred because they hap-

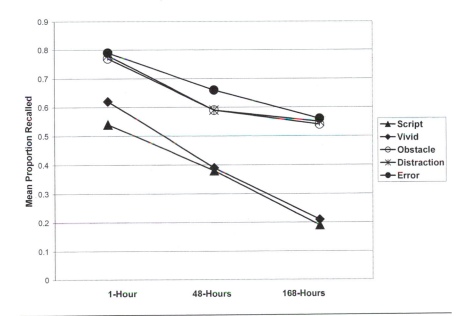

FIGURE 8.9 Mean recall proportions for script, script-irrelevant, and script-interruptive (uncorrected errors, obstacles, distractions) actions by adults. From Davidson, 1994. (Copyright 1994 by Elsevier. Reprinted with permission.)

pened. As Graesser et al. (1994) note, there is a coherence break when an incoming clause cannot be readily explained by prior text or background information. When a coherence break occurs, the reader is often compelled to piece together an explanation of the text. It may be this extra processing of text that leads to its subsequent better recall.

These results also are compatible with text research that has shown that the relationship between recall and number of connections to other story actions may be more complicated than originally believed. Sentence pairs with the strongest causal relations do not necessarily produce the best memory (e.g., Duffy, Shinjo, & Myers, 1990; Myers, Shinjo, & Duffy, 1987). Instead, recall appears to be better for moderately related pairs than for highly related pairs. According to Myers et al.'s (1987) elaboration hypothesis, readers more readily generate an elaboration, or causal bridging inference, between moderately related pairs, and it is this extra elaboration that presumably aids recall. In contrast, the highly related pairs are unlikely to elicit further elaboration or inferences from the reader, and hence are not as well recalled. Within the context of our research, readers would have had to infer that the uncorrected script-interruptive actions were corrected in some way or were temporary. A causal bridge inference may have then been made between these uncorrected interruptions and future story events.

This explanation is compatible with working-memory models of text processing. Fletcher and his colleagues have argued that an ideal working-memory management strategy for narrative comprehension should accomplish two goals (Fletcher & Bloom, 1988; Fletcher, Briggs, & Linzie, 1997). First, it should minimize the occurrence of causal coherence breaks—situations in which attention is focused on an event that has no causal relation to the following sentence. Second, it should maximize the number of causal connections in a narrative that can be uncovered by the reader without maximum effort. Thus, one might be compelled to infer how an uncorrected interruption was corrected in a story in order to minimize the causal coherence break. In doing so, the likelihood that the uncorrected interruption was better connected to ongoing and preceding story events would increase. Likewise, it is possible that bizarre information leads to coherence breaks. As most text-processing models assume, strategic inferences are constructed when local coherence cannot be established during the interpretation of a clause (e.g., McKoon & Ratcliff, 1992).

The Role of Emotions and Memory for Text

Further research has suggested additional reasons for the enhanced recall of atypical actions. For example, interruption effects were found to be more pronounced in children when the interruption was of greater consequence (Davidson & Jergovic, 1996). Thus, children more readily remembered the interruption "At the grocery store he dropped a carton of eggs" than "At the grocery store he dropped an apple." Note that the consequences of each interruption would have to be inferred by the children, a sophisticated feat given that the youngest children in the study were 6 years of age.

Interruptions that lead to consequences of an emotional nature, even when these consequences have to be inferred by the reader, also lead to better memory for the action. For example, young children generated not only more consequences for the interruption "At the grocery store he dropped a carton of eggs" than for the interruption "At the grocery store he dropped an apple," but also generated more consequences of an emotional nature, "The eggs would make a mess and his mom would be mad at him," "He would feel funny (embarrassed) and turn red," "He would get in trouble and he would be sad." Sometimes these consequences, while not in the story, would be given in children's recall.

In order to more closely examine the effects of emotion on memory for text, we recently conducted a series of studies that presented first-, third-, and fifth-grade children stories that consisted of emotional information (i.e., an action leading to emotion), nonemotional information, and the emotional label for the action (Davidson, Luo, & Burden, 2001). Although not all of the emotional actions were interruptions, nor were the stories script-based, we used actions that were often interruptive in nature (e.g., "That night, Maria dropped a carton of eggs in the kitchen and her parents got mad at her") and assessed children's memory not only for the action, "dropping a carton of eggs," but for the emotional label as well, "her parents got mad at her." It was found that children recalled emotional information (i.e., the actions) better than the emotion label and nonemotional information. In addition, actions that were emotionally significant—"A child was sad because her puppy was not well"—were better recalled than when the same information was presented in a less significant, but still "emotional" form: "The child was sad when her plant did not look well." While children recalled emotional information better than nonemotional information even when the emotion label was removed, recall for the action was not as well recalled as when the action was explicitly labeled with the emotion.

Perhaps the most important finding of this research, however, was that fewer developmental differences were found in younger and older children's memory for emotional information. That is, while older children recalled significantly more nonemotional information than did younger children, younger and older children's recall of emotional information was similar. These results suggest that information that is distinct in some way, particularly if it is emotional, should be used to assess differences in younger and older children's memory. These results are also compatible with past assumptions about what makes text more distinctive. As Schmidt (1991) notes, "Distinctiveness has been defined in terms of the emotional response to the stimuli, a comparison of the stimulus with other recent stimuli, a comparison of the stimulus with the contents of long-term memory, and the types of processes employed to encode the stimulus" (p. 534).

CONCLUSIONS

As noted in the introduction to this chapter, it was surprising to find that atypical actions in text can be well recalled across individuals (children, college students, and older adults) and across delay intervals. Continual work examining memory for script-based text, as well as research using other techniques such as the list format, have provided some answers as to what makes certain types of atypical actions distinct and, subsequently, well recalled. Although it is easy to allude to a distinctiveness explanation to explain bizarreness and interruption effects, it is clear that this explanation cannot fully explain differences in memory for common and less common information without considering the factors that lead to distinctiveness. This was noted by Hunt (1995, and Chapter 1 this volume) and others (e.g., Schmidt, 1991), who have well described why a distinctiveness explanation, in and of itself, cannot explain these findings. As research on bizarreness effects has shown, the factors underlying memory for bizarre information, whether in lists or in stories, are far ranging and complex. It is hoped, however, that by examining these effects using a range of experimental materials (as described in this book), and by applying models such as text-processing models to distinctiveness explanations, a more complete understanding of these memory findings can be obtained.

ACKNOWLEDGMENTS

Portions of this paper were presented at the 49th Annual Meeting of the Southwestern Psychological Association, New Orleans, LA.

REFERENCES

Bower, G. H., Black, J. B., & Turner, T. J. (1979). Scripts in comprehension and memory. *Cognitive Psychology, 11,* 177–220.

Cox, S. D., & Wollen, K. A. (1981). Bizarreness and recall. *Bulletin of the Psychonomic Society, 18,* 244–245.

Davidson, D. (1994). Recognition and recall of irrelevant and interruptive atypical actions in script-based stories. *Journal of Memory and Language, 33,* 757–775.

Davidson, D., & Hoe, S. (1993). Children's recall and recognition memory for typical and atypical actions in script-based stories. *Journal of Experimental Child Psychology, 55,* 104–126.

Davidson, D., & Jergovic, D. (1996). Children's memory for atypical actions in script-based stories: An examination of the disruption effect. *Journal of Experimental Child Psychology, 61,* 134–152.

Davidson, D., Larson, S. L., Luo, Z. & Burden, M. J. (2000). Interruption and bizarreness effects in the recall of script-based text. *Memory, 8,* 217–234.

Davidson, D., Luo, Z., & Burden, M. J. (2001). Children's recall of emotional behaviours, emotional labels, and nonemotional behaviours: Does emotion enhance recall? *Cognition and Emotion, 15,* 1–26.

Davidson, D., Malmstrom, T., Burden, M. J., & Luo, Z. (2000). Younger and older adults' recall of typical and atypical actions from script-based text: Evidence for interruption and bizarreness effects. *Experimental Aging Research, 26,* 409–430.

Dopkins, S., Klin, C., & Myers, J. L. (1993). Accessibility of information about goals during the processing of narrative texts. *Journal of Experimental Psychology: Learning, Memory, and Cognition, 19,* 70–80.

Duffy, S. A., Shinjo, M., & Myers, J. L. (1990). The effect of encoding task on memory for sentence pairs varying in causal relatedness. *Journal of Memory and Language, 29,* 27–42.

Einstein, G. O., & McDaniel, M. A. (1987). Distinctiveness and the mnemonic benefits of bizarreness. In M. A. McDaniel & M. Pressley (Eds.), *Imagery and related mnemonic processes: Theories, individual differences, and applications* (pp. 78–102). New York: Springer-Verlag.

Einstein, G. O., McDaniel, M. A., & Lackey, S. (1989). Bizarre imagery, interference, and distinctiveness. *Journal of Experimental Psychology: Learning, Memory and Cognition, 15,* 137–146.

Farrar, M. J., & Goodman, G. S. (1992). Developmental changes in event memory. *Child Development, 63,* 173–187.

Fivush, R. (1984). Learning about school: The development of kindergartners' school scripts. *Child Development, 55,* 1697–1709.

Fletcher, C. R., & Bloom, C. P. (1988). Causal reasoning in the comprehension of simple narrative texts. *Journal of Memory and Language, 27,* 235–244.

Fletcher, C. R., Briggs, A., & Linzie, B. (1997). Understanding the causal structure of narrative events. In P. W. van den Broek, P. J. Bauer, & T. Bourg (Eds.), *Developmental spans in event comprehension and representation: Bridging fictional and actual events* (pp. 343–360). Mahwah, NJ: Lawrence Erlbaum Associates.

Graesser, A. C., Gordon, S. E., & Sawyer, J. D. (1979). Memory for typical and atypical actions in scripted activities: Test of a script pointer and tag hypothesis. *Journal of Verbal Learning and Verbal Behavior, 18,* 319–332.

Graesser, A. C., Singer, M., & Trabasso, T. (1994). Constructing inferences during text comprehension. *Psychological Review, 101,* 371–395.

Graesser, A. C., Woll, S. B., Kowalaski, D. J., & Smith, D. A. (1980). Memory for typical and atypical actions in script activities. *Journal of Experimental Psychology: Human Learning and Memory, 6,* 503–515.

Green, R. T. (1956). Surprise as a factor in the Von Restorff effect. *Journal of Experimental Psychology, 52,* 340–344.

Grice, H. P. (1975). Logic and conversation. In P. Cole & J. L. Morgan (Eds.), *Syntax and semantics: Speech acts* (Vol. 3, pp. 41–58). San Diego, CA: Academic Press.

Hess, T. M. (1990). Aging and schematic influences on memory. In T. M. Hess (Ed.), *Aging and cognition: Knowledge organization and utilization* (pp. 93–160). Amsterdam, North Holland.

Hess, T. M., & Tate, C. S. (1992). Direct and indirect assessments of memory for script-based narratives in young and older adults. *Cognitive Development, 7*, 467–484.

Hirshman, E., Whelley, M. M., & Palij, M. (1989). An investigation of paradoxical memory effects. *Journal of Memory and Language, 28*, 594–609.

Hudson, J. A. (1988). Children's memory for atypical actions in script-based stories: Evidence for a disruption effect. *Journal of Experimental Child Psychology, 46*, 159–173.

Hunt, R. R. (1995). The subtlety of distinctiveness: What von Restorff really did. *Psychonomic Bulletin & Review, 2*, 105–112.

Hunt, R. R., & Lamb, C. A. (2001). What causes the isolation effect? *Journal of Experimental Psychology: Learning, Memory and Cognition, 21*, 1359–1366.

Hunt, R. R., & McDaniel, M. A. (1993). The enigma of organization and distinctiveness. *Journal of Memory and Language, 32*, 421–445.

Maki, R. H. (1990). Memory for script actions: Effects of relevance and detail expectancy. *Memory and Cognition, 18*, 5–14.

McDaniel, M. A., & Einstein, G. O. (1986). Bizarreness: Mnemonic benefits and theoretical implications. In R. H. Logie & M. Denis (Eds.), *Mental images in human cognition* (pp. 183–192). Amsterdam: Elsevier Science Publishers.

McDaniel, M. S., Einstein, G. O., DeLosh, E. L., May, C. P., & Brady, P. (1995). The bizarreness effect: It's not surprising, it's complex. *Journal of Experimental Psychology: Learning, Memory, and Cognition, 21*, 422–435.

McKoon, G., & Ratcliff, R. (1992). Inference during reading. *Psychological Review, 99*, 440–466.

Myers, J., Shinjo, M., & Duffy, S. A. (1987). Degree of causal relatedness and memory. *Journal of Memory and Language, 26*, 453–465.

Nelson, K. (Ed.) (1986). *Event knowledge: Structure and function in development*. Hillsdale, NJ: Lawrence Erlbaum Associates.

Poon, L. W., & Walsh-Sweeney, L. (1981). Effects of bizarre or interacting imagery on learning and retrieval in the aged. *Experimental Aging Research, 7*, 65–70.

Schank, R. C., & Abelson, R. (1977). *Scripts, plans, goals, and understanding*. Hillsdale, NJ: Lawrence Erlbaum Associates.

Schmidt, S. R. (1991). Can we have a distinctive theory of memory? *Memory & Cognition, 19*, 523–542.

Smith, D. A., & Graesser, A. C. (1981). Memory for actions in scripted activities as a function of typicality, retention interval, and retrieval task. *Memory and Cognition, 9*, 550–559.

Smith, R. E., & Hunt, R. R. (2000). The effects of distinctiveness require reinstatement of organization: The importance of intentional memory strategies. *Journal of Memory and Language, 43*, 431–446.

Trabasso, T., & van den Broek, P. (1985). Causal thinking and the representation of narrative events. *Journal of Memory and Language, 24,* 612–630.

van den Broek, P. (1988). The effects of causal relations and hierarchial position on the importance of story statements. *Journal of Memory and Language, 27,* 1–22.

Wallace, W. P. (1965). Review of the historical, empirical, and the theoretical status of the von Restorff phenomenon. *Psychological Bulletin, 63,* 410–424.

Weir, D., & Richman, C. L. (1996). Subject-generated bizarreness: Imagery or semantic processing. *American Journal of Psychology, 109,* 173–185.

Worthen, J. B. (1997). Resiliency of bizarreness effects under varying conditions of verbal and imaginal elaboration and processing mode. *Journal of Mental Imagery, 21,* 167–194.

Worthen, J. B., Garcia-Rivas, G., Green, C. R., & Vidos, R. A. (2000). Tests of a cognitive resource allocation account of the bizarreness effect. *Journal of General Psychology, 127,* 117–144.

Worthen, J. B., & Marshall, P. H. (1996). Intralist and extralist distinctiveness and the bizarreness effect: The importance of contrast. *American Journal of Psychology, 109,* 239–263.

Worthen, J. B., Marshall, P. H., & Cox, K. B. (1998). List length and the bizarreness effect: Support for a hybrid explanation. *Psychological Research/Psychologische Forschung, 61,* 147–156.

Worthen, J. B., & Wood, V. V. (2001a). A disruptive effect of bizarreness on memory for relational and contextual details of self-performed and other performed acts. *American Journal of Psychology, 114,* 535–546.

Worthen, J. B., & Wood, V. V. (2001b). Memory discrimination for self-performed and imagined acts: Bizarreness effects in false recognition. *Quarterly Journal of Experimental Psychology: Human Experimental Psychology, 54,* 49–67.

III

DISTINCTIVENESS AND IMPLICIT MEMORY TESTS

9

Conceptual Implicit Memory and the Item-Specific–Relational Distinction

Neil W. Mulligan

Research on distinctiveness and memory has largely focused on explicit, or recollective, aspects of memory. However, memory also affects behavior in ways unaccompanied by conscious recollection. The present chapter discusses research on distinctiveness and implicit memory, within the framework of item-specific and relational information. The present chapter begins with a brief overview of implicit and explicit memory, describes the utility of the item-specific–relational framework, and reviews recent empirical results supporting this analysis.

IMPLICIT AND EXPLICIT MEMORY

Traditional memory tests, such as recognition and free or cued recall, require the participant to think about some prior (usually, experimenter-provided) event and report on it. Such tests are referred to as *explicit memory tests* and may be contrasted with tests of unintentional or incidental retrieval, known as *implicit memory tests*. On implicit tests, participants are asked to perform a task such as the identification of perceptually degraded stimuli, the completion of word fragments, or the generation of category examples, without reference to any prior experience. Memory for prior events is inferred from the increased ease in identifying, completing, generating, or otherwise processing previously experienced information. This enhanced performance is referred to as priming. As typically conceived, explicit tests measure primarily intentional or deliberate recollection, whereas implicit tests assess unintentional or unconscious manifestations of memory (Mulligan, 2003).

The principles that govern implicit and explicit memory appear to differ in important ways (for reviews, see Roediger & McDermott, 1993;

Schacter, 1987). For example, compared to healthy control subjects, amnesics are profoundly impaired on explicit memory tests but often not on implicit tests (Shimamura, 1993). Several other populations (such as people with depression or schizophrenia and older adults) show a similar pattern: deficient explicit memory tests coupled with normal, or near-normal, priming on implicit memory tests (e.g., Denny & Hunt, 1992; Light, 1991; Schwartz, Rosse, & Deutsch, 1993). Pharmacological treatments produce similar dissociations. For example, administering benzodiazepine (a class of drugs including alprazolam, triazolam, diazepam, and midazolam) prior to a study session produces poor explicit memory but equivalent performance on implicit tests compared to a placebo control group. Thus, pharmacological amnesia produces a dissociation like that produced by organic amnesia: it affects conscious recollection but appears to have no effect on unconscious influences of memory (see Curran, 2000, for a review). Recent neuroimaging research (e.g., Gabrieli, 1998; Schacter & Badgaiyan, 2001) provides converging evidence for separable components of memory underlying implicit and explicit memory phenomena.

Experimental manipulations also produce dissociations between priming and performance on explicit tests. These are referred to as *functional dissociations* and a large number have been documented (Roediger & McDermott, 1993). For instance, variation in the amount of semantic processing at encoding has a marked effect on many explicit tests but little effect on many implicit tests. Conversely, the similarity between the physical features of the stimuli as presented at the time of study and test has a strong impact on many implicit tests but little effect on many explicit tests (e.g., Craik, Moscovitch, & McDowd, 1994; Roediger & Blaxton, 1987).

THE DISTINCTION BETWEEN PERCEPTUAL AND CONCEPTUAL IMPLICIT MEMORY

One important theoretical account of implicit and explicit memory, and the most successful in accounting for functional dissociations, is based on the general principle of transfer-appropriate processing (TAP). The central tenet of this view is that performance on a memory test benefits to the extent that the cognitive processes carried out during encoding are reengaged during retrieval (e.g., Morris, Bransford, & Frank, 1977). In applying this general principle to implicit and explicit memory tests, Roediger and colleagues (e.g., Roediger, 1990; Roediger, Buckner & McDermott, 1999; Roediger & McDermott, 1993) distinguished between perceptual (or data-driven) processes, which refer to analyses of a stimulus's physical or surface-level features, and conceptual processes, which refer to analyses of a stimulus's semantic content or significance.

Under the TAP view, it is proposed that explicit and implicit memory tests often rely differentially on conceptual and perceptual processing, and thus benefit from different types of encoding conditions. Because the most commonly used implicit tests (e.g., perceptual identification, fragment and stem completion) require the identification of perceptually degraded or incomplete stimuli, these tests are assumed to rely heavily on perceptual retrieval processes. In contrast, many of the commonly used explicit tests (e.g., free and cued recall, recognition) are assumed to rely heavily on conceptual retrieval processes (because, it has been argued, explicit memory instructions encourage the re-engagement of conceptual or elaborative retrieval processes; e.g., Craik et al., 1994; Roediger, Weldon, Stadler, & Reigler 1992).

Although the most commonly used implicit tests are perceptual in nature, the TAP view argues that implicit tests are not necessarily perceptual, nor are explicit tests exclusively conceptual. According to the TAP view, functional dissociations are only indirectly attributable to test instructions (implicit vs. explicit); the type of memory cues in conjunction with test type, rather than test type per se determines whether a test engages primarily conceptual or perceptual retrieval processes. Given the appropriate combination of memory cues and task instructions, conceptual implicit tests and perceptual explicit tests can be constructed. Furthermore, because the TAP framework focuses on the type of retrieval processes engaged by a test, the TAP view predicts dissociations between perceptual and conceptual tests whether the tests are implicit or explicit. In addition, the TAP view predicts similar effects of encoding manipulations (i.e., associations rather than dissociations) on an implicit and an explicit test provided that both tests are of the same type (either perceptual or conceptual).

An example of a conceptual implicit test is category-exemplar generation. In each trial of this test, participants are presented with a category name and asked to generate as many examples as possible in a short period of time (e.g., 20 seconds) or, in another variant, asked to produce the first eight examples that came to mind as rapidly as possible. Although the participant is not informed, examples from some of the categories were presented in an earlier (study) portion of the experiment. It is typically found that these "old" examples are more likely to be produced than control examples from other (new) categories, indicating priming (or implicit memory). Importantly, successful retrieval of an example in this task is not mediated by perceptual information. Unlike implicit tests that make use of degraded perceptual stimuli (like fragment completion or perceptual identification), there is no particular perceptual match in the category-exemplar generation task between the provided cue (a category name: e.g., *animal*) and a retrieved example (e.g., *tiger*). Obviously, the category name leads to retrieval of an example via their conceptual relationship and not through any shared perceptual features. Consequently, enhanced performance on this task is considered to be conceptual in nature. Empirical evidence for this classification comes from studies finding that semantic encoding manipulations affect this form of priming (as they affect explicit tests) whereas perceptual encoding manipulations (such as study modality) do not (Roediger & McDermott, 1993).

PROBLEMATIC DISSOCIATIONS AMONG CONCEPTUAL TESTS

Although the TAP framework has had great success accounting for functional dissociations between implicit and explicit memory (Roediger & McDermott, 1993), recently obtained dissociations within the class of conceptual tests have produced important challenges to the TAP view. The most compelling dissociations occur between matched conceptual implicit and explicit tests. Mulligan (1996) observed one such dissociation in a study of the perceptual-interference effect, the finding that interfering with the perception of a word can enhance later memory for the word (Nairne, 1988; Hirshman & Mulligan, 1991). Because this effect is important for later discussion, it will be described in some detail. The perceptual-interference manipulation consists of two encoding conditions. In the perceptual-interference condition, the study word is very briefly presented (e.g., for 100 milliseconds) on a computer screen followed by a backward mask (e.g., a row of Xs) which is left on the screen until the end of the trial (e.g., 2400 milliseconds). The participant's task is to read the quickly presented word (usually aloud, so that identification rates can be assessed). The presentation time is just long enough to allow successful identification of almost all of the words in this condition. In the intact condition, the study words are presented unmasked for the entire study trial (e.g., 2500 milliseconds) and can be easily identified. On a subsequent explicit memory test (e.g., recognition, free recall), the perceptual-interference items produce better performance than the intact items. As an aside, this phenomenon is referred to as the *perceptual-interference effect* because it appears to arise during the initial perception of the word. That is, if the mask is delayed until after perception is complete (e.g., 266 milliseconds; reading research indicates that identification times for a single common word is on the order of 200 milliseconds; see Mulligan, 2000a, for discussion), the perceptual interference effect does not occur. Evidence that the mask disrupts perception comes from the longer identification times and slightly lower identification rates at study in the perceptual-interference condition compared to intact condition (Hirshman, Trembath & Mulligan, 1994).

Mulligan (1996) investigated the effect of perceptual interference on conceptual implicit and explicit memory as follows. In the study portion of the experiment, examples from various categories were presented in either the perceptual-interference or intact conditions. After a distracter task, half the participants were tested with the implicit test of category-exemplar production and the other half were tested with its explicit counterpart, category-cued recall. In the implicit task, half of the categories corresponded to examples that were presented on the study list and the other categories did not (the latter half corresponded to a control set of examples that were used to assess baseline production rates). Of course, the participants were not informed of the relationship between this task and the preceding study list. Rather, they were told that the task was a norming study, designed to measure association strength between categories and examples. In the explicit test, the same category cues were presented but participants were instructed to use the category names to try to remember words from the study list.[1]

The cued-recall test exhibited the typical perceptual-interference effect: more words were recalled from the perceptual-interference than intact condition. In contrast, the amount of conceptual priming in the category-exemplar production task did not differ across the encoding conditions. Perceptual interference dissociated performance between two matched conceptual explicit and implicit tests, enhancing performance on the explicit but not the implicit test. Parenthetically, this pattern was found across several experiments that, in sum, yielded overwhelming power to detect a perceptual-interference effect on conceptual priming if one existed.

A similar dissociation was reported by Weldon and Coyote (1996) in their study of the picture-superiority effect. Generally, when study items are presented either as words or as pictures of the word's referent, the pictures produce better recall and recognition on subsequent memory tests. Weldon and Coyote examined this effect on category-exemplar production and category-cued recall, as well as on two other matched conceptual tests: word association and associate-cued recall. Word association is an implicit test in which participants are presented with a series of cue words (e.g., *doctor* . . .) and asked to generate the first word that comes to mind. Unbeknownst to the participant, associates of some of the cue words (e.g., *nurse*) were presented in the study portion of the experiment. The old associates are typically produced more often than associates from a control (unstudied) set (i.e., the task exhibits priming). The associate-cued recall task is the explicit counterpart, in which the same cues are presented and participants are asked to use the cues to try to recall words from the study list. For the explicit tests, Weldon and Coyote found the typical picture-superiority effect, but for the implicit tests no effect of study mode was found, although both words and pictures produce significant priming. Thus, Weldon and Coyote found a dissociation similar to that reported by Mulligan (1996): the picture-superiority effect was found on conceptual explicit tests but not on matched conceptual implicit tests.

An effect often associated with the picture-superiority effect is the word-concreteness effect. Concrete nouns (e.g., *football*) are typically better remembered than abstract nouns (e.g., *freedom*) on explicit tests like recognition and recall (Paivio, 1991). Hamilton and Rajaram (2001) investigated the effect of word concreteness on a conceptual implicit test, general knowledge questions, and its explicit counterpart, question-cued recall. In the general knowledge task, participants are presented with a set of questions (e.g., "What is the fastest land animal?"), presented as a trivia test. Unbeknownst to the participant, the answers to some of the questions (e.g., *cheetah*) were presented in the study portion of the experiment. The likelihood of correctly answering the question is higher for the recently experienced answers than for other, baseline questions, whose answers were not presented at study. In the explicit version, participants are explicitly told that answers to some of the questions were presented earlier, and they should use the questions to try to remember words presented in the study phase. Hamilton and Rajaram found the typical word-concreteness effect for the explicit test but not for its implicit counterpart.

A fourth dissociation was reported by Smith and Hunt (2000) in their analysis of distinctiveness effects in implicit and explicit memory. During each study trial, participants were presented with a set of five words, all examples from the same category. One of the words was set apart from the rest and participants were asked to find either a difference between the target word and the others or a similarity. Judging differences in the context of similarity (i.e., common category membership) is known to have a powerful impact on explicit memory (e.g., Hunt & Smith, 1996). In the present experiments, the effect of this manipulation was assessed with one explicit test, category-cued recall, and two conceptual implicit tests, category-exemplar production and word association. The items in the difference condition produced greater recall than did items in the similarity condition (this is the standard distinctiveness effect in recall), but no effect was found on the conceptual implicit tests.[2]

Mulligan and Stone (1999, Experiment 5) observed another dissociation between conceptual implicit and explicit memory. The study portion of this experiment consisted of a list of six examples from each of six categories, and all the examples from a given category were presented in sequence (i.e., a blocked list presentation). The focus of the experiment was on within-category serial position effects. Prior research indicated that the first one or two items from a new category produced superior recall on subsequent explicit memory tests (e.g., Mandler, 1979). Mulligan and Stone found the expected within-category primacy effect on category-cued recall. However, priming in the category-exemplar production task was somewhat lower (though nonsignificantly) in the initial within-category serial positions than in later positions. Thus, within-category serial position produced different effects on matched conceptual implicit and explicit tests.

A final dissociation is produced by the generation manipulation. As a general rule, self-generated information produces better explicit memory than merely perceiving the same information (Slamecka & Graf, 1978). For example, generating a word from its antonym (*north–s___*) produces better recall and recognition than reading the same word (*north–south*). Likewise, generating a word by transposing the first two letters (e.g., *osuth*) produces better explicit memory than reading the same word. Previous research indicates that generating words from semantic cues (e.g., antonyms, category names) enhances conceptual priming (Roediger & McDermott, 1993). Mulligan (2002) found that nonsemantic generation tasks, like letter transposition or word fragment generation, did not enhance conceptual priming in category-exemplar production, even though these generation manipulations enhanced recall on the matched explicit test of category-cued recall (more on this later).

A number of dissociations between matched conceptual implicit and explicit tests have been observed. Perceptual-interference, study mode (picture vs. word), word concreteness, similarity vs. difference encoding, within-category serial position, and nonsemantic generation all produce such dissociations. In addition, dissociations have been reported among conceptual implicit tests (e.g., Cabeza, 1994; Gabrieli et al., 1999; Vaidya et al., 1997) and among conceptual explicit tests (McDermott & Roediger, 1996).

ITEM-SPECIFIC VS. RELATIONAL INFORMATION

Dissociations within the class of conceptual tests are problematic for the TAP view and suggest that its continued viability requires further refinement (e.g., McDermott and Roediger, 1996; Mulligan, 1996; Weldon & Coyote, 1996; see Mulligan, 1998, for related discussion). Mulligan (1996) proposed one possibility: framing the difference between category-exemplar production and category-cued recall in terms of the distinction between item-specific and relational processing (e.g., Hunt & Einstein, 1981; Hunt & McDaniel, 1993). As defined by Hunt & Einstein (1981; Hunt & McDaniel, 1993; Smith & Hunt, 2000), relational information refers to features shared by to-be-retrieved items whereas item-specific information refers to features unique to an item. Relational information is important in the selection of effective retrieval strategies and the generation of potential responses, whereas item-specific information provides discriminative or distinctive information during retrieval (Hunt & Einstein, 1981; Hunt & McDaniel, 1993; Smith & Hunt, 2000). Hunt & Einstein (1981) describe memory retrieval as "a process of increasingly finer discriminations" (p. 511), beginning at a coarse level in which relational information delimits the class from which to-be-retrieved responses come and progressing to a more fine-grained level in which item-specific information permits discrimination between potential responses.

Mulligan (1996) argued that the item-specific–relational distinction provides a plausible account of the difference between category-exemplar production and category-cued recall (other results indicate the distinction applies to conceptual implicit and explicit memory more generally; Hamilton & Rajaram, 2001; Mulligan, Guyer, & Beland, 1999; Smith & Hunt, 2000; Weldon & Coyote, 1996). Specifically, category-cued recall, which calls for the production of words that are both members of the category and were on the study list, requires finer discriminations than category-exemplar production, which requires only producing examples from the category. Consequently, we might expect that category-cued recall is sensitive to both item-specific and relational encodings, whereas category-exemplar production is differentially reliant on relational encoding. Presumably, the relevant relational information for the category-exemplar production task is category-level information (e.g., Mulligan et al., 1999; Rappold & Hashtroudi, 1991).

Several findings (Hamilton & Rajaram, 2001; Mulligan, 1996, 2002; Mulligan et al., 1999; Mulligan & Stone, 1999; Smith & Hunt, 2000; Weldon & Coyote, 1996) indicate that, unlike category-cued recall, category-exemplar production is relatively insensitive to encoding effects mediated by item-specific information. In addition, priming in this task appears to be sensitive to relational encodings; generating category labels for studied exemplars increases category-exemplar priming (Cabeza, 1994), as does blocking studied examples by category (Mulligan et al., 1999; Rappold & Hashtroudi,1991), a manipulation which makes relational information highly salient (e.g., Hunt & Einstein, 1981). Finally, conceptual replication during study (i.e., following a target item with an associate) enhances conceptual priming under relational encoding instructions but not when participants encoded targets and associates in isolation (McDermott & Roediger, 1996).

PERCEPTUAL INTERFERENCE AND THE ITEM-SPECIFIC–RELATIONAL DISTINCTION

The foregoing analysis implies that perceptual interference enhances memory because it enhances item-specific processing and not relational encoding. A number of results support this implication. First, consider the initial studies of the perceptual-interference effect (Hirshman & Mulligan, 1991; Hirshman et al., 1994; Mulligan, 1996), which convincingly demonstrated that the effect is mediated by perceptual encoding processes and not by post-perceptual rehearsal. It has already been mentioned that the effect occurs if the word is presented very briefly prior to the mask onset (e.g., 100 milliseconds) but not if the mask is delayed (e.g., to 266 milliseconds). This indicates that the mask must interfere with ongoing perceptual analyses to have mnemonic effect. Additional evidence that the effect is mediated by perceptual rather than post-perceptual processes comes from experiments in which the duration of the entire study trial is varied (trial duration is word duration plus mask duration in the perceptual-interference condition, and simply word duration in the intact condition). If the perceptual-interference effect were mediated by post-perceptual rehearsal, then lengthening the study trials would lengthen the amount of time available for the differential rehearsal, which should increase the size to the effect. In contrast, if the effect arises as a consequence of perceptual encoding processes, then varying the amount of time for post-perceptual processing should not moderate the size of the effect. Hirshman et al. (1994) varied the study-trial duration (900 milliseconds vs. 2500 milliseconds) and found no difference in the size of the perceptual-interference effect on recall. This set of results implies that the locus of the perceptual-interference effect is in initial perceptual identification and not in subsequent, post-perceptual rehearsal (e.g., elaboration; see Hirshman et al., 1994; Mulligan, 1996, for converging evidence).

Mulligan (1996) argued that if the representations underlying the perceptual-interference effect are encoded during perception, then they are representations of the study item in isolation. That is, they do not include associative information about the study item as related to other ongoing events or stimuli. Such associative processing logically requires that one first decipher the present stimulus in order to find bases for association (i.e., associative processing is post-perceptual). This characterization meshes well with the item-specific–relational framework and suggests that perceptual interference is an item-specific effect.[3]

According to the item-specific–relational framework, item-specific information is important on all tests of item occurrence, such as recognition and free recall, and we have already seen that perceptual interference enhances performance on these tests. However, recognition is more sensitive than free recall to item-specific information (Hunt & McDaniel, 1993), implying that recognition should be more sensitive to the effects of perceptual-interference. This implication is borne out in the observation that the perceptual-interference effect is more readily demonstrated on recognition than on free-recall tests (cf. Hirshman & Mulligan, 1991; Nairne, 1988; see also Mulligan, 1999).

Whereas perceptual-interference appears to enhance item-specific processing, it does not enhance (and in some ways disrupts) relational or associative information in memory. One common way to assess the amount of relational processing during encoding is to use a study list consisting of several examples from each of a number of categories and then to examine the extent to which later recall exhibits category-clustering (members of the same category recalled in sequence). The clustering score is used as a measure of relational encoding. Mulligan (1999) found that, although perceptual interference enhanced overall recall, it produced less category clustering in recall than did the intact condition. This implies that perceptual-interference disrupts relational encoding. Relational and associative encoding have also been assessed with memory for the temporal order in which events occur. As with category clustering, perceptual interference generally impairs memory for order (Mulligan, 1999, 2000a). On a related note, Mulligan (1996) found that although perceptual interference enhanced recognition (item) memory, it did not enhance memory for contextual details.

A final bit of converging evidence comes from experiments using multiple recall tests (participants are asked to recall the study list multiple times without additional study trials). With multiple recall tests, some items are recalled on later tests that had not been recalled earlier (item gains), while other items that were successfully recalled earlier may not be recalled on later tests (item losses). Klein, Loftus, Kihlstrom, and Aseron (1989; see also Burns, 1993; McDaniel, Moore, & Whiteman, 1998) demonstrated that conditions fostering item-specific encoding increase the probability of item gains, whereas conditions fostering relational encoding protect against item losses. Mulligan (2000b) found that perceptual-interference produced both more item gains and more item losses than the intact condition, indicating enhanced item-specific encoding coupled with reduced relational encoding.

As a set, these results support the notion that perceptual interference enhances item-specific processing and either disrupts or at least fails to enhance relational encoding.[4] This in turn bolsters the item-specific–relational account of conceptual implicit and explicit memory. Perceptual-interference enhances category-cued recall but not conceptual priming, indicating that the former test is sensitive to a manipulation of item-specific encoding whereas the latter test is not.

THE EFFECTS OF GENERATION ON CONCEPTUAL PRIMING

The item-specific–relational analysis also sheds light on the effects of generation on conceptual priming. The effects of generation are similar in many ways to the effects of perceptual interference. Like perceptual interference, generation typically enhances item memory on explicit tests such as recognition and free and cued recall. In contrast, measures of relational and order encoding often produce negative or null effects of generation. Both perceptual interference and generation disrupt order memory (e.g., Burns, 1996; Nairne, Reigler, & Serra, 1991). In addition, generation generally does not enhance category clustering scores (McDaniel, Waddill, & Einstein, 1988). When order information is an important determinant of recall, both the generation and perceptual-interference effects can reverse, with the read or intact condition leading to better recall than the generate or perceptual-interference condition (Mulligan, 1999; Nairne et al., 1991). In explicit memory, both the generation and perceptual-interference effects are sensitive to the type of stimulus materials, occurring with words but typically not with nonwords (e.g., McElroy & Slamecka, 1982; Westerman & Greene, 1997). Generation and perceptual interference produce similar patterns of item gains and losses across multiple recall tests (Mulligan 2000b, 2001). A final similarity is that the effects of both perceptual interference and generation are more readily observed on tests of recognition than on free recall, especially for between-subjects designs (Hirshman & Bjork, 1988; Mulligan, 1999; Slamecka & Katsaiti, 1987).[5]

Mulligan (2002) investigated whether the similarity between generation and perceptual interference extended to their effects on conceptual priming. It should be noted that this possibility confronts an immediate problem because it suggests that generation ought to enhance conceptual explicit memory while leaving conceptual priming unaffected. The empirical picture is

unclear. Srinivas and Roediger (1990) found that generating words from semantic cues (sentence frames) enhanced conceptual priming in the category-
exemplar production task (a finding replicated by Maki & Knopman, 1996).
In contrast, Kinoshita (1989) found that words generated by letter transposition (e.g., *rgass* for *grass*) failed to enhance conceptual priming even
though they enhanced free recall. From the current perspective, it may be
that generation from semantic cues (sentence frames) elicited some amount
of categorical-relational processing in addition to enhancing item-specific
encoding. Mulligan (2002) pursued the idea that nonsemantic generation
tasks (e.g., letter transposition, word fragment generation) behave like the
perceptual-interference manipulation, enhancing recall without increasing
conceptual priming. In addition, Mulligan (2002) used category-cued recall
as the explicit test to determine if nonsemantic generation dissociates
matched conceptual implicit and explicit tests (Kinoshita, 1989, used free
recall as the explicit test, which differs from category-exemplar production
in ways other than the operative implicit vs. explicit instructions).

Mulligan (2002): experiments 1a and 1b

In the study portion of the experiment, participants read or generated a set
of words. The generation task was letter transposition in Experiment 1a
and word-fragment generation in Experiment 1b. In the latter manipulation, words are presented as fragments to be generated (e.g., *gra_s*) or as
intact words to be read. After a brief distracter task, half the participants
were tested with category-exemplar production and the other half with
category-cued recall. Finally, participants in the implicit condition were
given an awareness questionnaire designed to determine the extent of explicit contamination and to allow for an analysis excluding participants reporting test awareness (a common approach; Hamilton & Rajaram, 2001;
Smith & Hunt, 2000).

The test results are presented in Figures 9.1 and 9.2. First, consider the
results of the category-cued recall (Fig. 9.1), in which the proportion of
study words recalled is presented as a function of the two encoding conditions (generate vs. read). It can be seen that the typical generation effect
was found for explicit memory: the generate condition enhanced recall in
both experiments. This is consistent with a good deal of research indicating that nonsemantic as well as semantic generation tasks enhance recall
(see Mulligan, 2002, for discussion).

Next, consider the results of the category-exemplar production task
(Fig. 9.2). Here, the proportion of study words produced in the two encoding conditions is juxtaposed with the proportion of critical baseline examples produced for the new categories (those categories with no examples
in the study list). The higher proportions for examples from the old (generate and read) conditions than the new condition indicates that priming
was obtained for both encoding conditions. More important, the amount

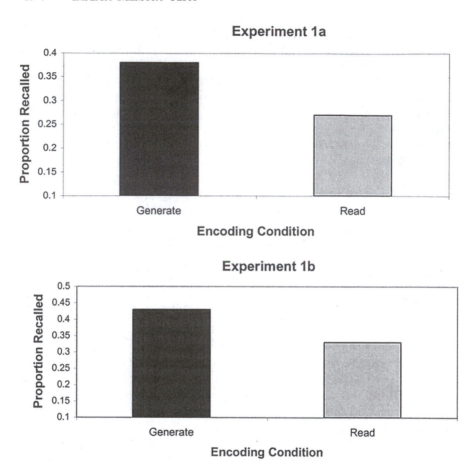

FIGURE 9.1 Mulligan (2002) Experiments 1a and 1b: Category-cued recall as a function of encoding condition (letter transposition generation task in Experiment 1a; word-fragment generation task in Experiment 1b).

of priming did not differ across the generate and read conditions. It should be noted that the results presented in the figures represent all of the implicit participants. The same pattern of results was found when participants reporting test awareness were excluded.

The two nonsemantic generation tasks dissociated matched conceptual implicit and explicit tests, affecting the latter but not the former. In such a case, it is important to consider the power of the implicit test to detect the sought-after effect. In the present experiments, there were relatively large numbers of participants in the implicit condition (40 and 36 in Experiment 1a and Experiment 1b, respectively). In the combined analysis, the power to detect an effect of generation on conceptual priming just one-half the size of the effect detected on cued recall exceeded .99. The power to detect an effect one third that size was .88. The present experiments provided

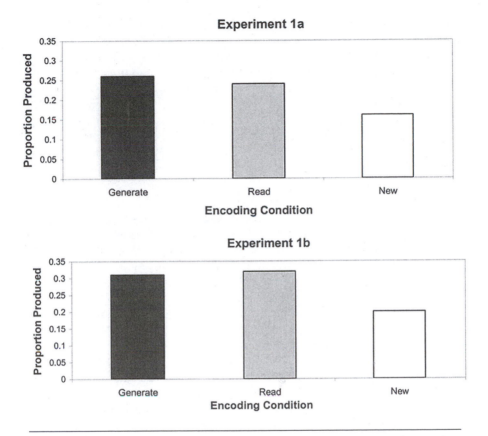

FIGURE 9.2 Mulligan (2002) Experiments 1a and 1b: Category-exemplar production as a function of encoding condition (letter transposition generation task in Experiment 1a; word-fragment generation task in Experiment 1b).

overwhelming power to detect an effect of generation on conceptual priming even if the effect was one half the size produced in recall, rendering a power artifact unlikely.

Mulligan (2002): Experiment 3

To further explore the effects of generation on conceptual priming, it is useful to juxtapose the present account of conceptual priming with the multifactor account of the generation effect, the most successful theoretical account of generation and one that is also based on the item-specific–relational distinction (e.g., Hunt & McDaniel, 1993; McDaniel et al., 1988; Mulligan, 2001). The multifactor account indicates that under certain conditions, nonsemantic generation manipulations, like the letter-transposition task, ought to impact conceptual priming.

According to the multifactor account, generation always enhances the processing of item-specific features of the target item, differentiating the item from other items in the list and increasing item distinctiveness (e.g., Begg, Snider, Foley, & Goddard, 1989; Gardiner & Hampton, 1988; Nairne et al., 1991). However, generation may also enhance relational information if it is useful in the process of generation. That is, the multifactor account views generation as a problem-solving task (Jacoby, 1978) in which any relevant information will be exploited (and its encoding enhanced) in the act of generation (McDaniel et al., 1988). In the present case, the sentence frames used in experiments exhibiting the generation effect on conceptual priming (Maki & Knopman, 1996; Srinivas & Roediger, 1990) presumably induced more categorical processing in the generate than in the read condition in addition to whatever item-specific encoding advantage accrued to the generate condition. However, for the letter-transposition and word-fragment tasks used in the prior experiment, the generate condition provided only item-specific information and no semantic or categorical information. Thus, the generate condition enhanced item-specific encoding but not relational encoding, producing an effect on cued recall but not on the category-exemplar production test.

The multifactor account proposes that the structure of the study list may provide useful information for generation. For example, if the study items are members of a common category and this is made obvious at encoding, then processing their common characteristics would assist generation. Under these conditions, generation leads to higher levels of category clustering than the read condition, providing evidence for enhanced categorical-relational processing (deWinstanley & Bjork, 1997; McDaniel et al., 1988; Mulligan, 2001). When study items are unrelated or categorical information is not salient, relational processing is not as useful and is neglected in favor of item-specific processing. Under these conditions, generation is expected to enhance item-specific but not categorical-relational processing.

Mulligan (2002, Experiment 3) investigated these issues by using the letter transposition task and list structures that make categorical information more or less salient. Study lists consisted of several examples from each of a number of categories. Categorical information was either made salient by presenting examples from the same category in sequence (the blocked condition) or less salient by presenting the examples in a pseudo-random order in which no two members from the same category occurred in sequence. As in the preceding experiments, the study list was followed by a brief distracter task, which in turn was followed by either category-cued recall or category-exemplar production. The implicit test was again followed by the post-test awareness questionnaire.

The random condition is similar to Experiment 1a and is expected to produce the same results: a generation effect in cued recall but not in category-exemplar production. In the blocked condition, however, categorical information provides a salient basis for generation. Under these conditions, the multifactor account predicts that generation enhances categorical-relational as well as item-specific processing. Thus, in contrast to the

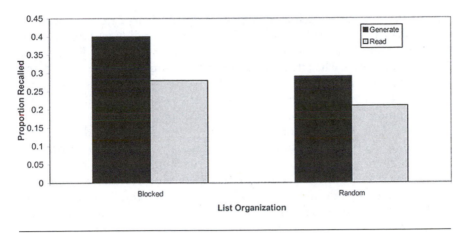

FIGURE 9.3 Mulligan (2002) Experiment 3: Category-cued recall as a function of encoding condition and list organization.

random condition, the blocked condition is expected to induce a generation effect in conceptual priming. For cued recall, the generation effect is expected regardless of list organization.

The results are presented in Figures 9.3 and 9.4, and conform to the expectations of the item-specific–relational analysis. Category-cued recall (Fig. 9.3) exhibited effects of list organization and encoding condition, with no interaction. The effect of list organization was expected and reflects greater recall in the blocked than in the random condition. Presenting materials in

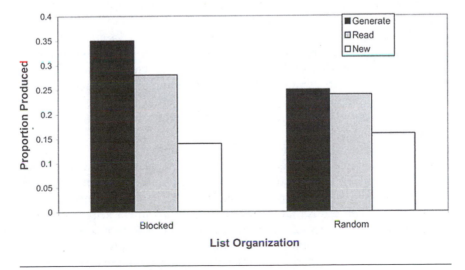

FIGURE 9.4 Mulligan (2002) Experiment 3: Category-exemplar production as a function of encoding condition and list organization.

an organized fashion (such as blocking study words by category membership) enhances later recall, an effect found in free recall (e.g., Hunt & Einstein, 1981) and category-cued recall (Mulligan et al., 1999; Rappold & Hashtroudi, 1991). The effect of encoding condition was also expected and reflects the typical generation effect. The lack of an interaction indicates that the generation effect was obtained regardless of list condition, an important point as we proceed to the conceptual priming results.

Figure 9.4 presents performance in category-exemplar production as a function of the study condition (generate, read, new) and list organization. First, production of critical examples is significantly higher in the two old conditions than in the new condition for both blocked and random lists. This indicates significant priming in all of the old conditions. Next, an analysis of the conceptual priming scores revealed two effects. First, there was a main effect of list organization, reflecting greater priming in the blocked than in the random condition. This replicates earlier research (Mulligan et al., 1999; Rappold & Hashtroudi, 1991) and is consistent with the current theoretical framework: presenting the list in an organized manner facilitates categorical-relational encoding, boosting performance on category-exemplar production—a test assumed to be sensitive to this type of information. Even more central for current concerns is the second effect, an interaction between encoding condition (generate vs. read) and list organization. This interaction reflects a significant generation effect in the blocked condition and no effect of generation in the random condition. An analysis excluding the test-aware participants produced the same pattern of results.

The results of this experiment are consistent with the item-specific–relational analysis provided earlier. Specifically, in the random list condition, in which generation produces enhanced encoding of item-specific but not relational information, generation enhanced cued recall but not conceptual priming (replicating the results of Experiments 1a and 1b). However, when categorical-relational information is made salient and becomes a relevant basis for generation, the generation effect emerged in conceptual priming. These results demonstrate that, depending on the structure of the encoding environment, an apparently nonsemantic generation task can enlist categorical-relational information and produce a generation effect on conceptual priming.

The present experiment is important for another reason. The present analysis was initially developed to account for dissociations in which a purported item-specific effect (like perceptual interference or picture superiority) was observed on a conceptual explicit test but not on a conceptual implicit test. The concern is that this pattern of results might arise simply due to differential sensitivity of the tests; perhaps both tests assess the same type of memorial information but the implicit test is simply a weaker measure of this common underlying information. Power analyses go some way toward alleviating this concern. If the implicit test has substantial power to detect an effect a fraction of the size of that observed on the explicit test, and if the effect is still not observed, then the differential-sensitivity alternative seems less plausible (as was the case in Experiments 1a and 1b). However, stronger evidence for the item-specific–relational analysis is garnered in the present experiment because the theory does not simply predict a null effect for conceptual priming but, rather, predicts when the generation effect will and will not be observed. In a similar way, the account makes predictions about the effects of semantic encoding on conceptual priming, foreseeing the conditions under which the levels-of-processing effect will and will not occur. This research is discussed next.

LEVELS-OF-PROCESSING AND CONCEPTUAL PRIMING IN THE CATEGORY-EXEMPLAR PRODUCTION TASK

The item-specific–relational analysis also motivated a re-examination of one of the most important encoding manipulations in the study of implicit and explicit memory. The effects of levels-of-processing (LOP) have been central to research in this area. Foundational studies indicated that although semantic encoding produces dramatic effects on explicit memory, it produces little effect on perceptual implicit tests (e.g., Jacoby & Dallas, 1981). The effects of LOP were equally important in the development of the TAP framework when it was reported that the levels manipulation did, in fact, enhance implicit memory, at least for conceptual priming tasks (Hamann, 1990; Srinivas & Roediger, 1990). This result is part of the groundwork of the TAP distinction between perceptual and conceptual priming.

Mulligan et al. (1999) investigated the effects of the LOP manipulation in light of the item-specific–relational analysis. More specifically, this study investigated how priming in the category-exemplar production task is affected by simultaneous manipulations of semantic elaboration and list organization. To manipulate semantic elaboration, a traditional LOP manipulation was used, in which some study items were encoded semantically (using a pleasantness-rating task) and others nonsemantically (using a vowel-counting task). It should be noted that typical semantic encoding tasks, such as the pleasantness-rating task, appear to induce item-specific processing (e.g., Hunt & Einstein, 1981; Hunt & McDaniel, 1993). In contrast, the manipulation of list organization, as in the prior experiment, affects relational encoding (e.g., Hunt & Einstein, 1981; Rappold & Hashtroudi, 1991).

One implication of the item-specific–relational analysis is that effects of semantic encoding should be greater when encoding takes place in a relational context. In particular, for the category-exemplar production task, LOP effects should be greater when category-level information is highly salient, as in the categorized study condition. An even stronger interpretation of this view suggests that priming in this task is not affected by all forms of semantic encoding but only by those that emphasize relational information—in this case, categorical information. In particular, if the relevant relational information is not salient and the semantic task emphasizes item-specific information (like the pleasantness-rating task), we may observe no effect of semantic elaboration at all. This strong interpretation is at odds with the TAP view, which makes an unqualified prediction of LOP effects on conceptual tests.

The strong version of the item-specific–relational analysis is challenged by findings of LOP effects on the category-exemplar production test (Hamann, 1990; Srinivas & Roediger, 1990; Weldon & Coyote, 1996). These studies typically used pleasantness (Srinivas & Roediger, 1990; Weldon & Coyote, 1996) or liking ratings (Hamann, 1990) as the semantic encoding task. According to the strong interpretation of the item-specific–relational account, because these tasks emphasize item-specific encoding, they should be less likely to enhance priming in the category-exemplar production task. However, there are two potential reasons, consistent with the strong hypothesis, that LOP effects were observed. First, the relevant relational information may have been salient at study, inducing relational rather than item-specific encoding. For instance, if many of the study words were examples from the same category, this fact may have become apparent to the participants and induced relational encoding of the common category information. Second, the observed LOP effects may have been due to explicit contamination. The results of post-test questionnaires indicate that some level of explicit contamination is likely with the category-exemplar production task. For example, in the preceding experiments, the percentage of participants reporting an awareness of the connection between the study and test portions of the experiment ranged from 36% to 46%. Other experiments report even higher levels of explicit contamination (e.g., Light & Albertson, 1989; Mulligan & Hartman, 1996). Post-test questionnaires were not used in the studies demonstrating LOP effects on conceptual priming, so the number of test-aware participants is unknown. However, it is plausible that some level of explicit contamination was present in these studies.

In Mulligan et al.'s (1999) experiments, study lists consisted of multiple examples from each of a number of categories. Study lists were either organized by category (the blocked condition), rendering the categorical structure of the list salient, or presented in a pseudo-random order (barring members of the same category from appearing in sequence), rendering the categorical structure less salient. Each item was encoded with either a semantic (pleasantness rating) or a nonsemantic (vowel-counting) task. Later, participants were tested with either category-exemplar production or category-cued recall. In the implicit condition, the test was followed by an awareness questionnaire.

Mulligan et al. (1999) implemented this general design in three experiments, which varied the type of experimental design (within-subjects vs. between-subjects) and used two variants of the category-exemplar production task. Regardless, the experiments produced consistent results. The analysis of the priming data (which included all of the participants) revealed several important effects. First, the main effect of LOP was significant, indicating that semantic encoding produced greater conceptual priming than did non-semantic encoding. Second, the LOP effect was larger in the blocked than in the random condition (i.e., LOP interacted with list organization), although the LOP effect was significant within both conditions. This indicates that semantic elaboration was more effective in a relational context. Finally, as expected based on previous research, blocked list organization generally enhanced conceptual priming compared to random list presentation.

The next set of analyses made use of the test-awareness classification from the post-test questionnaire. The item-specific–relational account of conceptual priming makes a prediction regarding the influence of explicit contamination. Explicit contamination should make the category-exemplar production task more like category-cued recall, rendering it more sensitive to item-specific encoding. Consequently, reducing explicit contamination by restricting analysis to test-unaware participants should largely reduce the influence of item-specific encoding on this task. This generates different implications for LOP effects depending on whether semantic elaboration occurred under conditions of item-specific processing, as in the random condition, or relational processing, as in the categorized condition. Specifically, eliminating test-aware participants should reduce the LOP effect in the random condition but not in the categorized condition, where relational processing predominates. The results of the experiments were in accord with these expectations. That is, removing test-aware subjects reduced LOP effects in the random condition, in which item-specific encoding dominates, but not in the categorized condition, in which relational encoding predominates.

The final set of analyses was restricted to the test-unaware participants and produced three important results. First, consistent with the full analysis, the LOP effect was larger in the categorized than in the random list condition, indicating that the LOP by list condition interaction is not an artifact of explicit contamination. Second, in contrast to the analysis of all participants, there was no effect of LOP in the random list condition, even though the effect was still robust in the blocked condition. This is consistent with the strong as well as the weaker version of the item-specific–relational account, and is reminiscent of the results of Smith and Hunt (2000). The difference judgments of Smith and Hunt, and LOP in the random list condition, are both considered item-specific manipulations, and both effects are eliminated in conceptual priming when the test-aware participants are removed from the analysis.

Finally, the results of the category-cued recall test were consistent with expectations. Recall exhibited a robust LOP effect in both the random and the blocked conditions, although the effect was somewhat larger in the latter case (significantly so in one experiment with only a trend in the other).

The conceptual priming results are in accord with the item-specific–relational analysis, in both its weaker and stronger forms. The LOP manipulation was more effective in a relational encoding context (the blocked condition) than when categorical-relational information was not salient (the random condition). In addition, removing test-aware participants eliminated the LOP effect in the random condition but not in the blocked condition.

DISTINCTIVENESS, ITEM-SPECIFIC PROCESSING, AND EXTENDING THE ANALYSIS TO OTHER IMPLICIT TESTS

The item-specific–relational analysis has been useful in accounting for dissociations between conceptual implicit and explicit memory tests. This chapter applied the general framework to the most commonly used conceptual implicit test—category-exemplar production—and its explicit counterpart—category-cued recall—arguing that the latter test is sensitive to both item-specific and relational information, whereas the former test is relatively insensitive to item-specific information, relying instead on relational (particularly categorical-relational) information. Consistent with the analysis, encoding variables thought to affect item-specific encoding (e.g., perceptual interference, pictures vs. words, word concreteness, difference judgments) affect category-cued recall but not category-exemplar production. In addition to accounting for existing dissociations, this account has also motivated reanalysis of the effects of generation and of LOP on category-exemplar production, successfully predicting the conditions under which these effects are and are not observed. In a similar manner, Mulligan and Stone (1999) applied this account to clarify the effects of divided attention on conceptual priming. These dissociations do not fit easily within the TAP account of implicit and explicit memory. Thus, the item-specific–relational framework appears to be a useful way to extend the analysis of implicit and explicit memory.

Two points should be made about the present analysis. First, it is not framed directly in terms of distinctiveness, but rather in terms of the item-specific–relational framework. The encoding variables of interest (such as generation and perceptual interference) are not prima facie distinctiveness manipulations in the same sense as are isolation or bizarreness manipulations. Rather, the connection between these manipulations and distinctiveness is indirect, mediated by evidence that these manipulations enhance memory via processing of the item's features in isolation and not by enhanced processing of the item's features in relation to other items. Other researchers who have used similar analyses have framed the issues more directly in terms of distinctiveness (e.g., Geraci & Rajaram, 2002; Hamilton & Rajaram, 2001; Smith & Hunt, 2000), concluding that distinctiveness effects emerge as a consequence of direct or explicit test instructions.

Second, this chapter has focused primarily on one measure of conceptual implicit memory: the category-exemplar production task. This raises the question of whether the analysis applies to perceptual implicit tests or even to other conceptual priming tasks. Several researchers have argued that it does. Regarding other conceptual tasks, several of the "distinctive-ness" dissociations reported earlier were obtained with conceptual priming tasks other than category-exemplar production. Weldon and Coyote (1996) found a picture-superiority effect for associate-cued recall but not for word association. Hamilton and Rajaram (2001) found a concreteness effect on question-cued recall test but not on the implicit version of the task, the general knowledge test. Finally, Smith and Hunt (2000) failed to find an effect of difference judgments on priming in word association (among test-unaware participants), even though this manipulation enhanced cued recall. These results indicate that the dissociative power of distinctiveness extends to other conceptual priming tests.[6]

The notion that distinctiveness effects are mediated by explicit retrieval, and its corollary, that implicit tests are insensitive to distinctiveness, may also hold for perceptual implicit tests. Geraci and Rajaram (2002) present one suggestive result. These authors examined the effects of orthographic distinctiveness on implicit and explicit memory. Previous research had shown that orthographically unusual words (e.g., *subpoena*) are better recalled than orthographically common words (e.g., *sailboat*; Hunt & Elliott, 1980). Geraci and Rajaram contrasted the effects of this distinctiveness variable on matched perceptual implicit and explicit tests—word fragment completion and word-fragment cued recall, respectively. Orthographic distinctiveness enhanced recall on the explicit test. In contrast, among the test-unaware participants, there was no distinctiveness effect on perceptual priming. Similarly, orthographic distinctiveness failed to affect priming in the perceptual identification task (Hunt & Toth, 1990). Orthographic distinctiveness produces a dissociation between perceptual implicit and explicit tests similar to the dissociations found between conceptual implicit and explicit tests. Although more research is needed on distinctiveness and perceptual implicit memory, initial results imply that perceptual implicit and explicit tests may exhibit the same differential sensitivity to distinctiveness (or item-specific effects) as conceptual implicit and explicit tests.

ACKNOWLEDGMENTS

Portions of this chapter were presented to the Southwestern Psychological Association, New Orleans, LA 2003.

NOTES

1. In fact, two versions of the category-cued recall tests were used and produced the same results. In the first, only the old categories were presented; in the second, both the old and new categories were presented and participants were additionally informed that some of the categories corresponded to studied words and others did not.

2. More specifically, no effect was found for test-unaware participants. Smith and Hunt (2000) gave participants a post-test questionnaire to assess test-awareness. The difference manipulation failed to affect conceptual priming among participants who claimed no awareness of the study-test relationship, whereas those claiming awareness exhibited the distinctiveness effect on the priming tasks. By the logic of the post-test questionnaires, the former group provides a purer assessment of implicit memory, ideally, uncontaminated by explicit retrieval strategies.

3. The exact nature of this information (item-specific representations that arise during word perception) is not critical to the rest of our discussion. Hirshman et al. (1994) characterized it as higher level (but nonvisual) perceptual information that plays a role in word perception, presumably phonological or semantic in nature (also see Mulligan, 1996, for discussion).

4. It should be noted that several researchers have made similar arguments regarding other manipulations of distinctiveness (e.g., generation, bizarreness), providing evidence that distinctiveness can have negative effects on relational information despite its enhancement of item-specific encoding (e.g., McDaniel, Einstein, DeLosh, May, & Brady, 1995; Nairne et al., 1991; Schmidt, Chapter 3 this volume; Worthen, Chapter 7 this volume).

5. The result summarized obtain primarily for lists of unrelated words. When the study words are related to one another (e.g., examples from the same taxonomic category), the situation differs as discussed shortly.

6. Although conceptual implicit tests may be alike in their relatively insensitivity to distinctiveness effects, other important differences might be found within the class of conceptual implicit test (e.g., Gabrieli et al., 1999). For example, category-exemplar production is not only insensitive to item-specific manipulations, it appears to be quite sensitive to categorical-relational information. Other conceptual priming tasks, such as word association and general knowledge questions, are presumably much less sensitive to categorical information.

REFERENCES

Begg, I., Snider, A., Foley, F., & Goddard, R. (1989). The generation effect is no artifact: Generating makes words distinctive. *Journal of Experimental Psychology: Learning, Memory, and Cognition, 15,* 977–989.

Burns, D. J. (1993). Item gains and losses during hypermnesic recall: Implications for the item-specific-relational information distinction. *Journal of Experimental Psychology: Learning, Memory, & Cognition, 19,* 163–173.

Burns, D. J. (1996). The item-order distinction and the generation effect: The importance of order information in long-term memory. *American Journal of Psychology, 109,* 567–580.

Cabeza, R. (1994). A dissociation between two implicit conceptual tests supports the distinction between types of conceptual processing. *Psychonomic Bulletin & Review, 1,* 505–508.

Craik, F. I. M., Moscovitch, M., & McDowd, J. M. (1994). Contributions of surface and conceptual information to performance on implicit and explicit tasks. *Journal of Experimental Psychology: Learning, Memory and Cognition, 20,* 864–875.

Curran, H. V. (2000). Psychopharmacological perspectives on memory. In E. Tulving & F. I. M. Craik (Eds.), *The Oxford handbook of memory* (pp. 539–554). New York: Oxford University Press.

Denny, E. B., & Hunt, R. R. (1992). Affective valence and memory in depression: Dissociation of recall and fragment completion. *Journal of Abnormal Psychology, 101,* 575–580.

deWinstanley, P. A., & Bjork, E. L. (1997). Processing instructions and the generation effect: A test of the multifactor transfer-appropriate processing theory. *Memory, 5,* 401–421.

Gabrieli, J. D. E. (1998). Cognitive neuroscience of human memory. *Annual Review of Psychology, 49,* 87–115.

Gabrieli, J. D. E., Vaidya, C. J., Stone, M., Francis, W. S., Thompson-Schill, S. L., Fleischman, D. A., Tinklenberg, J. R., Yesavage, J. A., & Wilson, R. S. (1999). Convergent behavioral and neuropsychological evidence for a distinction between identification and production forms of repetition priming. *Journal of Experimental Psychology: General, 128,* 479–498.

Gardiner, J. M., & Hampton, J. A. (1988). Item-specific processing and the generation effect: Support for a distinctiveness account. *American Journal of Psychology, 101,* 495–504.

Geraci, L., & Rajaram, S. (2002). The orthographic distinctiveness effect on direct and indirect tests of memory: Delineating the awareness and processing requirements. *Journal of Memory and Language, 47,* 273–291.

Hamann, S. B. (1990). Level-of-processing effects in conceptually driven implicit tasks. *Journal of Experimental Psychology: Learning, Memory and Cognition, 16,* 970–977.

Hamilton, M., & Rajaram, S. (2001). The concreteness effect in implicit and explicit memory. *Journal of Memory and Language, 44,* 96–117.

Hirshman, E., & Bjork, R. A. (1988). The generation effect: Support for a two-factor theory. *Journal of Experimental Psychology: Learning, Memory and Cognition, 14,* 484–494.

Hirshman, E., & Jackson, E. (1997). Distinctive perceptual processing and memory. *Journal of Memory and Language, 36,* 2–12.

Hirshman, E., & Mulligan, N. W. (1991). Perceptual interference improves explicit memory but does not enhance data-driven processing. *Journal of Experimental Psychology: Learning, Memory and Cognition, 17,* 507–513.

Hirshman, E., Trembath, D., & Mulligan, N. W. (1994). Theoretical implications of the mnemonic benefits of perceptual interference. *Journal of Experimental Psychology: Learning, Memory and Cognition, 20,* 608–620.

Hunt, R. R., & Einstein, G. O. (1981). Relational and item-specific information in memory. *Journal of Verbal Learning and Verbal Behavior, 19,* 497–514.

Hunt, R. R., & Elliott, J. M. (1980). The role of nonsemantic information in memory: Orthographic distinctiveness effects on retention. *Journal of Experimental Psychology: General, 109,* 49–74.

Hunt, R. R., & McDaniel, M. A. (1993). The enigma of organization and distinctiveness. *Journal of Memory & Language., 32,* 421–445.

Hunt, R. R., & Smith, R. E. (1996). Accessing the particular from the general: The power of distinctiveness in the context of organization. *Memory & Cognition, 24,* 217–225.

Hunt, R. R., & Toth, J. P. (1990). Perceptual identification, fragment completion, and free recall: Concepts and data. *Journal of Experimental Psychology: Learning, Memory, and Cognition, 16,* 282–290.

Jacoby, L. L. (1978). On interpreting the effects of repetition: Solving a problem versus remembering a solution. *Journal of Verbal Learning and Verbal Behavior, 17,* 649–667.

Jacoby, L. L., & Dallas, M. (1981). On the relationship between autobiographical memory and perceptual learning. *Journal of Experimental Psychology: General, 110,* 306–340.

Kinoshita, S. (1989). Generation enhances semantic processing? The role of distinctiveness in the generation effect. *Memory & Cognition, 17,* 563–571.

Klein, S. B., Loftus, J., Kihlstrom, J. F., & Aseron, R. (1989). Effects of item specific and relational information on hypermnesic recall. *Journal of Experimental Psychology: Learning, Memory and Cognition, 15,* 1192–1197.

Light, L. L. (1991). Memory and aging: Four hypotheses in search of data. *Annual Review of Psychology, 42,* 333–376.

Light, L. L., & Albertson, S. A. (1989). Direct and indirect tests of memory for category exemplars in young and older adults. *Psychology and Aging, 4,* 487–492.

Maki, P. M., & Knopman, D. S. (1996). Limitations of the distinction between conceptual and perceptual implicit memory: A study of Alzheimer's disease. *Psychology and Aging, 10,* 464–474.

Mandler, J. M. (1979). Categorical and schematic organization in memory. In C. R. Puff (Ed.), *Memory organization and structure* (pp. 259–299). New York: Academic Press.

McDaniel, M. A., Einstein, G. O., DeLosh, E. L., May, C. P., & Brady, P. (1995). The bizarreness effect: It's not surprising, it's complex. *Journal of Experimental Psychology: Learning, Memory, and Cognition, 21,* 422–435.

McDaniel, M. A., Moore, B. A., & Whiteman, H. L. (1998). Dynamic changes in hypermnesia across early and late tests: A relational/item-specific account. *Journal of Experimental Psychology: Learning, Memory, and Cognition, 24,* 173–185.

McDaniel, M. A., & Wadill, P. J. (1990). Generation effects for context words: Implications for item-specific and multifactor theories. *Journal of Memory and Language, 29,* 201–211.

McDaniel, M. A., Wadill, P. J., & Einstein, G. O. (1988). A contextual account of the generation effect: A three-factor theory. *Journal of Memory and Language, 27,* 521–536.

McDermott, K. B., & Roediger, H. L. (1996). Exact and conceptual repetition dissociate conceptual memory tests: Problems for transfer appropriate processing theory. *Canadian Journal of Experimental Psychology, 50,* 57–71.

McElroy, L. A., & Slamecka, N. J. (1982). Memorial consequences of generating nonwords: Implications for semantic-memory interpretations of the generation effect. *Journal of Verbal Learning and Verbal Behavior, 21,* 243–259.

Morris, C. D., Bransford, J. D., & Franks, J. J. (1977). Levels of processing versus transfer appropriate processing. *Journal of Verbal Learning and Verbal Behavior, 16,* 519–533.

Mulligan, N. W. (1996). The effects of perceptual interference at encoding on implicit memory, explicit memory, and memory for source. *Journal of Experimental Psychology: Learning, Memory and Cognition, 22,* 1067–1087.

Mulligan, N. W. (1998). The role of attention during encoding on implicit and explicit memory. *Journal of Experimental Psychology: Learning, Memory and Cognition, 24,* 27–47.

Mulligan, N. W. (1999). The effects of perceptual interference at encoding on organization and order: Investigating the roles of item-specific and relational information. *Journal of Experimental Psychology: Learning, Memory and Cognition, 25,* 54–69.

Mulligan, N. W. (2000a). Perceptual interference and memory for order. *Journal of Memory and Language, 43,* 680–697.

Mulligan, N. W. (2000b). Perceptual interference at encoding enhances item-specific encoding and disrupts relational encoding: Evidence from multiple recall tests. *Memory & Cognition, 28,* 539–546.

Mulligan, N. W. (2001). Generation and hypermnesia. *Journal of Experimental Psychology: Learning, Memory and Cognition, 27,* 436–450.

Mulligan, N. W. (2002). The effects of generation on conceptual implicit memory. *Journal of Memory and Language, 47,* 327–342.

Mulligan, N. W. (2003). Memory: Implicit versus explicit. In L. Nadel (Ed.), *Encyclopedia of cognitive science* (pp. 1114–1120). London: Nature Publishing Group/Macmillan.

Mulligan, N. W., Guyer, S., & Beland, A. (1999). The effects of levels-of-processing and organization on conceptual priming. *Memory & Cognition, 27,* 633–647.

Mulligan, N. W., & Hartman, M. (1996). Divided attention and indirect memory tests. *Memory & Cognition, 24,* 453–465.

Mulligan, N. W., & Stone, M. V. (1999). Attention and conceptual priming: Limits on the effects of divided attention in the category-exemplar production task. *Journal of Memory and Language, 41,* 253–280.

Nairne, J. S. (1988). The mnemonic value of perceptual identification. *Journal of Experimental Psychology: Learning, Memory and Cognition, 14,* 244–255.

Nairne, J. S., Reigler, G. L., & Serra, M. (1991). Dissociative effects of generation on item and order retention. *Journal of Experimental Psychology: Learning, Memory and Cognition, 17,* 702–709.

Paivio, A. (1991). Dual coding theory: Retrospect and current status. *Canadian Journal of Psychology, 45,* 255–287.

Rappold, V. A., & Hashtroudi, S. (1991). Does organization improve priming? *Journal of Experimental Psychology: Learning, Memory and Cognition, 17,* 103–114.

Roediger, H. L. (1990). Implicit memory: Retention without remembering. *American Psychologist, 45,* 1043–1056.

Roediger, H. L., & Blaxton, T. A. (1987). Retrieval modes produce dissociations in memory for surface information. In D. S. Gorfein & R. R. Hoffman (Eds.), *Memory and cognitive processes: The Ebbinghaus centennial conference* (pp. 349–379). Hillside, NJ: Lawrence Erlbaum Associates.

Roediger, H. L., Buckner, R. L., & McDermott, K. B. (1999). Components of processing. In J. K. Foster & M. Jelicic (Eds.), *Memory: Systems, process, or function* (pp. 31–65). New York: Oxford University Press.

Roediger, H. L., & McDermott, K. B. (1993). Implicit memory in normal human subjects. In F. Boller & J. Grafman (Eds.), *Handbook of neuropsychology* (Vol. 8, pp. 63–131). Amsterdam: Elsevier.

Roediger, H. L., Weldon, M. S., Stadler, M. A., & Reigler, G. H. (1992). Direct comparison of two implicit memory tests: Word fragment and word stem completion. *Journal of Experimental Psychology: Learning, Memory and Cognition, 18,* 1251–1269.

Schacter, D. L. (1987). Implicit memory: History and current status. *Journal of Experimental Psychology: Learning, Memory and Cognition, 13,* 501–518.

Schacter, D. L., & Badgaiyan, R. D. (2001). Neuroimaging of priming: New perspectives on implicit and explicit memory. *Current Directions in Psychological Science, 10,* 1–4.

Schwartz, B. L., Rosse, R. B., & Deutsch, S. I. (1993). Limits of the processing view in accounting for dissociations among memory measures in a clinical population. *Memory and Cognition, 21,* 63–72.

Shimamura, A. P. (1993). Neuropsychological analyses of implicit memory: History, methodology, and theoretical interpretations. In P. Graf & M. E. J. Masson (Eds.), *Implicit memory: New directions in cognition, development, and neuropsychology* (pp. 265–285). Hillside, NJ: Lawrence Erlbaum Associates.

Slamecka, N. J., & Graf, P. (1978). The generation effect: Delineation of a phenomenon. *Journal of Experimental Psychology: Human Learning and Memory, 4,* 592–604.

Slamecka, N. J., & Katsaiti, L. T. (1987). The generation effect as an artifact of selective displaced rehearsal. *Journal of Memory & Language, 26,* 589–607.

Smith, R. E., & Hunt, R. R. (2000). The effects of distinctiveness require reinstatement of organization: The importance of intentional memory instructions. *Journal of Memory and Language, 43,* 431–446.

Srinivas, K., & Roediger, H. L. (1990). Classifying implicit memory tests: Category association and anagram solution. *Journal of Memory and Language, 29,* 389–412.

Vaidya, C. J., Gabrieli, J. D. E., Keane, M. M., Monti, L. A., Gutierrez-Rivas, H., & Zarella, M. M. (1997). Evidence for multiple mechanisms of conceptual priming on implicit memory tests. *Journal of Experimental Psychology: Learning, Memory and Cognition, 23,* 1324–1343.

Weldon, M. S., & Coyote, K. C. (1996). Failure to find the picture superiority effect in implicit conceptual memory tests. *Journal of Experimental Psychology: Learning, Memory and Cognition, 22,* 670–686.

Westerman, D. L., & Greene, R. L. (1997). The effects of visual masking on recognition: Similarities to the generation effect. *Journal of Memory and Language, 37,* 584–596.

10

The Distinctiveness Effect in Explicit and Implicit Memory

Lisa Geraci and Suparna Rajaram

Much research supports the intuitive belief that people have very good memory for unusual or distinct information. This phenomenon has been called the *distinctiveness effect*. The majority of this research comes from studies using explicit memory tests on which people make a deliberate effort to remember past events. However, there is very little research examining the distinctiveness effect using different probes of memory, known as implicit tests. On implicit memory tests, people do not intend to remember, but nonetheless memory shows its effects behaviorally. In this chapter, our goal is to understand the role of awareness in mediating superior memory for unusual information. To do this, we will synthesize a select group of studies in which distinctiveness effects have been examined using explicit and implicit memory measures. In short, we ask, Can distinctiveness influence memory when one is not trying to remember? The answer to this question has important implications for current theories of distinctiveness that posit a prominent role for the reinstatement of the study context in producing the distinctiveness effect.

We begin the body of this chapter by describing the distinction between explicit and implicit memory tests. We then describe studies that demonstrate the effects of distinctiveness in explicit memory as well as those studies that show that distinctiveness is closely related to the vivid and recollective component of explicit memory. We focus on the processes that might be critical in producing the distinctiveness effect (independent of conscious recollection) and make the case that the effect can be obtained without conscious access to the study episode if these critical processes are reinstated at the time of test. Lastly, we provide empirical evidence for this claim; evidence that highlights some of the critical processes that produce the distinctiveness effect on both explicit and implicit memory tests.

EXPLICIT AND IMPLICIT MEMORY TESTS

Most common memory tests, such as recall and recognition, are designed to measure explicit memory. These tests require intentional (or explicit) reference to the episode to perform the task (e.g., recalling all the words presented on the study list). As such, these tests measure memory when one is attempting to retrieve information. In contrast, implicit memory tests are designed to measure the unintentional and unaware use of memory. These tests measure retention indirectly by having participants perform an ostensibly unrelated task, such as naming fragmented words or pictures, or generating items that belong to a category. For example, participants may study a list of words and then be given a series of word fragments (_ p _ l _) or word stems (*app___*), or a category cue (fruit) and be asked to either complete the fragments or stems with the first word that comes to mind or to simply list examples from the category. These tests are called implicit, or indirect, tests. Thus, the crucial procedural difference between explicit and implicit tests has to do with test instructions; explicit tests make a reference to the study episode and implicit tests do not (Graf & Schacter, 1985.)

One of the most influential accounts of processes underlying explicit and implicit test performance is the transfer appropriate processing framework (Roediger, 1990; Roediger, Weldon, & Challis, 1989). According to this framework, memory performance benefits to the extent that the conceptual or perceptual processing during the test recapitulates the same conceptual or perceptual processing that occurred at study, regardless of whether the test requires conscious reference to the study episode. The main contention is that the match in processing at study and during the test determines memory performance. Indeed, a large body of work supports this hypothesis (see Roediger & McDermott, 1993, for a review). According to this framework, there are two main classes of tests: perceptual and conceptual. Perceptual tests typically require participants to identify a degraded or fast presentation of a stimulus. Performance on these tests typically benefits from having previously performed similar perceptual analysis of the test items. For instance, the word-fragment and word-stem completion tests would fall into this category because performance on these tests benefits from having studied the item in that same physical format (e.g., studying the item as a word rather than as a picture). Similarly, the picture-fragment test would be considered a perceptual test because performance on this test benefits from previous study of the same format (in this case, studying the item as a picture rather than as a word; Weldon & Roediger, 1987). In both cases, the overlap across study and testing in the perceptual processing of physical features aids performance. Similarly, other changes in stimulus format, such as modality (visual versus auditory) of presentation influence performance on implicit tests that rely on the perceptual features of the stimulus (Blaxton, 1989; Graf & Mandler, 1984; Jacoby & Dallas, 1981; Rajaram & Roediger, 1993; Srinivas & Roediger, 1990).

In contrast, these perceptual manipulations do not generally influence performance on the other class of implicit tests, called *conceptual tests* (Blaxton, 1989; Challis & Sidhu, 1993; Srinivas & Roediger, 1990). The category production test described earlier (in which participants are presented with category labels and asked to list examples of the category) is considered a conceptual implicit memory test because performance on this and other similar tests is largely influenced by enhanced conceptual analysis of the items at study. For example, studying items for their meaning aids performance on conceptual implicit tests but not on perceptual tests described previously (e.g., Blaxton, 1989; Hamann, 1990; Srinivas & Roediger, 1990). With both types of implicit tests, though, memory is measured by the benefit in performance that results from recent study of the word or picture on the task of interest. This benefit in performance is called *priming* (Graf & Schacter, 1985; Tulving, Schacter, & Stark, 1982). We use this framework to organize and understand the body of data examining the distinctiveness effect in explicit and implicit memory.

THE DISTINCTIVENESS EFFECT ON EXPLICIT MEMORY TESTS

Several chapters in this book review research that shows that distinctiveness influences explicit memory test performance. Therefore, we will not cover all of this research here. Instead, we list just a few representative findings to illustrate the ubiquity of this phenomenon. The isolation, or von Restorff, effect (superior memory for isolated items) is perhaps the best-known example of the distinctiveness effect in memory. (We describe this effect in greater detail in a later section, and details of von Restorff's dissertation can be found in Hunt, 1995.) There are other results that have also been categorized as distinctiveness effects. These include the bizarreness effect (superior memory for bizarre sentences; McDaniel, Dunay, Lyman, & Kerwin, 1988) and the orthographic distinctiveness effect (superior memory for words with unusual orthographies; Hunt & Elliott, 1980; Hunt & Mitchell, 1978, 1982; Hunt & Toth, 1990). Several classic memory effects have also been attributed to distinctiveness. These include the levels-of-processing effect (better memory for items processed for meaning than for surface characteristics; Craik & Lockhart, 1972), the picture superiority effect (better memory for pictures than for words; Madigan, 1983; Nelson, 1979; Paivio, 1971; Shepard, 1967), and the imagery effect (better memory for imagined items than for perceived words; Paivio, 1971, 1991; see also Craik & Tulving, 1975; Weldon & Coyote, 1996; Marschark & Hunt, 1989, for respective interpretations of these effects in terms of distinctiveness). Similarly, the generation effect (better memory for generated items at study than for read items; Slamecka & Graf, 1978) and the concreteness effect (better memory for concrete nouns, such as *house*, than for abstract nouns, such as *humility;* see Paivio, 1971, for a review) have been interpreted in terms of distinctiveness (see Gardiner & Hampton, 1988; Hamilton & Rajaram, 2001, and Murdock, 1960, for interpretation of the respective effects). One can continue this list, and indeed by doing so the concept of distinctiveness could become too expansive and might seem underspecified. However, a careful consideration of the similarities and differences between these various effects also has the potential to advance the theoretical understanding about the notion of distinctiveness. For this reason, we have included many of these effects in our discussion of distinctiveness.

Recent research shows that distinctiveness does not simply affect explicit memory performance; it is in fact associated with the conscious recollective component of explicit memory (see Rajaram, 1996, 1998). This evidence comes from studies that have used the remember/know paradigm (Tulving, 1985) to isolate the effects on the recollective and familiarity components of explicit memory. In this paradigm, participants assign "remember" or "know" judgments to items that they recognize from a previous study episode. A "remember" judgment is assigned to a recognized item when participants can vividly recall encountering it in the study episode, and a "know" response is assigned when the recognized item is familiar but participants cannot recollect any specific details associated with studying the item. As such, remembering is considered a pure measure of explicit memory because it arises from volitional retrieval and is associated with one's vivid awareness that an event occurred as part of one's personal past (Tulving, 1985; Hamilton & Rajaram, 2003). Knowing, on the other hand, is considered to reflect the contributions from implicit memory (Gardiner, 1988; Gardiner & Parkin, 1990).

The differential nature of remembering and knowing has recently been conceptualized within a distinctiveness/fluency framework (Rajaram, 1996, 1998) where remembering is assumed to be influenced by processing the distinctive properties of the material and knowing is assumed to be influenced by the fluency, or the ease with which materials are processed (Rajaram, 1993; Rajaram & Geraci, 2000).

The distinctiveness/fluency framework receives support from different lines of evidence. For example, noting the distinctive features of a face increases remembering (Mantyla, 1997) and not knowing. In this study, participants studied faces, and either examined the differences between faces by noting the facial distinctiveness of various features or categorized the faces together based on general stereotypes, such as "intellectual" or "partygoer." Results showed that distinctive processing of individual features increased "remember" responses, whereas categorizing faces (presumably leading to schematization of information), increased "know" responses.

A test of this framework for the distinctiveness component came from a study in which the effects of orthographic distinctiveness were examined on remember/know judgments. The *orthographic distinctiveness effect* refers to the finding that words with unusual letter combinations, such as *subpoena*, are remembered better than words with more common letter combinations, such as *sailboat* (Hunt & Elliott, 1980; Hunt & Mitchell, 1978, 1982; Hunt & Toth, 1990; Zechmeister, 1969, 1972). This effect was observed for "remember" responses and not for "know" responses (Rajaram, 1998). Participants studied a list of orthographically common and distinct words. Replicating the standard finding in the literature, the results are shown in Figure 10.1, and they demonstrate that people had superior recognition for the orthographically distinct words. Interestingly, this effect selectively affected "remember" responses, and not "know" responses (Rajaram, 1998), demonstrating that the distinctiveness of the studied words affects remember and not know judgments.

The notion that remember but not know judgments are sensitive to distinctiveness has recently been challenged by evidence that estimates of familiarity show a distinctiveness effect (Kishiyama & Yonelinas, Chapter 17 this volume). In that approach, the familiarity estimate is computed as know/(1-remember) on the assumption that know judgments underestimate the operation of familiarity process. However, it is crucial to note, as these researchers do, that the distinctiveness/fluency framework was proposed to account for the influence of variables on direct measures of experiential states (remember and know) and not on the derived estimates of familiarity.

Interestingly, Kishiyama and Yonelinas (2003) have also reported novelty effects from the von Restorff paradigm on know judgments as well as on estimates of familiarity. These findings seem more challenging to the notion that fluency, and not distinctiveness, affects know judgments. However, only the know false alarms in this study were influenced by novelty, whereas the hit rates for know judgments were equivalent for novel and nonnovel items, and this complicates the interpretation of a distinctiveness

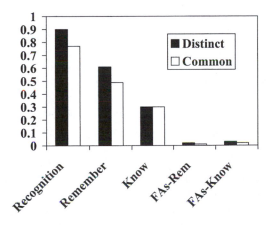

FIGURE 10.1 The effect of orthographic distinctiveness on remember responses, but not know responses. From Rajaram, 1998, p. 76. (Copyright 1998 by the Psychonomic Society. Reprinted with permission.)

effect on know judgments. Thus, it would be important to see whether these effects extend beyond know false alarms for nonnovel items to better understand their implications for the distinctiveness/fluency hypothesis. Findings from studies with amnesic participants are also relevant in the consideration of recollection and familiarity effects. Both recollection and familiarity processes are impaired in amnesia, but familiarity is reported to be less so (Yonelinas, Kroll, Dobbins, Lazzara, & Knight, 1998). To the extent that familiarity may be less impaired, a lack of a novelty effect on the familiarity process in amnesic participants (reported in Kishiyama & Yonelinas, Chapter 17 this volume) seems problematic for the idea that novelty affects familiarity.

Nevertheless, novelty effects reported by Kishiyama and Yonelinas raise interesting questions about the influence of distinctiveness on different forms of memory. As we later describe in this chapter, distinctiveness may not be limited to conscious recollection or explicit memory. Our reports of distinctiveness effects on measures of conceptual implicit memory may converge on the suggestion that distinctiveness effects can be associated with the automatic, familiarity-driven component of recognition (Kishiyama & Yonelinas, Chapter 17 this volume) to the extent that specific implicit measures can be shown to rely on automatic processes. For now, we return to our discussion of proposals that theoretically and experimentally tie distinctiveness to recollection.

THE IMPORTANCE OF REINSTATING THE STUDY CONTEXT

The conclusion that distinctiveness is associated with explicit memory (and not implicit memory) is consistent with prominent theories of distinctiveness. One set of ideas proposes that the distinctiveness effect depends critically on retrieval processes that reinstate the encoding context (Hunt, 1995; Hunt & McDaniel, 1993; Hunt & Smith, 1996; Waddill & McDaniel, 1998). Another set of ideas emphasizes the specific role of conscious recollection in this process of reinstatement (Smith & Hunt, 2000). Both lines of thinking emphasize the need to reinstate the encoding context to obtain a distinctiveness effect. Within this framework, we describe research demonstrating the importance of context, the retrieval processes that reinstate context, and the specific role of conscious awareness in mediating the reinstatement of context.

Study context is important for producing the distinctiveness effect (see Hunt, Chapter 1 this volume). Take for example, von Restorff's original work showing better memory for isolated items as compared to nonisolated items (see Hunt, 1995, or Wallace, 1965). This research shows that items are distinct only with respect to their context (see also Hunt, 1995, for an explanation of this idea). In one experiment from her classic dissertation work, von Restorff presented participants with a list of items on which all but one of the items was similar. Participants might see a list of numbers (9, 12, 3, 6 . . .) with one three-letter nonsense string (*QXK*) in the set. Or they might see the reverse, a list of nonsense three-letter stings (*QXK*) and one number (9) in the set. In both cases, people had superior memory for the isolated item, either the number or the three-letter nonsense string. The example makes it abundantly clear that study context is important. The number, 9, is not distinct at all unless it is presented in a list of letter strings. This type of distinctiveness may be contrasted with other effects where the item appears to be inherently distinct, such as the bizarreness effect (superior memory for bizarre sentences); the sentence "The dog rode the bicycle down the street" seems distinct regardless of the nature of the other sentences in the study list. Would the study context be important for this type of distinctiveness effect as well?

The difference between these two types of distinctiveness is captured nicely by Schmidt's (1991) distinction between primary and secondary distinctiveness effects. Using this classification, the isolation effect can be considered a primary distinctiveness effect because the isolated item differs from other items in its immediate context, or the study list, in this case. The bizarreness effect, on the other hand, can be considered a secondary distinctiveness effect because the sentence differs from the general set of items in its class stored in long-term memory (normal sentences). From this distinction, one might propose that only primary, not secondary, distinctiveness would rely on study context. Interestingly, it appears that even secondary distinctiveness effects, including the bizarreness effect, depend to some extent on study context.

Evidence for the importance of the study context comes from work showing that secondary distinctiveness effects depend critically on study-list construction. For example, the orthographic distinctiveness effect is obtained only when mixed-list designs are used and not between-subject designs (see Hunt & Elliott, 1980; Hunt & Mitchell, 1982). This finding contrasts with the idea that orthographically distinct words are inherently odd. Similarly, although bizarre sentences also appear to be inherently odd, this effect is typically obtained only using mixed-list designs (Waddill & McDaniel, 1998; see also McDaniel and Geraci, Chapter 4 this volume) and not between-list designs. The fact that even these distinctiveness effects typically occur only when people study lists that also include common items suggests that the distinctiveness effect, in general, depends on the study context. If this is true, then the distinctiveness effect may necessarily require direct reference to the study context at the time of retrieval.

According to one theory (Hunt & Smith, 1996; Matthews, Smith, Hunt, & Pivetta, 1999; Smith & Hunt, 2000), the study context is critical at test because it specifies a particular item in a particular setting. This idea can be captured in an everyday example; it is not sufficient to ask someone how his or her talk went without asking how the individual's talk went at the Southwestern Psychological Association (SWPA). Here, the name of the conference provides contextual information that, along with the target—

"your talk"—is highly diagnostic of the event. Thus, the context serves as a common cue that specifies the study episode (Hunt & Smith, 1996).

In a similar vein, the processing of contextual information is often described in terms of relational processing, and the processing of the target information is often described in terms of item-specific processing (Hunt, 1995; Hunt & Einstein, 1981; Hunt & McDaniel, 1993). Relational information results from processing the way in which items in a set are similar to each other (e.g., all events occurring at SWPA). Item-specific information results from processing the properties that are unique to a specific item (e.g., your talk). At retrieval, the two types of information act in concert to aid memory (Hunt, Ausley, & Schultz, 1986; Hunt & McDaniel, 1993; Hunt & Seta, 1984; Einstein & Hunt, 1980; Epstein, Phillips, & Johnson, 1975). Relational information helps to distinguish one episode from another and item-specific information helps to distinguish one item from another within that context. So, relational information may help people to generate possible candidates for recall, which may be defined by the particular episode; and item-specific information may help people discriminate between theses candidates (Hunt & Mitchell, 1982). These two types of information, in turn, provide highly diagnostic information that benefits memory performance (Hunt & McDaniel, 1993).

Recent research shows that it is critical to cue the relational information at retrieval to obtain the distinctiveness effect. In one experiment (Hunt & Smith, 1996), participants studied categorized lists and indicated either how an item is different or how it is similar to the other items in the list. For example, participants might have studied a list of fish including the category-exemplar *salmon*. In the difference-judgment condition, a participant might list "red" as a feature unique to salmon. In the similarity-judgment condition, a participant might list "swims" as a feature shared by all items. Results showed that memory was best when participants had provided a difference judgment (e.g., "red") at study and were given either their own difference cue again at test or another participant's common cue (e.g., "swims") at test.

Receiving one's own difference judgment aids memory, but importantly so does receiving another's common cue. Hunt and Smith (1996) suggest that the common cue (the similarity judgment) aids memory because it provides the context against which the distinctive processing becomes highly diagnostic of the particular item. The cue "swims" establishes the study episode (the list of fish) and the processing of difference (that one item is red) narrows the search to *salmon*. Therefore, Hunt and Smith (1996) suggest that the shared cue (that the items all swim) provides access to both the episode and the processing therein (that one of the items is red).

Thus, we see that the organizational context is critical at the time of retrieval. It is critical to reinstate the organizational information to be able to benefit from the distinctive information. There are various ways to reinstate the encoding context, but the most obvious way is to explicitly cue the context, "How did the talk you gave at SWPA go?" or its memory ex-

periment analog, "Was this word on the study list you saw earlier?" Because implicit tests, by definition, do not make reference to the study context, it is less likely that the encoding context is reinstated in these tests
and, as a result, they should not show the effects of distinctiveness.

THE LACK OF A DISTINCTIVENESS EFFECT ON IMPLICIT MEMORY TESTS

In a direct test of this hypothesis, Smith and Hunt (2000) provide evidence
that the distinctiveness effect influences explicit but not implicit memory
performance. In this study, distinctiveness was manipulated at study by
having participants judge how a category exemplar (e.g., *table*) was different from, or similar to, other exemplars (e.g., *chair, desk, couch . . .*).
At test, participants were given either an explicit test of cued recall or an
implicit test of word association or category-exemplar production. In the
explicit cued-recall test, participants saw a category label, such as *furniture*
and were asked to recall all the items from that category presented at study.
In the implicit word-association test, participants simply wrote 8 words
that were associated with the category label (e.g., *furniture*), and in the implicit category-exemplar test, participants listed 8 exemplars in response to
the cue. Results demonstrated a distinctiveness effect (i.e., better memory
for exemplars processed for difference than for similarity) only on the explicit test of cued recall and not on the implicit tests of word association
or category-exemplar production. Thus, these results provide direct evidence that the distinctiveness effect cannot be obtained using implicit tests,
and they further suggest that this is because the effect depends on explicitly reinstating the encoding context.

Other researchers have similarly proposed that the distinctiveness effect can be obtained only on explicit, and not on implicit, memory tests
(Weldon & Coyote, 1996). Weldon and Coyote suggested that explicit
memory tests benefit from intentional efforts to distinguish between studied and nonstudied information based on distinctive aspects of the studied information. They proposed this idea to explain the lack of a picture-superiority effect (better memory for pictures than words) on a
conceptual implicit test. According to leading theories, pictures are remembered better than words because pictures require more elaborative
processing of the item's meaning than does simply reading a word (Nelson, Reed, & McEvoy, 1977; Paivio, 1971,1991). Thus, a transfer-
appropriate processing view (Roediger, 1990; Roediger et al., 1989) of
memory would predict that the picture-superiority effect should occur
on all memory tests that require conceptual processing. This would include most explicit tests such as recall and recognition, and the data are
consistent with this hypothesis. Importantly, this view predicts that the
picture-superiority effect should be obtained on implicit tests that require

conceptual processing as well. In contrast to this prediction, Weldon and Coyote failed to find the picture-superiority effect on both conceptual tests of category production and word association. Results showed that pictures and words produced equivalent amounts of priming. However, when the same two tests were given with explicit instructions to produce only studied items, the picture-superiority effect emerged.

Weldon and Coyote interpreted the lack of a picture-superiority effect on the conceptual implicit tests by appealing to the notion of distinctiveness. They suggested that the picture-superiority effect is mediated by the visual distinctiveness of pictures. Because implicit tests typically have more than one possible answer, and people do not access particular episodes to discriminate studied items from other possible answers on these tests, performance does not benefit from distinctive processes or attributes. Other researchers have agreed that the distinctiveness of pictures, rather than conceptual processing of pictures, is critical, and this may explain the lack of a picture-superiority effect in conceptual priming. These researchers have applied this reasoning to explain the lack of a concreteness effect, yet another image-based "conceptual" effect, in conceptual priming (Hamilton & Rajaram, 2001).

Similarly, Mulligan (1996, 2002; Mulligan & Stone, 1999) has suggested that certain distinctiveness effects are not obtained on implicit tests because these tests require only relational processing and not relational and item-specific processing. The idea is that conceptual implicit tests, such as category production, simply require category knowledge—for example, as is represented by relational processes. However, explicit tasks show distinctiveness effects because these tests require both types of processes, item-specific and relational. For example, successful performance on category-cued recall requires access to both the relational category information and the specific studied item. Implicit tests do not typically show the effects of distinctive processing because they do not require item-specific information.

Other support for the idea that distinctiveness influences explicit memory but not implicit memory performance comes from studies examining the orthographic distinctiveness effect. This effect (superior memory for words like *subpoena* and *sphinx* that have unusual orthographies) is not obtained on the implicit test of word-fragment completion (Geraci & Rajaram, 2002). In this experiment, participants studied a list of orthographically common words (e.g., *sailboat*) and orthographically distinct words (e.g., *subpoena*). Half the participants were given the implicit test of word-fragment completion, in which they were asked to complete fragmented words (e.g., *s _ i l_ _ a t*) with the first word that comes to mind. The other half of the participants were given the same task with explicit instructions to complete the fragments with studied words. The data are shown in Figure 10.2. Results from the explicit version of the task replicated previous work using recall and recognition tests (Hunt & Elliott, 1980; Hunt & Mitchell, 1978, 1982; Hunt & Toth, 1990; Zechmeister,

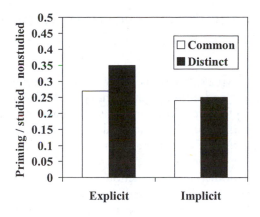

FIGURE 10.2 Results showing the effect of orthographic distinctiveness on an explicit test of word-fragment cued recall, but not on the implicit test of word-fragment completion. From Geraci and Rajaram, 2002, *Journal of Memory and Language, 47,* p. 281. (Copyright 2002 by Elsevier. Adapted with permission.)

1969, 1972) and showed superior memory for the orthographically distinct words: the distinctiveness effect. However, no such effect was obtained on the task when participants were given the same task with implicit instructions and were unaware of the connection between study and test (interestingly, those participants who reported being aware of the connection between study and test, despite our instructions, did show superior memory for the orthographically distinct words).

The orthographic distinctiveness effect is also not obtained on another implicit test, that of perceptual identification (Hunt & Toth, 1990). In this experiment, again participants studied orthographically common and distinct words. At test, they were asked to quickly identify intact but briefly presented words. Results showed no benefit in identification for distinct over common words.

In summary, the body of research on the orthographic distinctiveness effect shows that the effect is obtained on explicit tests of free recall (Hunt & Mitchell, 1982; Hunt & Elliott, 1980; Hunt & Toth, 1990), recognition (Hunt & Elliott, 1980), and explicit word-fragment cued recall (Geraci & Rajaram, 2002), and is associated with remember judgments (Rajaram, 1998). However, the effect is not obtained on implicit tests of word-fragment completion (Geraci & Rajaram, 2002) or perceptual identification (Hunt & Toth, 1990). As such, these findings suggest that the orthographic distinctiveness effect is an explicit memory phenomenon. In general, the studies discussed in this section support the hypothesis that distinctiveness influences explicit memory but not implicit memory.

Delineating the Processing That Mediates the Distinctiveness Effect

There are at least two explanations for why distinctiveness effects are obtained using explicit and not implicit memory tests. One hypothesis is that the distinctiveness effect requires conscious awareness of the study context (see Smith & Hunt, 2000). We discussed this hypothesis in the previous section. An alternate idea is that the distinctiveness effect requires recapitulating the processes typically associated with conscious recollection. We will discuss this hypothesis in this section.

Specifically, we have characterized the processes that mediate the distinctiveness effect in explicit memory as conceptual in nature on the assumption that they involve evaluating and comparing the different items to an established norm (Geraci & Rajaram, 2002). With the isolation effect discussed earlier, people may evaluate the isolated item as different from the standard item that is provided by the study list. With the orthographic distinctiveness effect, people may evaluate the odd-looking word as different from more common words in the English language. For the bizarreness effect, another distinctiveness effect we noted earlier, people may evaluate the bizarre sentence as strange compared to typical sentences, or they may evaluate the plausibility of the events described by the bizarre sentences. For other effects classified as distinctiveness effects, the type of conceptual processing may be different. We return to this issue later in our discussion of distinctiveness effects in implicit memory.

The idea that the critical processes that produce the distinctiveness effect are conceptual in nature is similar in some ways to previous theories of distinctiveness. Hunt and colleagues' theory of processing difference or item-specific information in the context of similarity suggests that the different item appears distinct against a background of similarity. Presumably the process that allows the different item to become distinct must have something to do with evaluating the item against this context. Thus, Hunt and colleagues' theory of processing difference in the context of similarity allows for the possibility that the process could be evaluative in nature. This idea of evaluative processing is also similar to some aspects to Schmidt's (1991) idea of incongruity. He describes the processing associated with incongruity and suggests that people engage in controlled memory processes that might include elaboration, rehearsal, or noting the relationships between the items in the study set. This last part, "noting the relationships between the items in the study set," could be taken as a similar notion to evaluating an item as different from some context. Building on these two ideas, we hypothesize that such processing is generally conceptual in nature, and to the extent the memory test capitalizes on this type of evaluative processing, the distinctiveness effect should be obtained.

Preliminary support for this idea has already been reported in some studies. For example, the orthographic distinctiveness effect is obtained only under study conditions that allow for higher level conceptual analysis, such as under full attention but not divided attention (Geraci & Rajaram, 2002). In this study, attention was divided using a digit-monitoring task that has been shown to selectively reduce conceptual processing (e.g., Culp & Rajaram, 1999; Craik, 1982; Jacoby, 1991). Participants studied a list of orthographically common and distinct words under either full or divided attention. Results from two experiments, which are shown in Figure 10.3, demonstrated that dividing attention at study selectively reduced memory for distinct words in free recall and further reduced it in word-fragment cued recall.

Results supported the hypothesis that the orthographic distinctiveness effect is mediated by conceptual processing to a considerable extent. Sim-

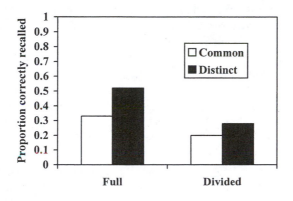

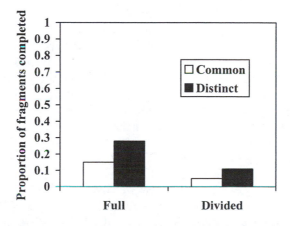

FIGURE 10.3 Results showing that divided attention reduces the effect of orthographic distinctiveness on explicit tests of free recall and word-fragment cued recall. From Geraci and Rajaram, 2002, p. 284. (Copyright 2002 by Elsevier. Reprinted with permission.)

ilarly, the orthographic distinctiveness effect is not obtained under test conditions that do not recapitulate these higher level processes, such as perceptual implicit memory tests that only benefit from low-level perceptual analysis (Geraci & Rajaram, 2002; Hunt & Toth, 1990). The lack of an orthographic distinctiveness effect on explicit memory tasks following encoding under divided attention, in conjunction with the lack of an effect in perceptual priming, provides converging evidence for the hypothesis that comparative, higher level processes are involved in mediating the distinctiveness effect. Note that the orthographic distinctiveness effect is obtained, however, when the study and testing conditions promote this type of analysis: under full-attention encoding followed by explicit testing conditions.

Supporting evidence for the hypothesis that conceptual processing is involved in the emergence of the distinctiveness effect also comes from an Event-related potential (ERP) study reported by Fabiani and Donchin (1995). This study examined the ERP components of the distinctiveness effect using an isolation manipulation in which one item was physically isolated (printed in large font) and one item was semantically isolated (from a different category). Results showed that only the P300 component, which is associated with encoding rare events, reliably predicted superior recall for both the physical and the semantic isolates. Fabiani and Donchin characterized the processing associated with P300 as conceptual in nature, and suggested that "the stimulus representation is compared with an ongoing memory representation" (p. 237), and that it is these comparative processes that predict superior memory for an isolated item. They further suggested that "the comparison-reorganization process that we believe is manifested by P300 would qualify as a conceptually driven process. Roediger et al. propose that direct memory tests, such as those used in the present study, would be particularly influenced by conceptually driven processes" (p. 237).

If this characterization of the conceptual processing that mediates the distinctiveness effect is correct, then a transfer-appropriate processing view of memory would also predict that the distinctiveness effect would be obtained on implicit memory tests as long as the tests recapitulate that critical conceptual process. To reiterate, according to the transfer-appropriate processing framework, memory performance on both explicit and implicit tests benefits to the extent that the test recapitulates the conceptual or perceptual processing from study (Roediger, 1990; Roediger et al., 1989). Here we refer to conceptual processes to include multiple types—evaluative processing as well as semantic analysis. Thus, our hypothesis requires that we differentiate between multiple conceptual processes as other researchers have recently done (see Cabeza, 1994; Hamilton & Rajaram, 2001; Vaidya et al., 1997; Weldon & Coyote, 1996). In the next section, we present evidence for our hypothesis showing a distinctiveness effect on conceptual implicit memory tests that recapitulate evaluative processes.

THE DISTINCTIVENESS EFFECT USING IMPLICIT MEMORY TESTS

Some indirect evidence demonstrates that the distinctiveness effect can be obtained on a conceptual implicit memory test. This evidence comes from research that was designed to assess the development of new conceptual associations in implicit memory (Srinivas, Culp, & Rajaram, 2000). In this study, participants saw pictures of common scenes that included many typical items as well as one critical congruent item and one critical incongruent item. For example, participants saw a picture of a restaurant scene containing a congruent item (e.g., *napkin*) and an incongruent item (e.g., *computer*). Participants also heard a dialog that clearly mentioned the congruent item and incorporated the incongruent item (e.g., "A student is writing a paper that is due tomorrow") into the scene without directly mentioning it. Then participants received either an explicit test of recognition or an implicit test of category verification. In this implicit test, the critical items in the scene were tested with verbal pairings of the ad hoc categories and target items (e.g., things found in a restaurant: computer) and by measuring the speed with which participants could indicate whether the items belonged to various ad hoc categories. Priming for the incongruent item was measured by the increase in reaction time to say no to the question "Does *computer* belong in the category of *things belonging in a restaurant*?" when *computer* was studied compared to when it was not studied.

On the explicit task of recognition, memory was superior for the incongruent item compared to the congruent item (a typical distinctiveness effect). Interestingly, the implicit test of category production also showed priming for the incongruent items: people were significantly slower to reject the once-incongruent item, *computer*, as belonging to the ad hoc category, *things found in a restaurant*, when it was studied compared to when it was not studied. These results provided evidence for the rapid development of new conceptual associations in implicit memory. Participants had learned to associate the incongruent item with the context, and were thus slowed down to reject it as a member of that context. The results also provide preliminary evidence that conceptual priming for incongruent items can be obtained.

A closer look at the procedure provides some insight into the factors that might be critical to producing priming for incongruent items. The category verification test required the participants to evaluate the target relative to its context. It required participants to evaluate whether *computer* belonged in the ad hoc category *things found in a restaurant* by having participants verify category membership. Unlike most distinctiveness manipulations, the incongruent item in this study had been integrated into the study scene via the accompanying dialog (explaining that the student had a paper due the next day). So, when participants studied the restaurant scene, for example, they integrated the computer into its context. Later, when given the category verification task, participants again had to evaluate whether the computer belonged in a restaurant. Because they had integrated the computer into the scene, they were slower to *disconfirm* that the computer belonged to the scene than they were to disconfirm that a nonstudied incongruent item belonged to a scene. Regardless of the direction of priming, this delay in disconfirming a studied incongruent item provides preliminary evidence for the idea that distinctive events can show conceptual priming.

We directly tested whether the distinctiveness effect could be obtained on a conceptual implicit memory test of category verification when the test recapitulated the distinctive process from the time of study (Geraci & Rajaram, 2003). Based on the discussion thus far, we characterize this process as evaluative in nature. This experiment used a classic isolation paradigm in which participants studied items that were either isolated in a study list (the word *table* was presented amid categorized items such as *salmon, trout, bass, tuna*) or not isolated (*table* was presented in a list of items all from different categories). Participants received either an explicit or an implicit test of category verification. We used this test to try to mimic the evaluative processes that participants presumably engage in at study after they encounter a list containing an incongruent item. For the implicit version of the test, participants were given the category *fish* and asked to verify or disconfirm whether *table* was a member of the category (note that regardless of whether *table* was studied in an isolated or nonisolated list, the correct response was always no). For the explicit version of the task, participants were given the same cues but asked to indicate whether they recognized the target item, *table*, as having been in the study list.

For the explicit version of the task, we predicted that people would show better recognition performance for items that were isolated in a list than items that were not isolated: the typical distinctiveness effect. For the implicit version of the task, we also predicted that we would obtain a distinctiveness effect. As in the study by Srinivas et al. (2000), we predicted that this effect would be present in reaction time and that accuracy would be at ceiling. However, unlike in the Srinivas et al. (2000) study, we predicted that participants would be *faster* to disconfirm category membership (to say no) for the isolated category members than the nonstudied and nonisolated members. We predicted a reaction-time advantage (instead of a disadvantage) for isolated category exemplars for the following reason. Unlike the Srinivas et al. (2000) study, the isolated category exemplars in the present study were not integrated into their study context. In the present study, participants did not have to learn to associate the isolated category member with the background items. Rather, they were simply required to read the items in the list. Because all but one item was from the same category, participants presumably evaluated this item as different or distinct. Note that the category verification test recapitulates this process by requiring participants to again disconfirm category membership for the critical items. Therefore, participants should be faster to engage in this same evaluation for the isolated items at test compared to the nonstudied and nonisolated items.

Results supported these predictions: people had better recognition for category exemplars that had been isolated in a list at study than those that had been presented in an unrelated list. We obtained the typical distinctiveness effect in explicit memory. Critically, we also obtained greater priming for isolated items as compared to nonisolated items on a category verification test. This study showed that reaction times to disconfirm category membership for the isolated items were significantly faster than reaction times to disconfirm membership for the nonisolated items. Thus, we also obtained the distinctiveness effect in implicit memory.

We have suggested that it is critical to reinstate the distinctive processing from study at the time of test to obtain the distinctiveness effect in implicit memory. For the isolation effect just discussed, we have characterized this processing as evaluative in nature—as the study context unfolds, people notice and evaluate the different item as distinct. Thus, it is critical to develop an implicit test that requires this same process for this distinctiveness effect to emerge. Similarly, for the orthographic distinctiveness effect, it would be ideal to develop an implicit memory test that accesses the evaluation of the word as unusual with respect to typical words in the English language. This would be far more difficult but the same principle would apply.

In contrast to these two distinctiveness effects that appear to rely on a comparison against common items (e.g., both require mixed-list designs), other effects that have been classified as distinctiveness effects do not appear to gain their "distinctiveness" by comparison. Take, for example, the picture-superiority effect. Few people would argue that pictures gain their distinctiveness by a comparison against words. Indeed, people have superior memory for pictures in between-subjects designs where one group of participants studies only pictures and the other group studies only words (e.g., Hamilton & Geraci, in press; McDermott & Roediger, 1996; Paivio & Csapo, 1973; Paivio, Rogers, & Smythe, 1968; Shepard, 1967). Given this result, the processing that mediates the picture-superiority effect is likely not comparative in nature. Instead, the picture-superiority effect is typically thought to be mediated by elaborative processing that arises from increased perceptual detail (Paivio, 1971, 1991). The idea is that because pictures are more visually distinct, they provide more semantic information about the object than does studying its word label (Nelson et al., 1977).

As mentioned earlier, in contrast to the predictions of the transfer-appropriate processing theory, however, recent studies have demonstrated that the picture-superiority effect is difficult to obtain using conceptual implicit memory tests that are designed to access semantic processing (Hamilton, 2000; McDermott & Roediger, 1996; Weldon & Coyote, 1996; but see Vaidya & Gabrieli, 2000). Based on the failure to obtain a picture-superiority effect on a conceptual implicit memory test, some researchers have suggested that the picture-superiority effect may be better explained by the visual distinctiveness of the pictures (Hamilton & Rajaram, 2001;

Weldon & Coyote, 1996; see also Nicolas & Marchal, 1996, for failure to find a picture bizarreness effect on a conceptual implicit test). However, it may not be the visual distinctiveness per se that mediates the memory advantage for pictures. Instead, the visual information contributes to the *conceptual salience* of pictures. Take, for example, a picture of an owl. Everyone knows that owls have big eyes. In fact, this is probably the most salient visual information about an owl. However, it is not that the eyes provide physical information that aids memory performance. More likely, the eyes provide the perceptual basis for what it is that distinguishes owls from other animals. As such, this information is conceptually diagnostic of the item and likely aids memory in this way. By this view, pictures are remembered better than words because they provide conceptually distinctive information that discriminates them from other items in the list and other items from that category, whereas words do not.

To test this hypothesis, participants were given two conceptual implicit memory tests (Hamilton & Geraci, in press). Both tests accessed semantic information, but only one emphasized the conceptually distinctive information about pictures (e.g., the eyes). We measured the picture-superiority effect using both a standard general knowledge test (see Blaxton, 1989) and a version of this test that we created to emphasize the individuating features of pictures. In the standard general-knowledge test, people study words such as *owl*, which later serve as answers to general-knowledge questions such as, "What bird is the figurehead of Tootsie-Roll Pops?" In the "distinctive" version of the standard test that we created, people were given general-knowledge questions that accessed the distinctive information about the items: "What animal has big eyes?" Priming, or implicit memory, is measured by participants' increased likelihood of answering the question with the word *owl* when it was studied than when it was not studied. A picture-superiority effect on either implicit test would be obtained if priming were greater when people had studied a picture of an owl than when they had simply read the word *owl*.

Results from the standard general-knowledge test replicated earlier work and showed no benefit in priming for pictures over words (Hamilton, 2000; McDermott & Roediger, 1996; Weldon & Coyote, 1996). However, using the distinctive cues test, we obtained the picture-superiority effect: pictures showed greater priming than words using test cues that access the conceptually distinctive attributes of pictures. This finding not only reveals some of the critical processes that mediate picture processing, but it also suggests that the distinctiveness effect can be obtained in the absence of conscious awareness when the test recapitulates the distinctive processing from study.

CONCLUSIONS

As several contributions in this volume, as well as findings from our work show, distinctiveness ubiquitously aids explicit memory performance. In this chapter, we have shown that it can also aid implicit memory. The general point is that while conscious recollection is sufficient to produce a distinctiveness effect in memory, it is not necessary. However, in the absence of conscious awareness, it is critical to create test conditions that reinstate evaluative processes. We reported recent work that illustrates this point.

This work further suggests that implicit tests provide a way to identify the processes that give rise to the distinctiveness effect. For the isolation effect, we tested the hypothesis that this distinctive processing is conceptual and evaluative in nature. For the picture-superiority effect, we tested the hypothesis that this processing is conceptual in nature too, but that it involves an analysis of the discriminative features of the objects. For other effects, the processing may be different, but we believe that it is fruitful to examine the various effects attributed to distinctiveness using implicit memory tests. This line of inquiry would help distinguish among the underlying processes that mediate these various distinctiveness effects.

The work reported in this chapter has implications for theories of distinctiveness and for theories of implicit memory. One view of distinctiveness proposes that the effect depends critically on reinstating the organizational context provided by the study list. However, the effects we obtained in implicit memory suggest that it is not necessary to consciously reinstate this context. Instead, we propose that it is necessary to reinstate the distinctive processes from study when conscious reference to the encoding episode is not involved. This hypothesis has implications for views of explicit and implicit memory. First, it suggests that there are multiple types of conceptual processes (as opposed to just one unitary process) that are important to consider. This point reconciles two accounts of implicit and explicit test performance. One account suggests that distinctiveness (and not conceptual or perceptual processing) is the critical factor that distinguishes implicit and explicit test performance (see Smith & Hunt, 2000). Another account suggests that conceptual and perceptual processes determine performance on both types of tests (Roediger, 1990; Roediger et al., 1989), and a variant on this second view is that there are different types of conceptual processes. Our data suggest that both ideas are necessary to account for explicit and implicit memory performance.

ACKNOWLEDGMENTS

Suparna Rajaram was supported by NIH grant R29MH57345. Portions of this chapter were presented to the Southwestern Psychological Association, New Orleans, LA, April 2003.

REFERENCES

Blaxton, T. (1989). Investigating dissociations among memory measures: Support for a transfer-appropriate processing framework. *Journal of Experimental Psychology: Learning, Memory, and Cognition, 15,* 657–668.

Cabeza, R. (1994). A dissociation between two implicit conceptual tests supports the distinction between types of conceptual processing. *Psychonomic Bulletin & Review, 1,* 505–508.

Challis, B. H. & Sidhu, R. (1993). Dissociative effect of massed repetition on implicit and explicit measures of memory. *Journal of Experimental Psychology: Learning, Memory, & Cognition, 19,* 115–127.

Craik, F. I. M. (1982). Selective changes in encoding as a function of reduced-processing capacity. In F. Klix, J. Hoffman & E. van der Meer (Eds.), *Cognitive research in psychology* (pp. 152–161). Amsterdam: North-Holland.

Craik, F. I. M., & Lockhart, R. S. (1972). Levels of processing: A framework for memory research. *Journal of Verbal Learning and Verbal Behavior, 11,* 671–684.

Craik, F. I. M., & Tulving, E. (1975). Depth of processing and the retention of words in episodic memory. *Journal of Experimental Psychology: General, 104,* 268–294.

Culp, D., & Rajaram, S. (1999, November). *Divided attention at encoding and retrieval differentially affects conceptual priming.* Paper presented at the 40th Annual Meeting of the Psychonomic Society, Dallas, TX.

Einstein, G. O., & Hunt, R. R. (1980). Levels of processing and organization: Additive effects of individual item and relational processing. *Journal of Experimental Psychology: Learning, Memory, and Cognition, 6,* 588–598.

Epstein, M. L., Phillips, W. D., & Johnson, S. J. (1975). Recall of related and unrelated word pairs as a function of processing level. *Journal of Experimental Psychology: Learning, Memory, and Cognition, 1,* 149–152.

Fabiani, M., & Donchin, E. (1995). Encoding processes and memory organization: A model of the von Restorff effect. *Journal of Experimental Psychology: Learning, Memory, and Cognition, 21,* 224–240.

Gardiner, J. M. (1988). Functional aspects of recollective experience. *Memory & Cognition, 16,* 309–313.

Gardiner, J. M., & Hampton, J. A. (1988) Item-specific processing and the generation effect: Support for a distinctiveness account. *American Journal of Psychology, 101,* 495–504.

Gardiner, J. M., & Parkin, A. J. (1990). Attention and recollective experience in recognition memory. *Memory & Cognition, 18,* 579–583.

Geraci, L., & Rajaram, S. (2002). The orthographic distinctiveness effect on direct and indirect tests of memory: delineating the awareness and processing requirements. *Journal of Memory and Language, 47,* 273–291.

Geraci, L., & Rajaram, S. (2003). *The distinctiveness effect in the absence of conscious recollection: Evidence from conceptual priming.* Manuscript submitted for publication.

Graf, P., & Mandler, G. (1984). Activation makes words more accessible, but not necessarily more retrievable. *Journal of Verbal Learning and Verbal Behavior, 23,* 553–568.

Graf, P., & Schacter, D. L. (1985). Implicit and explicit memory for new associations in normal and amnesic subjects. *Journal of Experimental Psychology: Learning, Memory, & Cognition, 11,* 501–518.

Hamann, S. (1990). Level-of-processing effects on conceptually driven implicit tasks. *Journal of Experimental Psychology: Learning, Memory, & Cognition, 16,* 970–977.

Hamilton, M. (2000). *Accessing meaning in implicit conceptual memory.* Doctoral dissertation, State University of New York, Stony Brook. *Dissertation abstracts international, 60,* 4265.

Hamilton, M., & Geraci, L. (in press). The picture superiority effect on a conceptual implicit memory test with distinctive cues. *American Journal of Psychology.*

Hamilton, M., & Rajaram, S. (2001). The concreteness effect in implicit and explicit memory tests. *Journal of Memory and Language, 44,* 96–117.

Hamilton, M., & Rajaram, S. (2003). States of awareness across multiple memory tasks: Obtaining a "pure" measure of conscious recollection. *Acta Psychologica, 112,* 43–69.

Hunt, R. R. (1995). The subtlety of distinctiveness: What von Restorff really did. *Psychonomic Bulletin & Review, 2,* 105–112.

Hunt, R. R., Ausley, J. A., & Schultz, E. E. (1986). Shared and item-specific information in memory for even descriptions. *Memory and Cognition, 14,* 49–54.

Hunt, R. R., & Einstein, G. O. (1981). Relational item-specific information in memory. *Journal of Verbal Learning and Verbal Behavior, 19,* 497–514.

Hunt, R. R., & Elliott, J. M. (1980). The role of nonsemantic information in memory: Orthographic distinctiveness effects on retention. *Journal of Experimental Psychology: General, 109,* 49–74.

Hunt, R. R., & McDaniel, M. A. (1993). The enigma of organization and distinctiveness. *Journal of Memory and Language, 32,* 421–445.

Hunt, R. R., & Mitchell, D. B. (1978). Specificity in nonsemantic orienting tasks and distinctive memory traces. *Journal of Experimental Psychology: Human Learning & Memory, 4,* 121–135.

Hunt, R. R., & Mitchell, D. B. (1982). Independent effects of semantic and nonsemantic distinctiveness. *Journal of Experimental Psychology: Learning, Memory, and Cognition, 8,* 81–87.

Hunt, R. R., & Seta, C. E. (1984). Category size effects in recall: The roles of relational and individual item information. *Journal of Experimental Psychology: Learning, Memory, and Cognition, 10,* 454–464.

Hunt, R. R., & Smith, R. E. (1996). Accessing the particular from the general: The power of distinctiveness in the context of organization. *Memory and Cognition, 24,* 217–225.

Hunt, R. R., & Toth, J. P. (1990). Perceptual identification, fragment completion, and free recall: Concepts and data. *Journal of Experimental Psychology: Learning, Memory, and Cognition, 16,* 282–290.

Jacoby, L. L. (1991). A process dissociation framework: Separating automatic from intentional uses of memory. *Journal of Memory and Language, 30,* 513–541.

Jacoby, L. L. & Dallas, M. (1981). On the relationship between autobiographical memory and perceptual learning. *Journal of Experimental Psychology General, 110,* 306–340.

Kishiyama, M. M. & Yonelinas, A. P. Novelty effects on recollection and familiarity in recognition memory. *Memory & Cognition, 31,* 1045–1051.

Madigan, S. (1983). Picture memory. In J. C. Yuille (Ed.), *Imagery, memory and cognition: Essays in honor of Allan Paivio* (pp. 65–89). Hillsdale, NJ: Lawrence Erlbaum Associates.

Mantyla, T. (1997). Recollections of faces: Remembering differences and knowing similarities. *Journal of Experimental Psychology: Learning, Memory, and Cognition, 23,* 1–14.

Matthews, T. D., Smith, R. E., Hunt, R. R., & Pivetta, C. E. (1999). Role of distinctive processing during retrieval. *Psychological Reports, 84,* 904–916.

Marschark, M., & Hunt, R. R. (1989). A reexamination of the role of imagery in learning and memory. *Journal of Experimental Psychology: Learning, Memory, & Cognition,15,* 710–720.

McDaniel, M. A., Dunay, P. K., Lyman, B. J., & Kerwin, M. E. (1988). Effects of elaboration and relational distinctiveness on sentence memory. *American Journal of Psychology, 101,* 357–369.

McDermott, K. B., & Roediger, H. L. (1996). Exact and conceptual repetition dissociate conceptual memory tests: Problems for transfer appropriate processing theory. *Canadian Journal of Experimental Psychology, 50,* 57–71.

Mulligan, N. W. (1996). The effects of perceptual interference at encoding on implicit memory, explicit memory, and memory for source. *Journal of Experimental Psychology: Learning, Memory, and Cognition, 22,* 1067–1087.

Mulligan, N. W. (2002). The effects of generation on conceptual implicit memory. *Journal of Memory and Language, 47,* 327–342.

Mulligan, N. W., & Stone, M. V. (1999). Attention and conceptual priming: limits on the effects of divided attention in the category-exemplar production task. *Journal of Memory and Language, 41,* 253–280.

Murdock, B. B. (1960). The distinctiveness of stimuli. *Psychological Review, 67,* 16–31.

Nelson, D. L. (1979). Remembering pictures and words: Appearance, significance, and name. In L. S. Cermak & F. I. M. Craik (Eds.), *Levels of processing in human memory* (pp. 45–76). Hillsdale, NJ: Lawrence Erlbaum Associates.

Nelson, D. L., Reed, V. S., & McEvoy, C. L. (1977). Learning to order picture and words: A model of sensory and semantic encoding. *Journal of Experimental Psychology: Learning, Memory, and Cognition, 3,* 485–497.

Nicolas, S., & Marchal, A. (1996). Picture bizarreness effect and word association. *Current Psychology of Cognition, 15,* 629–643.

Paivio, A. (1971). *Imagery and verbal processes.* Oxford: Holt, Rinehart & Winston.

Paivio, A. (1991). Dual coding theory: Retrospect and current status. *Canadian Journal of Psychology, 45,* 255–287.

Paivio, A., & Csapo, K. (1973). Picture superiority in free recall: Imagery or dual coding? *Cognitive Psychology, 5,* 176–206.

Paivio, A., Rogers, T. B., & Smythe, P. C. (1968). Why are pictures easier to recall than words? *Psychonomic Science, 11,* 137–138.

Rajaram, S. (1993). Remembering and knowing: Two means of access to the personal past. *Memory & Cognition, 21,* 89–102.

Rajaram, S. (1996). Perceptual effects on remembering: Recollective processes in picture recognition memory. *Journal of Experimental Psychology: Learning,Memory, and Cognition, 22,* 365–377.

Rajaram, S. (1998). The effects of conceptual salience and perceptual distinctiveness on conscious recollection. *Psychological Bulletin & Review, 5,* 71–78.

Rajaram, S., & Geraci, L. (2000). Conceptual fluency selectively influences knowing. *Journal of Experimental Psychology: Learning, Memory, & Cognition, 26,* 1070–1074.

Rajaram, S. & Roediger, H. L. (1993). Direct comparison of four implicit memory tests. *Journal of Experimental Psychology: Learning, Memory, & Cognition, 19,* 765–776.

Roediger, H. L. III (1990). Implicit memory: retention without remembering. *American Psychologist, 45,* 1043–1056.

Roediger, H. L. III., & McDermott, K. B. (1993). Implicit memory in normal human subjects. In F. Boller & J. Grafman (Eds.), *Handbook of neuropsychology* (Vol. 8, pp. 63–131). Amsterdam: Elsevier.

Roediger, H. L., Weldon, M. S., & Challis, B. H. (1989). Explaining dissociations between implicit and explicit measures of retention: A processing account. In H. L. Roediger & F. I. M. Craik (Eds.), *Varieties of memory and consciousness: Essays in honor of Endel Tulving* (pp. 3–41), Hillsdale, NJ: Lawrence Erlbaum Associates.

Schmidt, S. R. (1991). Can we have a distinctive theory of memory? *Memory and Cognition, 19,* 523–542.

Srinivas, K. & Roediger, H. L. (1990). Classifying implicit memory tests: Category association and anagram solution. *Journal of Memory and Language, 29,* 389–412.

Shepard, R. N. (1967). Recognition memory for words, sentences, and pictures. *Journal of Verbal Learning & Verbal Behavior, 6,* 156–163.

Slamecka, N. J., & Graf, P. (1978). The generation effect: Delineation of a phenomenon. *Journal of Experimental Psychology: Human Learning and Memory, 4,* 592–604.

Smith, R. E., & Hunt, R. R. (2000). The effects of distinctiveness require reinstatement of organization: The importance of intentional memory instructions. *Journal of Memory and Language, 43,* 431–446.

Srinivas, K., Culp, D., & Rajaram, S. (2000). On associations between computers and restaurants: Rapid learning of new associations on a conceptual implicit memory test. *Memory & Cognition, 28,* 900–906.

Tulving, E. (1985). Memory and consciousness. *Canadian Psychologist, 26,* 1–12.

Tulving, E., Schacter, D. L., & Stark, H. A. (1982). Priming effects in word-fragment completion are independent of recognition memory. *Journal of Experimental Psychology: Human Learning and Memory, 8,* 336–342.

Vaidya, C. J., & Gabrieli, J. D. E. (2000). Picture superiority in conceptual memory: Dissociative effects of encoding and retrieval tasks. *Memory and Cognition, 28,* 1165–1172.

Vaidya, C. J., Gabrieli, J. D. E., Keane, M. M., Monti, L. A., Gutierrez-Rivas, H., & Zarella, M. M. (1997). Evidence for multiple mechanisms of conceptual priming on implicit memory tests. *Journal of Experimental Psychology: Learning, Memory and Cognition, 23,* 1324–1343.

Waddill, P. J., & McDaniel, M. A. (1998). Distinctiveness effects in recall: Differential processing or privileged retrieval? *Memory and Cognition, 26,* 108–120.

Wallace, W. P. (1965). Review of the historical, empirical, and theoretical status of the von Restorff phenomenon. *Psychological Bulletin, 63,* 410–424.

Weldon, M. S., & Coyote, K. C. (1996). Failure to find the picture superiority effect in implicit conceptual memory tests. *Journal of Experimental Psychology: Learning, Memory and Cognition, 22,* 670–686.

Weldon, M. S. & Roediger, H. L. (1987). Altering retrieval demands reverses the picture superiority effect. *Memory & Cognition, 15,* 269–280.

Yonelinas, A. P., Kroll, N. E. A., Dobbins, I., Lazzara, M., & Knight, R. T. (1998). Recollection and familiarity deficits in amnesia: Convergence of remember-know, process dissociation, and receiver operating characteristic data. *Neuropsychology, 12,* 323–339.

Zechmeister, E. B. (1969). Orthographic distinctiveness. *Journal of Verbal Learning and Verbal Behavior, 8,* 754–761.

Zechmeister, E. B. (1972). Orthographic distinctiveness as a variable in word recognition. *American Journal of Psychology, 85,* 425–430.

IV

DISTINCTIVENESS AND MEMORY ACROSS THE LIFE SPAN

11

Distinctiveness Effects in Children's Memory

Mark L. Howe

All of the research discussed in this volume leaves little doubt about the importance of distinctiveness in memory. Given this impressive body of evidence, it is fair to conclude that unusual or unique information tends to be better learned and remembered than more commonplace information. Of course, what we mean by unusual or unique is often difficult to define in any absolute sense (see Hunt, Chapter 1 this volume; Schmidt, 1991). Instead, it is often necessary to restrict its definition to the processing of those aspects of stimuli (memory lists, events, etc.) that are unusual or unique relative to some specified context (Medin, Goldstone, & Gentner, 1993). Here, two type of contexts are relevant: (1) the immediate or primary context in which the distinctive information appears and (2) the more global or secondary context in which the individual's greater knowledge base defines which information is distinctive. In proposing these contextually driven definitions of distinctiveness, Schmidt (1991) reasoned that unique (distinctive) items are conceptually incongruous if they do not fit currently active cognitive structures or contain salient features not present in active memory. Accordingly, *primary distinctiveness* occurs when there is a mismatch between the features of an item and the features active in primary memory as defined by other recently presented items. In contrast, *secondary distinctiveness* involves a mismatch between the features of an item and those that are already stored in long-term (or secondary) memory derived from the larger context of previous experiences. Although secondary distinctiveness can be viewed as independent of the primary context, the reverse is not true. This is because distinctiveness in the local context is dependent on the more general context that the individual brings to the situation. Thus, an animal exemplar is distinctive in a given primary context of a list of clothing exemplars only if the individual brings with them the knowledge that animal and clothing categories are different. This point is especially important when considering distinctiveness effects in children's memory, as they must understand the relevant conceptual distinctions before they can use them to integrate similar information into well-organized and cohesive wholes, and then use distinctiveness to discriminate unique and novel information.

Using definitions like this one, researchers have developed a diverse array of manipulations to extort distinctiveness effects in human memory, including varying the semantic (e.g., Hunt & Mitchell, 1982; Schmidt, 1985) and orthographic properties of individual words (e.g., Hunt & Elliot, 1980), the visual properties associated with facial features (e.g., Winograd, 1981), emotional components of flashbulb (Brown & Kulik, 1977) or traumatic events (Loftus & Burns, 1982), olfactory properties of odor-evoked memories (e.g., Herz, 1997; Herz & Cupchik, 1995), memory for humorous text (Kintsch & Bates, 1977), and bizarre images (e.g., Cox & Wollen, 1981; Einstein, McDaniel, & Lackey, 1989; Fritsch & Larsen, 1990; O'Brien & Wolford, 1982; for a review, see Worthen, Chapter 7 this volume), and so forth. This operational definition of distinctiveness is also useful in the study of autobiographical memories where particularly well-remembered events include those that are personally consequential (e.g., Conway, 1996), are change points or formative periods (e.g., Rubin & Schulkind, 1997), or are unique with respect to the self (e.g., Csikszentmihalyi & Beattie, 1979).

Because these facts are now so well documented, at least in the literature on adult memory, in this chapter I focus on a significant gap in this literature—namely, the importance of distinctiveness in the development of memory in childhood. In what follows, I outline what research does exist in children's memory and distinctiveness, both in more traditional paradigms (e.g., isolation effects, bizarre imagery, and similarity and difference judgments) and in some less traditional areas (e.g., intentional forgetting, recoding, and false memories). These data will be reviewed in two contexts—namely, immediate memory and long-term retention of information over protracted periods of time. Having described the extant database, I then consider the theoretical importance of distinctiveness effects in memory development and briefly describe two recent theories that can account for these developments. Finally, I discuss the importance of localizing distinctiveness effects in basic memory processes of encoding, storage, and retrieval.

ESTABLISHING THE IMPORTANCE OF DISTINCTIVENESS IN MEMORY DEVELOPMENT

Extant Data

As noted, although the role of distinctiveness in memory is well established in adults, the same cannot be said for its role in children's memory. Given the large body of evidence that shows that many of the mechanisms and processes that govern storage and retrieval in young children are the same as those that regulate memory processes in older children and adults (e.g., Howe, 2000), it might be tempting to conclude that the effects of distinctiveness should translate easily to children's memory. Unfortunately, such an assumption has not always panned out, largely because of the significant developmental advances in memory that occur across childhood (e.g., faster encoding, storage, and retrieval; greater ability to maintain information in storage for longer periods of time), ones that are contingent on advances in related cognitive processes (e.g., knowledge, attention, strategies, metamemory; see Howe, 2000). It is this latter set of changes that occur in children's semantic processing that may be particularly critical to our understanding of how distinctiveness effects change with development.

On the one hand, there is evidence that distinctiveness, broadly defined, is important from birth. Indeed, there is considerable evidence that shows that even in infancy, children, like adults, focus on features or elements of events that are surprising, unique, or novel—ones that violate their expectations (for recent reviews, see Howe, 1998a, 1998b). Children also respond (perceive and recognize) more favorably to distinctive information in faces (Rhodes & Moody, 1990) and caricatures (Chang, Levine, & Benson, 2002), with older children being more responsive than younger children. On the other hand, research on the use of distinctiveness to enhance children's *memory performance* (rather than attention and possibly encoding) is rare. When these effects have been obtained, it is clear that children (particularly older children) can remember atypical information better than information that conforms to their current expectations. Moreover, atypical information is especially well recalled if it disrupts current expectations or if it is implausible rather than simply irrelevant (i.e., the so-called disruption effect; Hudson, 1988). Irrelevant, atypical information is also better recalled if it is vivid rather than pallid (Davidson & Jergovic, 1996).

Distinctiveness effects in children's memory have also been examined in studies of bizarre imagery (see Howe, Courage, Vernescu, & Hunt, 2000, for a review). For example, in a study by Emmerich and Ackerman (1979), kindergarten children learned a list of paired associates that were elaborated using either common or unusual (bizarre) interactions. Using a cued-recall procedure at test, they found that like adults', children's memory performance was not enhanced by the bizarre nature of the interaction. However, when children were instructed to imagine the items interacting in either a common or unusual manner, and were tested using free recall, older children (12- and 13-year-olds), like adults, exhibited superior memory performance for the bizarre than for the common items (Merry & Graham, 1978). Younger, preschool children (i.e., 3½-year-olds) have been shown to perform more poorly with bizarre items than older preschool children (i.e., 4½-year-olds) who showed no differences in their cued recall of common and bizarre items (Tomasulo, 1982–83). Unfortunately, these latter two studies are difficult to interpret owing to a number of well-known methodological confounds.

In a more recent study (Howe et al., 2000, Experiment 2), kindergarten and Grade 2 children were presented with pairs of toys[1] representing everyday objects, and the experimenter illustrated either a common or a bizarre interaction between the objects in a mixed-list procedure. Testing was conducted using a free-recall procedure in which children were instructed to recall both nouns and the interaction between them (typically, children recalled the entire noun-verb-noun sequence or they recalled nothing). Each child learned a list of 8 noun pairs to a criterion of perfect recall on two consecutive test trials (acquisition) and were retested again three weeks later (long-term retention). Although older children outperformed younger children during the initial learning phase (made fewer errors, required fewer trials to reach an acquisition criterion of 100% correct), there were no performance differences at acquisition as a function of the nature (common or bizarre) of the interaction between items. However, tests during the long-term retention phase showed that although older children were again better than younger children at free recall, bizarre items were better retained than common items, regardless of age. Thus, under optimal conditions (free recall, mixed-list design), the distinctiveness of bizarre interactions among common objects facilitates younger and older children's long-term retention.

Interestingly, although many studies have been published in the adult literature concerning the isolation, or von Restorff, effect, only one such study has also been published with children (Howe et al., 2000, Experiments 1a and 1b). In this procedure, a prevailing context is established (e.g., a list of categorized words is presented) along with a distinctive item (e.g., a word not belonging to the same category as the prevailing context) or isolate. Typically, the isolate is easier to remember than the nonisolates or category members (for a review, see Hunt, 1995). In the experiments by Howe et al. (2000), kindergarten and Grade 2 children learned (to a criterion of perfect recall) a list of 11 black-and-white lines drawings, 8 of which depicted the most frequent exemplars from the *clothing* or the *animal* categories and the 3 remaining items were isolates (Experiment 1a). Specifically, each list contained a same-category item (*coat* or *rabbit*) that was printed on colored paper (red or blue), an item that was a typical exemplar from another category (*hammer* or *television*), and a numeral (2 or 3). Three weeks following acquisition, children were tested for long-term retention. The results at acquisition showed that older children were better at learning the lists than were younger children and that all children, regardless of age, learned the color and semantic isolates (but not the number isolates) more quickly than the nonisolates. At retention, controlling for differences at acquisition, a similar pattern of findings emerged. That is, older children remembered more than younger children and all of the children found the color and semantic isolates easier to retain than the nonisolates. Interestingly, the number isolates were more poorly remembered than the nonisolates for the kindergarten children, whereas there were no differences for the Grade 2 children.

In a second experiment (Experiment 1b) these latter effects were investigated in more detail. Here, lists contained only a single, number isolate. The results at acquisition indicated the usual main effect for age and an Age × Item interaction such that number isolates were easier than nonisolates for older, but not younger, children. At long-term retention, younger children found the numerical isolates more difficult to remember than the nonisolates, but older children found the numerical isolates easier than the nonisolates. Interestingly, when a numeral served as an item on an unrelated list, numbers were no harder to learn and retain than other items on that list.

Overall, then, children's performance is much like that of adults' performance: isolates and stimuli that are placed in bizarre juxtaposition are better recalled than nonisolates and items depicted in normal interactions. Although older children tend to be better at recalling than younger children, all children can take advantage of distinctiveness to aid immediate as well as later recollection. That numerical information was not used to memorial advantage by young children presents an interesting paradox. That is, perhaps such information was too distinct to be remembered. Here, because distinctiveness is derived relative to some context, and because in this case perhaps the number of differences generated between a numeral and the prevailing context (the category of animals or clothes) was potentially infinite, there was not sufficient overlap in the encoded features to make such distinctiveness memorable (see Howe et al., 2000). That is, if the comparison process that determines distinctiveness yields a potentially infinite set of differences—ones not diagnostic of the context from whence they were derived—they will not be useful in retrieving that information later. In fact, such extreme levels of distinctiveness may be similar to situations in which one had studied a list of completely unrelated items. "In contrast, if a subset of those featural contrasts yields a set of differences that links the distinctive item to the context and is diagnostic of the unique relationship between the isolate and the other items that constitute the context, then distinctiveness will aid recollection. What makes distinctiveness work, therefore, is that the dissimilarities detected among items are representative of contextually sensitive points of contrast—ones that are unique and distinctive to the context in which the comparisons occurred" (Howe et al., 2000, p. 789). I return to this later.

Distinctiveness effects are also thought to reduce the probability of creating false memories (Howe, 1998b). That is, confusions among memories are more likely as their degree of similarity increases. To the extent that memories are distinct, standing out against the background of other memories, they should not be confused with one another nor permit false elements to enter into their recollection. A procedure that has been used frequently to study spontaneous false memories with adults is the Deese-Roediger-McDermott (DRM) paradigm (Deese, 1959; Roediger & McDermott, 1995). In this procedure, subjects learn lists of words, all of which have a common semantic associate (e.g., *bed, rest, awake, tired, dream, wake, snooze, blanket, doze, slumber, snore, nap* all have the common associate *sleep*). After hearing all of the words except for the common associate, subjects either attempt to recall the list of words or are given a recognition test. The false memory in this case is the recall or recognition of the unpresented common associate.

It is well known in the DRM paradigm that when adults encode distinctive information (e.g., imaginal representations of objects on a word list), the production of spontaneous false memories declines (Israel & Schacter, 1997; Schacter, Israel, & Racine, 1999; Smith & Hunt, 1998). For adults, two distinctiveness mechanisms have been proposed that bring about the reduction of false memories: item distinctiveness and a distinctiveness heuristic. Concerning the former, Smith and Hunt (1998) suggest that discriminating items studied from nonstudied items when retrieving DRM lists depends on distinctive processing at encoding. Thus, at an item-specific level, an operation that confers distinctiveness to DRM list members should lead to improved discrimination between studied and nonstudied items. This, in addition to the fact that item-specific processing reduces relational processing (similarities across list members), should lead to a reduction in false memories, a prediction borne out in the Smith and Hunt (1998) studies.

Concerning the latter—distinctiveness heuristic conception of reducing false memories—Schacter et al. (1999) invoke a rather sophisticated metamemorial mechanism. Here, subjects are said to reduce false memories because they are aware that true recognition of studied items should be accompanied by a recollection of distinctive details associated with its presentation. For example, if each item on a DRM list is accompanied by a picture, subjects "know" that they should endorse items on a recognition list only where their recollection also includes the episodic recollection of having seen a picture. As we will see next, it is unlikely that this explanation is correct for young children, who show a similar decline in false memories when pictures accompany DRM lists but who are not as sophisticated as adults in their metamemorial skills.

Although few studies have been conducted on children's false memories using the DRM paradigm, what research has been conducted shows that false memories generally increase with age (see Brainerd, Reyna, & Forrest, 2002; Howe, Cicchetti, Toth, & Cerrito, 2004). It has been argued that false memories created using the DRM procedure increase rather than decrease with age in childhood because older children are better able to engage in relational processing, specifically extracting the gist across items (relational processing) in a list (Brainerd et al., 2002). In contrast, Ghetti, Qin, and Goodman (2002) found that younger, not older, children were more susceptible to false memories in the DRM paradigm using a measure of recall (but not recognition). More importantly for the purposes of this chapter, they found that distinctive information reduced these false memories regardless of age.

In their study, Ghetti et al. (2002) manipulated distinctiveness by presenting pictures along with words. Their results showed that distinctiveness reduced false memories and increased correct recognition of studied items in all age groups (5-year-olds, 7-year-olds, and adults 18 to 37 years old). Because the same distinctiveness effects were seen in the youngest (5-year-olds) and oldest (adults) subjects, Ghetti et al. (2002) argued that these effects were not due to the spontaneous use of a distinctiveness heuristic requiring sophisticated metamemorial skills like that proposed by Schacter et al. (1999). This is because it is well known that children this young have limited metacognitive abilities. Instead, the authors considered a number of basic-level memory mechanisms including item-specific processing (Smith & Hunt, 1998), fuzzy-trace theory's (FTT) correct rejection mechanism (e.g., Brainerd, Reyna, & Kneer, 1995; also see Brainerd, Reyna, Wright, & Mojardin, 2003) and a recall-to-reject mechanism where subjects evaluate whether the recognition item can be recalled and, if not, it is rejected (e.g., Rotello, Macmillan, & van Tassel, 2000). Although the data did not discriminate between these various mechanisms, it was clear that the reduction in false-memory rates was due to the effects of distinctiveness on children's basic memory mechanisms, not higher order metacognitive processes.

Finally, Brainerd et al. (1995) studied distinctiveness in children and adults' false recognition. Here, false-recognition rates declined for children (kindergarten and Grade 3 students) and adults when memory targets (items actually on the studied lists—e.g., *cat*) were used to prime related distractors (items not on the studied lists—e.g., *dog*). This reduction occurs, according to FTT, because target primes activate verbatim representations of the list items, which in turn promotes distinctive processing of individual list members (i.e., item-specific processing). Thus, whereas gist representations carry similarity information about features common to all members of the list (relational processing), verbatim representations carry distinctive information about the unique features associated with each specific input item (item-specific processing). Because similarity manipulations can improve memory in circumstances where distinctive information prevails but impair memory where similarity is already high; and conversely, distinctiveness manipulations can improve memory in circumstances where similarity prevails but impair memory where distinctiveness is already high (see Hunt & McDaniel, 1993), priming verbatim traces should lead to better discrimination of what was presented from what was not presented, leading to overall reductions in false memories. This, of course, is exactly what happened in the Brainerd et al. (1995) experiments, and these effects were robust for children as well as adults.

More About Long-Term Retention and Distinctiveness

A second gap in the distinctiveness literature concerns the importance of documenting the longevity of memory for distinctive as compared to routine events. Much of the research with both children and adults has been limited to immediate or relatively short-term retention. Recently, it has been suggested that children's memory, particularly autobiographical memory, is enhanced not by the positive or negative valence of the event per se, but by its *distinctiveness* (see Howe, 1998a, 1998b, 2000). Consistent with the earlier discussion of what constitutes distinctiveness, autobiographical events (or aspects of events) are considered distinctive inasmuch as they stand out against the background of one's previous experiences and knowledge and, thus, tend to be well remembered over time. Indeed, recent retrospective research on college students' memory for distinctive autobiographical events indicates that certain of these events were retained from the age of about 2 years (Eacott & Crawley, 1998; Usher & Neisser, 1993). There is also an emerging consensus in the adult literature that memory, particularly autobiographical memory, is enhanced by the distinctiveness of an event and that what tends to be recalled about one's life are those events that are distinctive especially as they are consequential (e.g., Conway, 1996), involve personally significant changes (e.g., Rubin & Schulkind, 1997), or are somehow distinctive with respect to one's conception of oneself (e.g., Csikszentmihalkyi & Beattie, 1979).

Clearly, if distinctive events are the ones best remembered autobiographically, then distinctiveness must benefit long-term retention and not just initial acquisition. Unfortunately, in the few cases in which distinctiveness effects have been examined at long-term retention (e.g., Kroll, Schepeler, & Angin, 1986; O'Brien & Wolford, 1982), item differences at acquisition were confounded with item differences at retention, thus clouding the interpretation of the effects of distinctiveness at long-term retention. That is, whenever a fixed number of trials is administered at acquisition (often only one), more difficult items tend not to be learned as well as the easier items. Measures at long-term retention are confounded with these item-difficulty outcomes from acquisition and hence do not provide uncontaminated measures of processes at retention. Further, in the memory-development literature, because younger children almost always learn any list more slowly than do older children, the item difficulty confound is further complicated by age confounds. What is needed is a procedure that removes these confounds. For example, if participants are required to learn all of the items equally well at the time of acquisition (e.g., to a criterion of perfect recall), regardless of age and item difficulty, then most of the contamination from acquisition processes would be removed from retention test scores (additional statistical procedures can also be used to assist with this decontamination of retention scores; e.g., see Howe, 2002). In this way, the effects of any manipulation (e.g., distinctiveness) can be measured at retention independently of its effects at acquisition (for a more detailed analysis of this problem, see Howe & Courage, 1997; Howe, Kelland, Bryant-Brown, & Clark, 1992).

The few studies in which these conditions pertain exist in the literature on children's memory. For example, the study by Howe et al. (2000) reviewed earlier in this chapter utilized this procedure. More recently, Howe

(2002, 2004) examined the effects of intentional forgetting and recoding on retroactive interference in children's long-term retention using a criterion learning paradigm and corrective statistical procedures at long-term retention. Although one might not think of intentional forgetting or recoding as distinctiveness effects, it turns out that both manipulations confer distinctiveness to the material to-be-forgotten or the material that is to be recoded. To explain, in both studies children (4-year-olds and 6-year-olds in the intentional forgetting study [Howe, 2002] and 7-year-olds and 9-year-olds in the recoding study [Howe, 2004]) learned either one or two stories (intentional forgetting) or one or two categorized lists (recoding) to a criterion of 100% correct recall. For the intentional forgetting study, children were instructed to forget the second story (the experimenter acted as if she had made a mistake and that the children were not to have learned the second story and so they should simply forget it). If children could forget this second story, subsequent recall of the first story should not be impaired by retroactive interference from this second story (note that both stories were similar inasmuch as they depicted a child going to the store to buy something; what varied was the type of store, the reason for the purchase, the items available for purchase, and the item eventually purchased). The results indicated that children given the intentional forgetting instruction showed significantly less retroactive interference than children in the standard retroactive interference condition who were not instructed to forget the second story. Indeed, recall of the first story 24 hours later was almost as good when children were instructed to forget the second story as that evinced by children in a control group who only learned the one story. Of course, the children did not really forget the second story, as evidenced by near perfect recall of that story when asked to do so after they recalled the first story. (In fact, in some unpublished studies we have varied whether the to-be-forgotten story was recalled first or second and the results are always the same; the to-be-forgotten story is always extremely well remembered and retroactive interference is minimized.) Thus, it was not that children forgot the interfering story but rather that they were able to use the forgetting instruction to discriminate between the two stories in memory so they did not interfere with each other (as I show later in this chapter, this discrimination was storage-based not retrieval-based).

In the recoding study (Howe, 2004), children learned two lists of concepts, both of which could be classified as *toys*. After learning these lists to criterion, some of the children were told about another way the second (but not the first) list could be classified (i.e., as *vehicles*). Like intentional forgetting, if children successfully recoded the second list, the amount of retroactive interference from that list should be substantially reduced when children attempted to recall the first list 24 hours later. This is exactly what happened; in fact, children's recall of the first list when given recoding instructions was significantly better than that of children in a standard retroactive interference condition who received no such instruction and was almost as good as that of children in a control group who only studied one list.

Finally, in a recent series of experiments in which the role of similarities and differences in children's learning and retention was examined (Howe, 2003), 5-year-olds and 7-year-olds learned a list of semantically related concept pairs. Children were informed that both items in a pair (presented orally as well as pictorially) belonged to a category (e.g., *dogs and cats are both animals*). In the first experiment, children in the similarity condition were given a concrete property on which the item pairs were the same (e.g., *both dogs and cats have 4 legs*) and children in the difference condition were given concrete properties on which the item pairs were different (e.g., *dogs bark, cats meow*). In the second experiment the procedure was the same except that, instead of the experimenter's providing the additional similarities and differences, the children made up their own. All of the children learned the 18-pair list to a criterion of perfect cued recall and long-term retention was tested 3 weeks later.

The results showed that both similarities and differences were important at acquisition, regardless of whether they were experimenter-generated or self-generated. That is, children reached criterion faster in these conditions than in a control condition where only the category names were provided. At retention, self-generated lists were better remembered than experimenter-generated lists, and regardless of who generated the differences, pairs that were made distinct were better retained than those receiving additional similarity processing. Thus, distinctive processing was important both at acquisition and at long-term retention, regardless of age.

In sum, like the study of distinctiveness effects at acquisition, these studies all show that making information distinctive either at the time it is encoded (e.g., isolation effects, bizarre imagery, learning of similarities or differences; see Howe, 2003; Howe et al., 2000) or after it has been encoded and stored (e.g., intentional forgetting, recoding; see Howe, 2002, 2004), increases in the durability of that information in memory over protracted retention intervals. Interestingly, when model-based analyses of these effects have been examined with an eye toward determining the locus (storage or retrieval) of distinctiveness effects at retention, the results overwhelmingly have reflected a storage interpretation. In the next section, the locus of these effects will be considered in somewhat greater detail in the context of current models and theories of children's memory development.

THEORETICAL PERSPECTIVES ON DISTINCTIVENESS AND MEMORY DEVELOPMENT

What the preceding summary has revealed is that distinctiveness effects are present very early in life, that their influence on memory performance increases with age, and that the effects of various distinctiveness manipulations can be seen both at children's acquisition and their retention. Importantly, this increase is not primarily quantitative but more qualitative in nature. That is, as children mature, they use more and more sophisticated (or abstract) dimensions to facilitate distinctive processing. In this section, I consider two theories of memory development that can account for these changes—FTT and the trace-integrity theory—and discuss the locus (storage or retrieval) of these effects across the course of development.

Fuzzy-Trace Theory

Proponents of fuzzy-trace theory (FTT; Brainerd & Reyna, 2001; Brainerd et al., 2003) have suggested that children's memory development consists of advances in encoding, storing, and retrieving two types of memory traces, a verbatim trace and a gist trace. The essential idea is that there are two fundamentally different types of memory representations that are extracted in parallel and that co-exist in memory: *verbatim* traces that represent the literal or factual aspects (e.g., surfaces forms, item-specific properties) of information and *gist* traces that are fuzzy and imprecise and represent the meaning aspects (e.g., semantic, relational, elaborative) of information. *Fuzzy* or *gist* representations differ in important ways from verbatim representations; for example, fuzzy, but not verbatim, traces are easier to access and use and, regardless of age, tend to be the preferred representation when it comes to problem solving. Although verbatim traces are more precise than gist traces, they tend to be more fragile, are more susceptible to interference, and are forgotten more rapidly.

Developmentally, although verbatim representations undergo considerable development, the main contributor to children's memory development is change in the encoding, storage, and retrieval of gist representations. Although young children are biased toward the extraction of verbatim information, they do extract gist. There is a verbatim-to-gist shift that generally occurs during the elementary school years when, like adults, older children show a bias toward the extraction of gist. Because this shift toward the encoding and processing of gist is largely knowledge driven, the use of gist representations in memory undergoes a more protracted period of development.

Although this theory pertains to many different aspects of cognitive and memory development, it is perhaps best exemplified in its unequalled and comprehensive account of false memories. Recall the discussion earlier about the DRM paradigm and the fact that much of the research shows that older children are more susceptible to false memories than are younger children. Although seemingly contradictory with the findings concerning children's suggestibility, in which younger children are more susceptible to false memories through suggestion than are older children and adults, there are unique aspects of the DRM procedure that, according to FTT, make the opposite developmental pattern sensible. Specifically, because false memories in the DRM paradigm are contingent not only on extracting the gist of each presented concept but also extracting the gist across all of the concepts (relational processing— something younger children are less likely to do than older children), false-memory effects should be more likely in older than in younger children (see Brainerd et al., 2002).

FTT also distinguishes between similarity and distinctiveness at an item-specific level as well as a relational level for verbatim and gist traces. At a relational level, the formation of false memories in the DRM paradigm, for example, arises because of the similarity in gist that is extracted across list items (relational processing of similarity). If this gist is dissimilar (distinctive), then false recollections based on gist representations are less likely to emerge. Alternatively, at an item-specific level, false recollection can occur for gist representations when featural similarity (overlap) is high between the test item and gist memory that has been retrieved. In this case, false-memory production is increased when inter-item similarity is high and it is decreased when inter-item distinctiveness is high. For verbatim representations, when individual items are accessed (item-specific information), children and adults are less likely to form false memories because verbatim representations are matched exactly with that which has been presented (see Brainerd et al., 1995). That is, verbatim comparisons follow an identity rule; if a test item's verbatim representation does not match exactly that of the retrieved verbatim memory, then it is rejected.

Trace-Integrity Theory

In the trace-integrity theory, storage and retrieval are viewed as processes lying on a continuum where traces consist of collections of primitive elements (e.g., features, nodes). Initial acquisition of memory traces consists of integrating features into a single, cohesive structure in memory. Retention of information is determined by the integrity of that cohesive structure over time. Traces that are not well integrated tend to disintegrate, and their stability (in terms of both availability [storage] and accessibility [retrieval]) is compromised. When this occurs, the trace no longer represents a stable and cohesive structure in memory; it loses its distinctiveness and fades into the background noise of other memory traces (see Howe, 2000). This view of how memory traces are formed and retained is consistent with and provides an integration of many other views of memory more generally as well as memory development specifically (e.g., Bauer, Wenner, Dropik, & Wewerka, 2000; Estes, 1988; Rovee-Collier, Hayne, & Colombo, 2001; Schneider & Bjorklund, 1998). One advantage of the trace-integrity theory is that it comes with an associated mathematical model, one that permits the extraction of these proposed theoretical processes (storage and retrieval) from empirical outcomes on memory tests (test trial errors and successes).

Like other good developmental theories, this one includes a mechanism whereby memory improvements that occur with age are accounted for either directly in terms of changes in basic memory processes (e.g., encoding, storage, retrieval) or indirectly in terms of changes in other cognitive factors that are correlated with age (e.g., knowledge, strategies). In terms of the acquisition of memory representations, like FTT, the trace-integrity theory suggests that trace integration improves as children's ability to organize features into cohesive patterns develops (e.g., through improved categorization and feature extraction; see Howe, 2000) as well as their ability to create traces that stand out against the background noise of other memories (e.g., creating traces that are distinctive). Retention of these traces also depends on these factors. That is, developmental advances in memory in general and retention in particular depend on corresponding developments in a host of cognitive factors that facilitate the cohesion of primitive trace elements or bundles of features in memory (e.g., knowledge, distinctiveness, strategies such as rehearsal, categorization, scripts), reduce the likelihood of their modification over time (e.g., through blending, recoding, reconstruction, reorganization) or disintegration (e.g., interference, trace decay), and that facilitate trace redintegration (e.g., reinstatement, testing, retrieval cuing). This theory accounts for memory development from birth onward; proposes that memory development, like other aspects of cognitive development, is continuous (also see Courage & Howe, 2002); and, in contrast to FTT, is a unitary trace model in which differences between verbatim and gist aspects of a trace or between implicit and explicit memory (or declarative and nondeclarative memory) are due to different task requirements, not different traces being available or accessible in memory (for a similar point of view, see Rovee-Collier et al., 2001). That is, what differs is not the type of trace that is formed in memory but rather the diversity of what is stored in a single cohesive structure in memory and the variety (and flexibility) of ways this information can be accessed.

Considerable evidence consistent with this theory has been reviewed elsewhere (e.g., Courage & Howe, 2004; Howe, 2000; Howe, Courage, & Edison, 2003). For current purposes, a major advantage of this theoretical approach is that it is consistent with the outcome reviewed earlier in which distinctiveness can have a negative effect on performance. In all other models, distinctiveness typically has either no effect or a positive effect on memory performance. In the trace-integrity theory, information that is too distinct from the current context can actually have a negative effect on children's memory performance (e.g., Howe et al., 2000) because that information cannot be used to augment the distinctiveness of traces in memory. That is, although children in the Howe et al. (2000) experiments were sensitive to numerical information, such information could not be used to enhance memory because there were too many differences between the prevailing context and the number information. When too many distinctions exist, there is no advantage conferred to memory for those items because the differences generated within the context are not diagnostic of the unique relationship between the distinctive item(s) and the context. Indeed, as was pointed out in that article (Howe et al., 2000), this explanation is consistent with discrepancy theory (Hunt, 1965; Kagan, 1967; McCall & McGhee, 1977). Here, the efficacy of discrepancy (distinctiveness) from a standard stimulus (prevailing context) is determined by an inverted-U function in which information that is not very discrepant (i.e., is highly similar) is not useful in memory, moderate discrepancies provide valuable information that aids retention, and information that is highly discrepant does not provide useful information and can have negative consequences in memory. "That is, moderate (physical or conceptual) discrepancies from highly familiar stimuli receive both the highest degree of attention and positive affect (and presumably retention), whereas stimuli that are quite familiar or extremely different from what the organism knows will receive relatively less attention and less positive—perhaps even negative—affective responses and evaluations" (McCall & McGhee, 1977, p. 179).

The results of these and other studies with children are consistent with the idea that young children can and do use distinctive information to their advantage in memory and long-term retention. However, these data also show that distinctiveness may not be linearly related to memory. That is, this relationship may be best described by an invert-U function in which highly discrepant information is not only difficult to encode in memory but also may have a negative effect. This is not because children do not understand the meaning of concepts being studied but because there are too many potential differences between the discrepant stimulus and the prevailing context such that no particular difference or set of differences is diagnostic of the unique relationship between the distinctive stimulus and the context that can be effectively encoded in memory.

Storage or Retrieval Loci of Distinctiveness Effects

Traditionally, at least in the adult-memory literature, an important question has arisen about the nature of distinctiveness effects—namely, what is the locus of these effects? This question has been cast in terms of whether distinctiveness improves encoding (and storage), improves retrieval, or improves both processes (see Hunt, Chapter 1 this volume). It has long been thought that distinctiveness benefits memory performance by exerting its effect at retrieval. This is because distinctiveness is said to facilitate discriminative processes (e.g., Smith & Hunt, 1998), something that affects information retrieval. However, it is important to note that these effects may extend to storage. That is, better discriminated traces may be better discriminated because they stand out against the background noise of other, highly similar traces in storage. If true, then distinctiveness may affect both storage and retrieval, something that those who study false memories have attempted to establish (e.g., storage of distinctive traces increases longevity in memory, leading to lowered susceptibility to false memories—stronger traces are more resistant to suggestion, etc.—see Howe, 1998b). Developmentally this is important because improvements in children's memory performance manifest themselves at both storage and retrieval, and when it comes to long-term retention, these improvements are mainly the result of better maintenance of traces in storage. It is of interest, therefore, to determine whether any performance differences across age due to distinctiveness selectively target storage, retrieval, or both storage and retrieval. In order to examine this issue, a formal model of long-term retention can be used to partition the storage and retrieval components of children's retention performance.

Research using the trace-integrity theory has provided some of the answers to these questions, at least insofar as the memory development literature is concerned. Indeed, the trace-integrity theory is particularly well poised to answer storage-retrieval questions regardless of age, as the associated mathematical model's parameters that measure storage and retrieval do so independently of the developmental status of the participant. Although space precludes a full discussion of this mathematical model (for recent descriptions, see Howe, 2000, 2002), the outcome of tests of this model are germane.

Because this model applies to the long-term retention of information, participants in these studies are given more than a single study-test sequence on the to-be-remembered material. In fact, as described earlier, children learn the information to a strict acquisition criterion of two consecutive errorless recall trials. There are three reasons for adhering to such a strict criterion. First, this avoids item-difficulty confounds discussed earlier in this chapter. That is, items that are easier to learn are not better represented in memory than more difficult items by the time criterion is achieved. Second, to the extent that distinctiveness effects may take time to emerge (especially with children), more than a single study-test opportunity may be necessary to observe such effects at initial acquisition. This is particularly relevant in studies in which children are presented with conceptual information, as categorical relations may be activated more slowly in children than in adults (e.g., see Bjorklund, 1988). As well, if distinctiveness is being measured at retention, failures to equate item differences at the end of acquisition will be confounded with item differences at retention. Third, when these item-difficulty confounds are left uncontrolled in developmental research, additional difficulties arise because age differences in learning rates will be confounded with age differences in forgetting rates (see earlier discussion in this chapter and Howe & Courage, 1997). Thus, in all of the experiments using the trace-integrity model, children learned the list information to a criterion of two consecutive errorless trials, ensuring both that (1) all of the information was stored in memory and was correctly retrieved at least twice in a row and (2) differences (itemwise as well as developmental) at retention could be evaluated independently of differences in initial learning difficulty.

Model-based analyses of the experiments described earlier in this chapter provide strong support for a storage-based interpretation of distinctiveness effects, at least in children. Specifically, in a previously unreported series of analyses using this model on children's isolation effects (Howe et al., 2000, Experiments 1a and 1b), it was clear that when improvements were obtained (i.e., in particular, the color isolate for kindergarten children and the color and semantic isolates for the Grade 2 children in Experiment 1a; the number isolate for the Grade 2 children only in Experiment 1b) these improvements were localized in the model's storage parameter. This parameter measures the rate at which traces fail in storage. Thus, the lower the failure rate, the better traces were retained in storage for later recollection. In these experiments, then, information about isolates was better maintained in storage following the retention interval. (No reliable differences in either storage or retrieval were found for the bizarreness effects in Experiment 2.) Similar storage-based effects were reported for intentional forgetting (Howe, 2002) and recoding (Howe, 2004). The only exception to these storage-based findings was obtained in the series of experiments in which experimenter- and child-generated similarities and differences were examined (Howe, 2003). Here, although retention was better when children generated their own relations between items as measured at storage across the retention interval than experimenter-generated relations, small but statistically reliable advantages were obtained at retrieval for items in which differences rather than similarities had been generated regardless of who generated them and regardless of age. One reason for this latter finding may be that, in this experiment, children used cued rather than free recall. Because cued recall provides more support for the retrieval component of locating traces in storage, more weakly represented information can be redintegrated in storage with the use of cues (see Howe, 2003). Regardless, the body of evidence accumulated to date with children is consistent with the idea that maintaining traces in storage is the primary locus of distinctiveness effects, at least for long-term retention.

CONCLUSION

Research reviewed here on the role of distinctiveness in children's memory has produced a number of important conclusions, ones that inform not only the memory-development literature but also the literature on the nature of distinctiveness effects in memory more generally. First, concerning developmental trends, what the preceding review has shown is that distinctiveness is important from the very earliest days of life, in terms of both guiding attention, perception, and encoding and probably improving memory performance and retention. Certainly beginning in toddlerhood, distinctive information plays an important role in memory performance, not only immediately (see Howe, 2000) but also across transitions into adulthood (e.g., Eacott & Crawley, 1998; Usher & Neisser, 1993). More importantly, these improvements are qualitative as well as quantitative. That is, the types of dimensions along which children can make distinctiveness judgments change as children's knowledge base expands (e.g., Howe, 2000), as their ability to extract gist across materials in a display or a list improves (e.g., Brainerd et al., 2002), and as their ability to retain information in storage over longer and longer retention intervals grows (e.g., Howe, 2000).

Second, and related to the first conclusion, the literature on distinctiveness effects in children's memory indicates that there may exist dimensions that in some contexts present too many opportunities for distinctive processing, leading to poorer rather than better memory performance. For example, recall that Howe et al. (2000) found that some information was so distinct that young children were unable to use it to their advantage at recall. This finding was linked to discrepancy theory, in which an individual is said to attend to and efficiently process new stimuli as an inverted-U function of the stimuli's physical or conceptual discrepancies from well-known standards (see McCall & McGhee, 1977). Moderate discrepancies receive the highest degree of attention, whereas stimuli that are quite familiar or extremely different receive less attention. Thus, stimuli that are new but processable recruit the most attention, and those that present no new information or require too much processing effort or cognitive restructuring receive less. This observation may be useful in understanding developmental (and individual) differences in the distinctiveness effects in memory. As children's knowledge structures develop, there should exist predictable and corresponding differences in the types of information that recruit distinctive processing. Thus, although distinctiveness effects exist at all ages, what constitutes distinctive information will vary developmentally.

ACKNOWLEDGMENTS

Preparation of this chapter was funded by Grant OGP0003334 to Mark L. Howe from the Natural Sciences and Engineering Research Council of Canada. Portions of this chapter were presented at the 49th Annual Meeting of the Southwestern Psychological Association, New Orleans, LA, April 2003.

NOTE

1. Toys were used to increase the salience and relevance of the items for the children, thereby increasing the probability of criterion learning. This was important because children's long-term retention was also assessed in this experiment and age differences in learning needed to be controlled so as not to confound the retention data. This point will be discussed in greater detail in the next section.

REFERENCES

Bauer, P. J., Wenner, J. A., Dropik, P. L., & Wewerka, S. S. (2000). Parameters of remembering and forgetting in the transition from infancy to early childhood. *Monographs of the Society for Research in Child Development*, 65(4, Serial No. 263).

Bjorklund, D. F. (1988). Acquiring a mnemonic: Age and category knowledge effects. *Journal of Experimental Child Psychology*, 45, 71–87.

Brainerd, C. J., & Reyna, V. F. (2001). Fuzzy-trace theory: Dual processes in memory, reasoning, and cognitive neuroscience. *Advances in Child Development and Behavior, 28,* 41–100.

Brainerd, C. J., Reyna, V. F., & Forrest, T. J. (2002). Are young children more susceptible to the false-memory illusion? *Child Development, 73,* 1363–1377.

Brainerd, C. J., Reyna, V. F., & Kneer, R. (1995). False recognition reversal: When similarity is distinctive. *Journal of Memory and Language, 34,* 157–185.

Brainerd, C. J., Reyna, V. F., Wright, R., & Mojardin, A. H. (2003). Recollection rejection: False-memory editing in children and adults. *Psychological Review, 110,* 762–784.

Brown, R., & Kulik, J. (1977). Flashbulb memories. *Cognition, 5,* 73–99.

Chang, P. P. W., Levine, S. C., & Benson, P. J. (2002). Children's recognition of caricatures. *Developmental Psychology, 38,* 1038–1051.

Conway, M. A. (1996). Autobiographical knowledge and autobiographical memories. In D. C. Rubin (Ed.), *Remembering our past: Studies in autobiographical memory* (pp. 67–93). New York: Cambridge University Press.

Courage, M. L., & Howe, M. L. (2002). From infant to child: The dynamics of cognitive change in the second year of life. *Psychological Bulletin, 128,* 250–277.

Courage, M. L., & Howe, M. L. (2004). Advances in early memory development research: Insights about the dark side of the moon. *Developmental Review, 24,* 6–32.

Cox, S. D., & Wollen, K. A. (1981). Bizarreness and recall. *Bulletin of the Psychonomic Society, 18,* 244–245.

Csikszentmihalyi, M., & Beattie, O. V. (1979). Life themes: A theoretical and empirical exploration of their origins and effects. *Journal of Humanistic Psychology, 19,* 45–63.

Davidson, D., & Jergovic, D. (1996). Children's memory for atypical actions in script-based stories: An examination of the disruption effect. *Journal of Experimental Child Psychology, 61,* 134–152.

Deese, J. (1959). On the prediction of occurrence of certain verbal intrusions in free recall. *Journal of Experimental Psychology, 58,* 17–22.

Eacott, M. J., & Crawley, R. A. (1998). The offset of childhood amnesia: Memory for events that occurred before age 3. *Journal of Experimental Psychology: General, 127,* 22–33.

Einstein, G. O., McDaniel, M. A., & Lackey, S. (1989). Bizarre imagery, interference, and distinctiveness. *Journal of Experimental Psychology: Learning, Memory, and Cognition, 15,* 137–146.

Emmerich, H. J., & Ackerman, B. P. (1979). A test of bizarre interaction as a factor in children's memory. *Journal of Genetic Psychology, 134,* 225–232.

Estes, W. K. (1988). Human learning and memory. In R. C. Anderson, R. J. Hernstein, G. Lindzey, & R. D. Luce (Eds.), *Steven's handbook of experimental psychology: Vol. 2 Learning and cognition* (2nd ed., pp. 351–415). New York: Wiley.

Fritsch, T., & Larsen, J. D. (1990). Image-formation time is not related to recall of bizarre and plausible images. *Perceptual and Motor Skills, 70,* 1259–1266.

Ghetti, S., Qin, J., & Goodman, G. S. (2002). False memories in children and adults: Age, distinctiveness, and subjective experience. *Developmental Psychology, 38,* 705–718.

Herz, R. S. (1997). The effects of cue distinctiveness on odor-based context-dependent memory. *Memory & Cognition, 25,* 375–380.

Herz, R. S., & Cupchik, G. C. (1995). The emotional distinctiveness of odor-evoked memories. *Chemical Senses, 20,* 517–528.

Howe, M. L. (1998a). Individual differences in factors that modulate storage and retrieval of traumatic memories. *Development and Psychopathology, 10,* 681–698.

Howe, M. L. (1998b). When distinctiveness fails, false memories prevail. *Journal of Experimental Child Psychology, 71,* 170–177.

Howe, M. L. (2000). *The fate of early memories: Developmental science and the retention of childhood experiences.* Washington, DC: American Psychological Association.

Howe, M. L. (2002). The role of intentional forgetting in reducing children's retroactive interference. *Developmental Psychology, 38,* 3–14.

Howe, M. L. (2003). *Distinctiveness in children's memory: The role of similarities and differences.* Manuscript submitted for publication.

Howe, M. L. (2004). The role of conceptual recoding in reducing children's retroactive interference. *Developmental Psychology, 40,* 131–139.

Howe, M. L., Cicchetti, D., Toth, S., & Cerrito, B. M. (2004). True and false memories in maltreated children. *Child Development, 75,* 1402–1417.

Howe, M. L., & Courage, M. L. (1997). Independent paths in the development of infant learning and forgetting. *Journal of Experimental Child Psychology, 67,* 131–163.

Howe, M. L., Courage, M. L., & Edison, S. C. (2003). When autobiographical memory begins. *Developmental Review, 23,* 471–494.

Howe, M. L., Courage, M. L., Vernescu, R., & Hunt, M. (2000). Distinctiveness effects in children's long-term retention. *Developmental Psychology, 36,* 778–792.

Howe, M. L., Kelland, A., Bryant-Brown, L., & Clark, S. L. (1992). Measuring the development of children's amnesia and hypermnesia. In M. L. Howe, C. J. Brainerd, & V. F. Reyna (Eds.), *Development of long-term retention* (pp. 56–102). New York: Springer-Verlag.

Hudson, J. A. (1988). Children's memory for atypical actions in script-based stories: Evidence for a disruption effect. *Journal of Experimental Child Psychology, 46,* 159–173.

Hunt, J. (1965). Intrinsic motivation and its role in psychological development. In D. Levine (Ed.), *Nebraska symposium on motivation* (pp. 189–282). Lincoln: University of Nebraska Press.

Hunt, R. R. (1995). The subtlety of distinctiveness: What von Restorff really did. *Psychonomic Bulletin & Review, 2,* 105–112.

Hunt, R. R., & Elliot, J. M. (1980). The role of nonsemantic information in memory: Orthographic distinctiveness effects on retention. *Journal of Experimental Psychology: General, 109,* 49–74.

Hunt, R. R., & McDaniel, M. A. (1993). The enigma of organization and distinctiveness. *Journal of Memory and Language, 32,* 421–445.

Hunt, R. R., & Mitchell, D. B. (1982). Independent effects of semantic and nonsematic distinctiveness. *Journal of Experimental Psychology: Learning, Memory, and Cognition, 8,* 81–87.

Israel, L., & Schacter, D. L. (1997). Pictorial encoding reduces false memory recognition of semantic associates. *Psychonomic Bulletin & Review, 4,* 577–581.

Kagan, J. (1967). On the need for relativism. *American Psychologist, 22,* 131–143.

Kintsch, W., & Bates, E. (1977). Recognition memory for statements from a classroom lecture. *Journal of Experimental Psychology: Human Learning and Memory, 3,* 150–159.

Kroll, N. E. A., Schepeler, E. M., & Angin, K. T. (1986). Bizarre imagery: The misremembered mnemonic. *Journal of Experimental Psychology: Learning, Memory, and Cognition, 12,* 42–53.

Loftus, E. F., & Burns, T. E. (1982). Mental shock can produce retrograde amnesia. *Memory & Cognition, 10,* 318–323.

McCall, R. B., & McGhee, P. E. (1977). The discrepancy hypothesis of attention and affect in infants. In I. Uzgiris & F. Weizmann (Eds.), *The structuring of experience* (pp. 179–210). New York: Plenum Press.

Medin, D. L., Goldstone, R. L., & Gentner, D. (1993). Respects for similarity. *Psychological Review, 100,* 254–278.

Merry, R., & Graham, N. C. (1978). Imagery bizarreness in children's recall of sentences. *British Journal of Psychology, 69,* 315–321.

O'Brien, E. J., & Wolford, C. R. (1982). Effect of delay in testing on retention of plausible versus bizarre mental images. *Journal of Experimental Psychology: Learning, Memory, and Cognition, 8,* 148–152.

Rhodes, G., & Moody, J. (1990). Memory representations of unfamiliar faces: Coding distinctive information. *New Zealand Journal of Psychology, 19,* 70–78.

Roediger, H. L., III, & McDermott, K. B. (1995). Creating false memories: Remembering words not presented on lists. *Journal of Experimental Psychology: Learning, Memory, and Cognition, 21,* 803–814.

Rotello, C. M., Macmillan, N. A., & Van Tassel, G. (2000). Recall-to-reject in recognition: Evidence from ROC curves. *Journal of Memory and Language, 43,* 67–88.

Rovee-Collier, C., Hayne, H., & Colombo, M. (2001). *The development of implicit and explicit memory.* Amsterdam: John Benjamins.

Rubin, D. C., & Schulkind, M. D. (1997). Distribution of important and word-cued autobiographical memories in 20-, 35-, and 70-year-old adults. *Psychology and Aging, 12,* 524–535.

Schacter, D. L., Israel, L., & Racine, C. (1999). Suppressing false recognition in younger and older adults: The distinctiveness heuristic. *Journal of Memory and Language, 40,* 1–24.

Schmidt, S. R. (1985). Encoding and retrieval processes in the memory for conceptually distinctive events. *Journal of Experimental Psychology: Learning, Memory, and Cognition, 11,* 565–578.

Schmidt, S. R. (1991). Can we have a distinctive theory of memory? *Memory & Cognition, 19,* 523–542.

Schneider, W., & Bjorklund, D. F. (1998). Memory. In W. Damon (Series Ed.) & D. Kuhn & R. S. Siegler (Vol. Eds.), *Handbook of child psychology: Vol. 2 Cognition, perception, and language* (5th ed.). New York: Wiley.

Smith, R. E., & Hunt, R. R. (1998). Presentation modality affects false memory. *Psychonomic Bulletin & Review, 5,* 710–715.

Tomasulo, D. J. (1982-83). Effects of bizarre imagery on children's memory. *Imagination, Cognition, and Personality, 2,* 137–144.

Usher, J. A., & Neisser, U. (1993). Childhood amnesia and the beginnings of memory for four early life events. *Journal of Experimental Psychology: General, 122,* 155–165.

Winograd, E. (1981). Elaboration and distinctiveness in memory for faces. *Journal of Experimental Psychology: Human Learning and Memory, 7,* 181–190.

12

Adult Age Differences in Episodic Memory: Item-Specific, Relational, and Distinctive Processing

Rebekah E. Smith

Younger adults often perform better than older adults do on tests of memory (e.g.. Anderson & Craik, 2000; Balota, Dolan, & Duchek, 2000; Burke & Light, 1981; Craik & Jennings, 1992; Kausler, 1994; Light, 1996; Salthouse, 1991; Zacks, Hasher, & Li, 2000). Researchers interested in these age-associated performance differences have at times drawn concepts from the "mainstream" research (i.e., research that focuses on younger adults) and applied these concepts to explain why older adults frequently do not remember as well as younger adults. This chapter looks at attempts to explain age-related differences in memory as a function of relational and item-specific processing, and in some cases both kinds of processing. The focus is on studies comparing intentional retrospective memory in healthy younger (generally less than 30 years of age) and older adults (generally 60 years of age and older). The chapter primarily addresses three questions. First, are there age-related differences in item-specific processing? Second, are there age-related differences in relational processing? And finally, are there age-related differences in distinctive processing? The chapter concludes by relating the three of the four points concerning distinctiveness raised by Hunt (Chapter 1 this volume) to the literature on memory and aging.

ITEM-SPECIFIC PROCESSING

Potential age-related deficits in item-specific processing, or processing of properties that are unique to individual items in an event, have been investigated in several different ways. The number of items recalled per category has been taken as an index of item-specific processing, and researchers have compared the performance of younger and older adults on this variable. Other researchers have examined whether older adults process information in a more general fashion using a variety of techniques, such as making contextual changes at retrieval, offering specific versus general cues, or asking participants to generate information at encoding. Another alternative is to apply manipulations that arguably encourage item-specific processing in younger adults and see if the manipulations have the same effects for older adults. Most of the studies that have applied manipulations of item-specific processing have done so in the context of relational processing, and thus they fall into the category of manipulations of distinctive processing, which will be discussed in the third section.

Items pe-Category

The number of items recalled per category (IPC) has been taken as an index of the accessibility of individual items (Tulving & Pearlstone, 1966). Item-specific processing should increase IPC by increasing item discriminability (Hunt & Seta, 1984). Although there are potential problems with using the IPC measure (Burns, Chapter 6 this volume; Burns & Brown, 2000), the findings regarding age effects are more consistent than, as we shall see, is the case with the measures of clustering.

Age differences in IPC in favor of younger adults have been found in at least nine studies using free recall (Basden, Basden, & Bartlett, 1993; Fisher & McDowd, 1993; Guttentag, 1988; Hultsch, 1975; Park, Smith, Dudley, & Lafronza, 1989; Riefer & Batchelder, 1991; Sanders, Murphy, Schmitt, & Walsh, 1980; Witte, Freund, & Brown-Whistler, 1993; Zivian & Darjes, 1983). Three of these studies also included a cued-recall condition (Basden et al., 1993; Fisher & McDowd, 1993; Hultsch, 1975). Younger adults had higher IPC scores than older adults and in no case did age and test type interact. In other words, providing category label cues at test did not affect the age difference in IPC.

There is one exception to the otherwise clear pattern in favor of younger adults in IPC scores. Worden and Meggison (1984) had participants sort 48 unrelated words into two, four, six, or eight categories. After participants had completed at least two sorting trials with 95% agreement in the sorting pattern (i.e., the same person sorted words into the same categories on two successive sorting trials), participants were given an oral free-recall test. In the case of two categories, older adults actually recalled more items per category than the younger adults recalled. This pattern is somewhat surprising, but perhaps less so in light of the fact that the main effect of age on overall recall performance was not significant. It is not entirely clear why the older adults had better IPC scores in the two-category condition. Worden and Meggison suggested that the older adults may have formed subcategories that they used to guide retrieval.

In any event, it is perhaps best not to invest too much in this one study, for two reasons. First, as mentioned in the previous paragraph, Worden and Meggison's (1984) one experiment produced a finding regarding IPC that is contrary to a number of other studies that have found consistent age differences in IPC in favor of younger adults. More important, the Worden and Meggison IPC finding was not replicated in a study using very similar procedures. Basden et al. (1993) also asked participants to sort unrelated words into categories using a 95% agreement criterion. Basden et al. used 100 words, rather than 48, and did not specify the number of categories that each person should use. Younger adults had significantly higher IPC scores than the older adults in the Basden et al. study.

In short, with one exception, younger adults recall more items per category on both free-recall tests and cued-recall tests. Thus, the literature on age effects in IPC scores indicates that older adults have a deficit in item-specific processing.

Evidence for More General Encoding on the Part of Older Adults: Cue and Context Manipulations

This approach to the question of whether older adults engage in less item-specific processing grew out of an application of the principles of levels of processing (LOP; Craik & Lockhart, 1972) to understanding age differences in memory performance (e.g., Eysenck, 1974). It was argued that older adults processed information in a more general, less elaborate way. For instance, Till and Walsh (1980) had participants read sentences that provided additional implied information. The implied information was not directly stated, and it was thought that older adults would be less likely to fully process the sentences and therefore would be less likely to process the implied information. Younger and older adults were asked to recall the sentences. When provided with cues that corresponded to the implied information, younger adults recalled more sentences than when given no cues. Older adults did not benefit from the cues.

In another study comparing the effects of cues, Simon (reported in Craik & Simon, 1980) presented younger and older adults with a list of unrelated words. Memory for the words was tested using either a free-recall test or a cued-recall test. The cues were either the first two letters of the target words or synonyms of the target words. Both younger and older adults recalled more words in the letter-cued condition than in free recall. Only the younger adults showed an improvement in recall with the semantic cues. Presumably, the older adults engaged in less elaborate processing and therefore did not process the meaning of the word as fully and therefore could not use the synonym cues effectively. In a similar experiment, Simon presented participants with the to-be-remembered words in sentences. Younger and older adults both improved, relative to free recall, when given letter cues, but only the younger adults were able benefit from representation of the sentences, without the target word, to use as cues for recall of the targets. While these experiments show that older adults engaged in less elaborate processing, the older adults were still able to benefit from the item-specific letter cues.

Rabinowitz, Craik, and Ackerman (1982) also examined the age effect as a function of cue type. Participants studied target words that were paired with strong associates or weak associates at encoding. For the cued recall, test participants received either the same cue (strong or weak) or a different cue (strong or weak associate of the target). Thus, there were four cue conditions: strong at encoding–same strongly related associate as a cue at test; weak at encoding–same weakly related associate as a cue at test; strong at encoding–weak at test; weak at encoding–strong at test. Younger adults showed the expected encoding specificity effect: a weakly associated cue that had been presented at study was better for recall of the target word than a strongly associated cue that had not been presented at study. The older adults were no better with a weak cue that had been present at encoding than a strong cue that had not been present at encoding. Older adults processed the general semantic information captured by the strong associate cues, but did not process the more specific relationship between the target and its weak associate. This study provides further evidence that older adults process information at a more general level.

In three experiments conducted by Hess and Higgins (1983) and Hess (1984), participants were provided with target homographs paired with another word at encoding that biased one or the other meaning of the target word. For instance, participants might see *copper iron* at encoding. During a subsequent recognition test, participants would see either *copper iron* (same context) or *clothes iron* (different context). When the same context pair was used there were no age differences in hit rates; however, older adults were less likely than the younger adults to correctly recognize target words presented in a different context. Older adults were also more likely than the younger adults to make false alarms when the same context condition was presented with a lure word. These experiments are consistent with the idea that older adults processed the general information provided at study, but inadequately processed the item-specific information that could help them to identify the correct target word.

In a fourth experiment, the same technique was used, but the target and context words had no obvious relationship (Hess, 1984). Target words were presented with an unrelated context word at study. At test the target words were presented either with the same context word (old context) or a different unrelated context word (new context). Younger adults had higher hit rates and higher false-alarm rates in the old context condition than in the new context condition. Older adults' hit rates and false-alarm rates were insensitive to the change in context. The pattern from this experiment suggests that older adults did not process the relational information provided by the context in this study as effectively as the younger adults because that information was not as obvious as it had been in the previous three experiments. The older adults' difficulties in item-specific processing are not evident unless one examines a situation that involves more readily apparent relational information. Taken together, the experiments conducted by Hess (1984) and Hess and Higgins (1983) indicate that when looking for age effects in item-specific processing, it is important to examine item-specific processing as it relates to relational processing.

In a more recent study, Hay and Jacoby (1999) also used homographs. The Hay and Jacoby study involved a training phase in which a homograph was biased toward a particular meaning and biased to a particular associated response. For instance, the homograph *organ* was biased toward its musical rather than its biological meaning during training. To make one response more typical than the other, *music* was paired with *organ* 75% of the time (typical response). On the remaining 25% of training trials the word *organ* was paired with a different word to create an atypical response. For half of the participants, *organ* was paired with *piano* on 25% of the training trials (same meaning-atypical response). For the other half of participants, *organ* was paired with *heart* for 25% of the training trials (different meaning). After the training session, participants completed several study-test trials. On each study trial, participants studied a list of word pairs in which the homographs were paired either with the typical response, the same meaning-atypical response, or the different meaning response. Following encoding of the study list, participants completed a cued-recall test in which they had to provide the response that had been paired with the homograph on the immediately preceding study list.

Younger adults were less likely to make errors (i.e., producing the typical response *music* instead of *heart* or *piano*) in the different-meaning response condition than in the same-meaning atypical response condition. The older adults did not differ in their error rates between the atypical and the different meaning conditions. When the homographs were presented at study with a more discriminable response, the older adults were less able to take advantage of the information for overriding the habitual response that had been established during training. Hay and Jacoby (1999) showed that the older adults' deficit in processing of item-specific information could be overcome. Older adults made fewer errors in the different-meaning condition relative to the same-meaning atypical condition when they were provided additional time for both encoding and retrieval along with instructions that focused attention on processing the item-specific information that defined the different meaning condition.

Evidence for More General Encoding on the Part of Older Adults: Asking Participants to Generate Information at Encoding

Another approach to potential age differences in item-specific processing is to ask participants to generate information that is then examined for specificity. In an incidental learning task, Rankin and Collins (1986) presented participants with base sentences such as "The *thin* dog knocked over the trash can." There were four different conditions determined by whether elaboration was provided to the participant or generated by the participant. Within each of these conditions there was a precise and an imprecise condition. In all cases the base sentence was provided. In the elaboration-provided condition, the sentence also provided information that either high-lighted the meaning of the target word (precise elaboration provided: "The *thin* dog knocked over the trash can that held the garbage") or informa-tion that was related, but that did not emphasize the target word (impre-cise elaboration provided: "The *thin* dog knocked over the trash can by the back porch"). In the generation-condition, participants provided their own elaboration in response to one of two questions, either "Why might this person be engaged in this particular type of activity?" in the precise condition, or "What else might happen in this context?" in the imprecise condition. Recall was tested by presenting the same sentences again with-out the target word.

In all conditions, younger adults recalled more target words than older adults recalled, but different patterns emerged for each age group. Younger adults recalled more target words when they generated their own precise elaboration than when they were provided with precise elaboration sen-tences. Older adults were better when they were provided with the precise sentences rather than generating their own. This would seem to suggest that older adults are not precisely processing the material when attempting to generate their own elaboration. In fact, older adults did generate less pre-cise elaborations than the younger adults. The definition of precision used by Rankin and Collins (1986) was information that uniquely related the target to other information in the sentence. Older adults were less likely to provide this kind of information. While the results suggest that older adults may have engaged in less item-specific processing, it may also have been that the older adults were processing item-specific information about the target words, but that item-specific information was not related to the con-text. In other words, what the older adults lacked was not necessarily item-specific information but distinctive information.

More direct evidence for an age difference in item-specific processing comes from a study by Mäntylä and Bäckman (1990) in which younger and older adults were presented with a list of unrelated words. Participants generated either two (Experiment 2) or three (Experiment 1) properties of each word. The property-generation task was completed a second time after a delay of three weeks. Younger adults were more internally consistent—that is, they were more likely than the older adults were to pro-duce the same properties for each word in both sessions. Importantly, the younger adults showed more variability across subjects. The increased over-lap between older adults could reflect their more general level of process-ing. Processing information at a more general level—for example, thinking of *bear* as *animal* versus thinking of *bear* as *wild animal*—will likely lead to more overlap among individuals, but at the expense in this case of item-specific processing. (See also Mäntylä & Craik, 1993; Rankin & Firnhaber, 1986; Brosseau, & Cohen, 1996).

Perhaps if older adults are directed to generate item-specific informa-tion in the context of explicit relational information, this will reduce age differences in the generality of encoding processes. Hunt and Smith (1996) presented a paradigm, based on the technique used by Mäntylä and Bäckman (1990), that requires participants to generate information that focuses on item-specific information within a relational context (see also Smith & Hunt, 2000a, 2000b). Smith, Hunt, and Dunlosky (2005) applied this paradigm to understanding age differences in memory. Younger and older adults were shown sets of five words from each of 30 taxonomic categories. The words were arranged in a vertical list with the top item marked with an asterisk. Participants were asked to provide a single word that denoted something that was different about the top word from the other four words. Inter-subject overlap did not differ as a function of age, indicating that older adults can process information at a specific level as well as younger adults when (1) they are directed to consider what makes an item unique, and (2) they consider the uniqueness of the item in the context of highly obvious relational information. Similarly, Rankin and Firnhaber (1986) found that younger and older adults generated equally distinct adjectives when specifically instructed to generate unique adjectives.

Item-Specific Processing: Summary

The findings concerning the number of items recalled per category clearly show an advantage for younger adults, suggesting an age-related deficit in item-specific processing. Studies investigating the nature of older adults' elaboration provide consistent evidence that older adults process information at a more general level. However, older adults did engage in some item-specific processing, and age differences in memory performance can be reduced by providing sufficient support, particularly when the support draws on relational information as a background for highlighting differences.

RELATIONAL PROCESSING

Relational processing is the detection of relationships among elements of an event, a process that allows discrete elements to be integrated into a whole. Although the findings concerning organization as a function of age are mixed (Salthouse, 1991), some order is achieved by examining the different methods that have been used to imply the effects of organization on performance. Three of these methods will be considered here. First, studies that have examined whether younger and older adults benefit in the same way from manipulations that support or encourage relational processing at encoding are discussed. Next, the review focuses on whether younger and older adults benefit to the same extent from support for relational processing at retrieval, in the form of category label cues. Finally, the confusing findings regarding age differences in clustering will be considered.

Support for Relational Processing at Encoding

If there is an age difference in relational processing, then it is possible that providing support for such processing at encoding—in the form of organized material, for instance—could potentially reduce or eliminate age differences. In this case, older adults would be expected to benefit more than younger adults from a manipulation that supports relational processing. Studies investigating relational processing at encoding have used a variety of manipulations and have produced mixed results concerning the relative effects of those manipulations for younger and older adults.

In tests of memories for scenes (detection of relocation or substitution of objects), Frieske and Park (1993) found better performance for both younger and older adults when the scenes were organized compared to unorganized scenes. However, provision of an organized scene did not reduce age differences in memory for the scene (see also Park, Cherry, Smith, & LaFronza, 1990; Sharps, 1991). Cherry and Jones (1999) also failed to find a reduction in age differences in memory for object location when the objects were organized at encoding compared to when the objects were distributed randomly. In contrast to these studies, a number of studies have found smaller age differences when encoding encourages relational processing. Using related study items can reduce age differences. In a study involving memory for actions, Norris and West (1993) found a smaller age difference when the actions were categorizable according to a particular body part, as opposed to random actions. Similarly, Weinert, Schneider, and Knopf (1988) found reduced age effects when using categorizable words than when using unrelated words.

Blocking similar items can also reduce age differences. In a study conducted by Schacter, Kaszniak, Khilstrom, and Valdiserri (1991), factual sentences were read aloud by different sources. The words were presented either all from one source and then the other or back and forth between sources. The older adults recalled more facts when the source presentation was blocked compared to when the sources were random. Younger adults recalled equally well regardless of whether the source was random or blocked. More recently, Stuss, Craik, Sayer, Franchi, and Alexander (1996) found that age differences in memory for words were smaller with a blocked categorized list relative to an unrelated list, but a categorized list that was not blocked did not reduce the age difference.

The Stuss et al. finding suggests that, in order to reduce age differences, the relational information must be fairly explicit. Consistent with this proposal, Hess, Flannagan, and Tate (1993) found that older adults benefited from schematic organization at encoding only when labels related to that organization were provided at study. Other studies produced findings that are consistent with the notion that support for relational processing at encoding is important for reducing age differences. Smith (1977) found no age difference in free or cued recall when the category label cue was available during encoding (see also Craik, Byrd, & Swanson, 1987; Shaw & Craik, 1989).

Another way to make relational information explicit is to ask participants to engage in a sorting task. A number of studies involve just such a request. For example, Hultsch (1971) found that older adults benefited more than younger adults when a sorting task was included at encoding. Several studies that used a sorting task at encoding will be discussed in the section on distinctiveness because these studies involved explicit manipulations of both relational and item-specific processing (Fisher & McDowd, 1993; Guttenttag, 1988; Luszcz, Roberts, & Mattiske, 1990). Still others studies used sorting tasks, but did not contrast sorting with a different encoding task (e.g., Basden et al., 1993; Worden & Meggison, 1984)

One study that examined the effect of relational processing at encoding is of particular interest because it provides a nice example of how it can be more productive to think of relational processing and item-specific processing working in a joint fashion. Byrd (1986) presented participants with a prose passage, in which the sentences were either in the normal original order or were randomized. Participants in the two randomized conditions had to sort the sentences into the correct order. The sentences were randomized in two different ways—within a paragraph, in which case the sentences were in the correct paragraph but out of order; or completely randomized, with the sentences in random arrangement throughout the passage. The results may at first appear counterintuitive: in the case in which the sentences were completely randomized, there was no age-difference memory for the text, while there were age differences in favor of younger adults in the other two conditions. The age difference was not present in the most demanding condition.

Byrd's (1986) findings make sense when interpreted in light of relational and item-specific information working together. In the case of the within-paragraph randomized presentation, participants had to examine each sentence carefully in order to place it in the correct order, inducing item-specific processing of each sentence. The item-specific information for each sentence in the within-paragraph sorting condition was related to each paragraph, but not to the story structure. Moreover, the paragraphs themselves were not necessarily processed with respect to the overall structure of the story. In contrast, in the case of the completely randomized condition, participants had to attend to the details of each sentence while also paying attention to the overall relational structure of the passage. Participants in the completely randomized condition had to relate the sentences to paragraph relationships and the paragraphs had to be related to the overall story structure. The completely randomized condition encourages item-specific processing of both sentences and paragraphs, thereby increasing the likelihood of engaging adequately in both relational and item-specific processing that could aid later recall. When the task demands that participants engage in both types of processing, performance benefited the most. In other words, when the task encourages distinctive processing of both sentences and paragraphs, viewed as the combination of item-specific and relational processing, older adults perform as well as younger adults. Similarly, Hess and Arnould (1986) found age differences when the encoding materials were organized and no age difference when the materials were unorganized. In the Hess and Arnould experiment, participants studied sentences for a later memory test. The sentences were presented in a story format (organized) or in a random fashion (unorganized). Hess and Arnould found an advantage for younger adults in memory for the explicit content of the sentences in the organized case only. There was no age difference when the sentences were randomly presented.

Summarizing the effects of relational processing at encoding on age differences is somewhat difficult given the variety of techniques used for inducing relational processing and the somewhat inconsistent findings. Overall however, it appears that when the encoding task and materials directly encourage and support relational processing, age differences are reduced. The Byrd (1986) and Hess and Arnould (1986) studies suggest that participants will benefit the most when the task also involves distinctive processing—that is, when the task involves processing particular items in light of how each item relates to the overall organization.

Category Label Cued Recall

Relational processing can be supported at test by provision of category label cues (e.g., Hunt & Seta, 1984). Again, the literature on the effects of label cues and aging is inconsistent, with some studies reporting a reduction of age differences with label cues (e.g., Erber, 1984; Shaw & Craik, 1989) and other studies reporting no effect of the cues on age differences (e.g., Basden et al., 1993; Hultsch, 1975; Rankin & Hinricks, 1983; Weible, Nuest, Welty, Pate, & Turner, 2002). Examination of the materials and procedures used in these different studies suggests that the inconsistency is due to differential relational processing at encoding.

Consider the studies in which the age difference in recall was not reduced or eliminated by provision of category label cues. In the Rankin and Hinricks (1983) study, participants studied unrelated words, one word from each of 20 categories. Before studying the list of words, participants were given a three-item practice list and test so they were aware of the type of cue that would be presented, but the category labels were not provided at study. In other words, there was no encouragement to engage in relational processing during the encoding phase of the Rankin and Hinricks study. Weible et al. (2002) used categorized words, but the words were presented in a random fashion. The Stuss et al. (1996) study mentioned above found that age differences in recall were reduced when categories were presented in a blocked fashion at study. Thus, the older adults in the Weible et al. study may have engaged in little relational processing at study, which then reduced their ability to use the category label cues appropriately at retrieval.

Light and Albertson (1989) also used categorized words, but there were only three words from each category, the words were presented in a random order at encoding, and participants performed a pleasantness rating task, none of which would have been optimal for supporting relational processing (Hunt & Seta, 1984). In all of these cases it can be argued that support provided at encoding for relational processing was insufficient, reducing the ability to benefit from relational support at retrieval.

The Basden et al. (1993) study poses a more complex problem. Participants were presented with 100 unrelated words, but unlike the Rankin and Hinricks (1983) study, participants in the Basden et al. experiment were asked to sort the words into categories, which the participants named. The category names were used for a cued-recall test. The age difference was no smaller in the cued-recall condition than in a free-recall condition. Participants were asked to sort the words into categories, but were not told how many categories they should use. Younger adults sorted the words into more categories than did the older adults, consistent with the idea that older adults process information in a more general and less specific fashion (Craik & Byrd, 1982). Interestingly, the older adults were more likely than the younger adults to fail to recall any items associated with a particular category, even in the case of category-cued recall. Basden et al. suggested that the older adults produced category labels that were "less well related to category instances" (Basden et al., p.36). Basden et al. interpreted this as indicating that the older adults were deficient in relational processing. An alternative interpretation follows from the idea that older adults encoded the information in a more general fashion, without attending to item-specific information—that is, the older adults formed a less distinctive encoding and therefore were less likely to recall the specific items in a category. In fact, older adults did recall fewer items per category in both cued and free recall, providing another indicator that the older adults were less able to process the appropriate item-specific information within a particular category context, leading to poorer recall when provided with the category information at retrieval.

Hultsch (1975) also failed to find a reduction in age differences when participants were given category label cues at test. Unlike Rankin and Hinricks (1983) and Weible et al. (2002), Hultsch did use a blocked categorized study list (four words from each of ten categories). Instructions for the study task focused attention on the category relationship and therefore encouraged relational processing at the expense of item-specific processing. In fact, older and younger adults had similar category access in the cued-recall test, but the older adults recalled fewer items per category. In other words, there may have been sufficient relational processing, but there was insufficient item-specific processing to eliminate the age difference.

The studies that show a reduction in age differences when using category-cued recall involved methods that encourage both relational and item-specific encoding. The study by Erber (1984) used an encoding technique that very likely encouraged both. In the Erber experiment, participants studied 24 unrelated words, one from each category. At encoding, participants made a category membership judgment. Half of the words were paired with the appropriate category label and half were paired with a different label. No age difference was found in cued recall of words that had been paired with the correct category label at study. Hunt and Seta (1984) demonstrated that participants benefit from sorting when the categories are small because the sorting task encouraged relational processing and the small category size leads to item-specific processing. In the Erber study, the categories were as small as possible, one item per category, and the category membership task encouraged processing of the appropriate relational information. When both relational and item-specific information processing was encouraged at study, and the relational information was reinstated at retrieval in the form of category label cues, the age difference was eliminated (see also Shaw & Craik, 1989).

In summary, the overall pattern suggests that age differences can be reduced through the use of category label recall cues, but the original encoding experience must encourage the processing of the relevant relational information as well as item-specific information.

Clustering

Another way to investigate potential age differences in relational processing is to look for differences in measures of output organization using various clustering measures. As pointed out by Burns (Chapter 6 this volume), clustering measures might not provide the best measure for tapping into the role of relational processing, and it is certainly the case that the literature is rather confusing with respect to whether there are age differences in clustering (Kausler, 1994; Smith, 1980; see Murphy, 1979, for a discussion of different measures of clustering). In an attempt to shed some light on this confusing aspect of the literature on memory and aging, this section focuses on 30 experiments that have employed word lists as the to-be-remembered stimuli and that have compared measures of output organization for younger and older adults (see Table 12.1). There are also studies that report clustering measures for younger and older adults' free recall of pictures (e.g., Laurence, 1966; Wingard, 1980), designs (e.g., Tubi & Calev, 1989), and actions (e.g., Guttentag & Hunt, 1988; Norris & West, 1993; Rönnlund, Nyberg, Bäckman, & Nilsson, 2003; see Rönnlund et al. for an extensive review of age differences in memory for subject-performed task).

One potential explanation for the range of findings concerning age effects on clustering measures was provided by Witte, Freund, and Sebby (1990). Witte et al. suggested that differences in list length could explain difference in the outcomes regarding age effects. For instance, Smith (1980), Hultsch (1974), and Witte et al. (1990) found age differences using study lists of 30 words or more. Jackson and Schneider (1982) used 16 words and found no age differences. Unfortunately this solution cannot accommodate the results of many other studies. For instance, Luszcz et al. (1990),

TABLE 12.1 Age Effects on Clustering Scores in Free Recall of Word Lists

	Basis of Clustering	Number of		
		Tests	Categories	Items/Cat.
No Advantage for Younger Adults				
Amrhein et al., 1999[a,d]*	Order	1	24	2
Basden et al., 1993[a]	Category	1	varied	varied
Fisher & McDowd, Exp. 1[a]	Category	1	5	5
Fisher & McDowd, 1993, Exp. 2[a]	Category	1	4	2,4,8,16
Guttentag, 1988, Exp. 1[a]	Category	1	4	2,6,10,14
Hertzog et al., 1990[a]	Category	1	6	5
Hess et al., 1993, Exp. 1 and Exp. 2[a]	Category	1	6	6
Howard et al., 1981[d]	Category	1	4	10
Hultsch et al., 1990[a]	Category	1	6	5
Luszcz et al., 1990[a,b], Exp. 2	Category	1	5	2,4,8,12,16
Mungas et al., 1991[d]*	Order	1	8	2
Park et al., 1989, Exp. 1, Full Attention[a]	Category	1	6	6
Rankin et al., 1984[d]*	Category	4	8	6
Tubi & Calev, 1989[d]	Category	1	6	4
Weinert et al., 1988[a]	Category	1	4	6
Witte et al., 1993[a,b,d]*	Category	5	8	5
Worden & Meggison, 1984[d]	Category	1	varied	varied
Worden & Sherman-Brown, 1983, Exp. 2[d]	Order	3	N/A	N/A
Zevian & Darjes, 1983[a]	Category	1	6	5
Higher Clustering Scores for Younger Adults				
Amrhein et al., 1999[a,d]*	Category	1	24	2
Hultsch, 1974[d]	Order	10	N/A	N/A
Jackson & Schneider, 1985[c]	Order	4	N/A	N/A
Macht & Buschke, 1983[d]	Order	4	N/A	N/A
Mungas et al., 1991[a]*	Category	1	8	2
Park et al., 1989, Exp. 1, Divided Attention[a]	Category	1	6	6
Rankin et al., 1984[c]*	Order	4	8	6
Riefer & Batchelder, 1991[b]	Category	1	16	2
Sanders et al., 1980[b]	Category	1	4	4
Sanders et al., 1980[d]	Order	1	4	4
Smith, 1980[c]	Order	5	N/A	N/A
Stuss et al., 1996[c]	Order	4	N/A	N/A
Stuss et al., 1996[c] }within-subjects	Order	4	4	4
Stuss et al., 1996[c] }manipulation	Order	4	4	4
Witte et al., 1990[c] }of list type	Order	6	N/A	N/A
Witte et al., 1993[c]*	Order	5	8	5
Worden & Sherman-Brown, 1983, Exp. 1[d]	Category	3	7	varied

Note: Superscript letters indicate which measure of organization was used. [a]ARC [b]ratio of repetition based on category [c]Sternberg and Tulving's (1977) pair frequency measure [d]other.

*Study includes measures based upon both order and category information in a single experiment.

Hertzog, Dixon, and Hultsch (1990), and Rankin, Karol, and Tuten (1984) found no age differences when using lists of 42, 30, and 48 items, respectively. Basden et al. (1993) found no age difference with 100 words.

Subsequently, Witte et al. (1993) presented an experiment concerned with age differences in both category and subjective organization. Witte et al. (1993) presented younger and older adults with an unblocked categorized list of 40 words (5 words from each of eight categories) one at a time for 3 seconds, each followed by a 3-minute written recall test. The study test trial was repeated four more times for a total of five tests. Younger adults recalled more words than did the older adults. Witte et al. used three measures of category-based clustering (ratio of repetition, modified ratio of repetition, and adjusted rate of clustering, or ARC), all of which produced the same pattern of results. Older adults actually showed higher levels of category-based clustering on the first trial than did the younger adults. The age difference in category-based clustering was not found on test trials two through five.

Witte et al. (1993) also examined the overlap between output order and input order, which they referred to as a seriation measure (Sternberg & Tulving, 1977). Younger adults showed greater seriation scores on the first test trial than on subsequent trials, and the seriation scores for younger adults were greater than the scores for older adults on the first trial. Witte et al. suggested that researchers frequently fail to find age differences in clustering on a single test trial, not because the older adults are equally good at relational processing but because the category-based clustering measures do not adequately capture the relational processing employed in the task. Because younger adults are more likely to engage in a seriation strategy on an initial recall trial, they will have reduced category-based clustering scores. Witte et al. (1993) suggested that in order to get a clear picture of potential age differences in relational information, one should use multiple test trials. Unfortunately, the earlier work by Witte and colleagues contradicts this claim.

Witte et al. (1990) also used repeated testing and examined output organization employing the same measure of seriation as was used in the Witte et al. (1993) study. In the 1990 experiment, age effects were demonstrated in seriation—but not on the first trial, only on later trials. Furthermore, in several other experiments, there was no benefit for younger adults on a measure of seriation on an initial or single recall trial (Amrhein, Bond, & Hamilton, 1999; Mungas, Ehlers, & Blunden, 1991; Worden & Sherman-Brown, 1983). Thus, it does not appear that younger adults will necessarily employ a greater seriation strategy on recall. Furthermore, this explanation cannot accommodate findings of an age difference in favor of younger adults on category-based measures of output organization (Amrhein et al., 1999; Mungas et al., 1991; Riefer & Batchelder, 1984; Sanders et al., 1980; Worden & Sherman-Brown, 1983).

The explanations provided by Witte et al. (1990, 1993) cannot explain the variations in age differences in clustering. However, there is an alternative explanation that relies on the interplay of relational and item-specific information. As can be seen in Table 12.1, the majority of studies that have failed to find an advantage for younger adults in clustering scores have used the measures based on category organization (Basden et al., 1993; Fisher & McDowd, 1993; Guttentag, 1988; Hertzog et al., 1990; Hess et al., 1993; Howard, McAndrews, & Lasaga, 1981; Hultsch, Hertzog, & Dixon, 1990; Luszcz et al., 1990; Park et al., 1989; Rankin et al., 1984; Tubi & Calev, 1989; Weinert et al., 1988; Witte et al., 1993; Worden & Meggison, 1984; Zivian & Darjes, 1983). In contrast, studies that have found age differences in favor of younger adults have frequently used measures of subjective organization that reflect the concordance between input and output orders or between output orders on successive recall trials (Hultsch, 1974; Jackson & Schneider, 1982; Macht & Buschke, 1983; Rankin et al., 1984; Smith, 1980; Stuss et al., 1996; Witte et al., 1990, 1993). However, the differences cannot be explained simply as a difference in category-based versus order-based measures. There are studies that used category-based measures in which younger adults showed more clustering (Amrhein et al., 1999; Mungas et al., 1991; Riefer & Batchelder, 1991; Sanders et al., 1980; Worden & Sherman-Brown, 1983).

Is there any obvious difference between the studies that use category-based measures that show no advantage for younger adults and studies that use category-based measures that have found an advantage for younger adults? Consider Hunt and Seta's (1984) study demonstrating that spontaneous relational processing is encouraged by category materials when the category size (number of items from a given category) is sufficiently large, but not when there are fewer than four items from each category.

Of the six studies using a category-based measure of output organization that have found age differences in clustering, three used only two items per category (Amrhein et al., 1999; Mungas et al., 1991; Riefer & Batchelder, 1991). The study by Worden and Sherman-Brown (1983) did not use a specified number of items in each category, but it is most likely that the number was small. In the Worden and Sherman-Brown study, participants were given index cards, each with one of 30 words, and asked to sort the words into seven categories. The sorting task was repeated until the participants could sort with 95% consistency on two trials. The average number of items per category was not reported, but assuming that the categories did not vary greatly in size, it is likely that each category consisted of fewer than four items on average.

Of the remaining two experiments that found higher clustering scores for younger adults using a category-based measure, the Sanders et al. (1980) experiment included a relatively small category size of four items in a category. Although there is one study that failed to find an age difference in a category-based measure using categories of four items (Tubi & Calev, 1989), all of the other studies that did not find an advantage for younger adults included categories that were larger than four. Thus, it appears that if categories are sufficiently large to encourage the use of relational processing of the category information, and if output organization is then evaluated using a category-based measure, age differences are not likely to be found. In other words, as suggested above in the discussion of relational information at encoding, the relational information must be readily accessible for older adults to utilize the information effectively. When categories involve small numbers of items, the materials do not encourage the use of relational information (Hunt & Seta, 1984), and it is more likely that age differences in output organization will be found.

The remaining study that found age differences in a category-based measure of output organization fits this explanation. In the Park et al. (1989) study, younger and older adults studied six words from each of six categories presented in a random order. For half of the participants attention was divided through the use of a secondary task during encoding. There was a significant interaction of age and the manipulation of attention at encoding. Older adults' clustering scores declined more (from .50 to .18) than did the scores for younger adults (from .42 to .27) when attention was divided at encoding. Given that the addition of a secondary task at encoding decreases output organization, this indicates that processing category-based relational information at encoding for use during retrieval is resource demanding. Older adults are assumed to have more limited cognitive resources (for reviews, see Light, 1996; Verhaeghen, Marcoen, & Goosens, 1993; Zacks et al., 2000). Therefore, if the relational information can be made more obvious through the use of larger categories, thereby reducing the resources required to process this relational information, then older adults may be able to benefit from the information to the same extent as do younger adults (unless attentions is divided). The Park et al. (1989) results are consistent with the argument that relational processing must be supported at encoding in order to benefit from this information.

Although the literature concerning the relationship between age and measures of clustering is a bit confusing, a pattern does emerge from the data. It appears that measures of clustering that are based on category information are less likely to show age differences in favor of younger adults as long as the studied categories are sufficiently large. In contrast, clustering scores based on item order are more likely to show a difference as a function of age in favor of younger adults. Two studies that measured both types of clustering for the same participants and the same stimuli are consistent with this summary. In both the Rankin et al. (1984) and Witte et al. (1993) experiments, younger adults scored higher than older adults on order-based measures but not on category-based measures. The experiments involved categories of six and five items, respectively. The Amrhein study showed the opposite pattern, but as mentioned above, there were only two items in each category in this experiment.

Is there a way to explain the difference in the effects of age on order-based and category-based measures of clustering? The order-based clustering scores are considered a reflection of relational information in that they tap into relationships among items. These relationships potentially reflect very small categories, with each category defined as the grouping of a few sequential items. Relational processing is less likely to be induced by small categories based on contiguity at presentation, as indicated by studies showing that clustering decreases as category size decreases for both younger (Hunt & Seta, 1984; Luszcz et al., 1990) and older adults (Luszcz et al., 1990). When the materials do not encourage the relevant relational processing, it is more likely that age differences in favor of younger adults will appear.

Relational Processing: Summary

Overall, the findings regarding relational processing suggest that older adults sometimes show deficits in relational processing, but that those deficits can be overcome when the encoding context encourages processing of the relevant relational information. Similarly, the use of category label cues can reduce age differences in memory performance, given sufficient support for processing of the related category information at the time of encoding. Age differences in clustering measures are eliminated when the to-be-remembered materials encourage processing of category information. When the measure of clustering focuses on less obvious category information or on order information, age differences in clustering are more often demonstrated. Thus, the clustering data also indicate that there are age differences in relational processing, but those differences can be overcome with adequate support for the relevant relational processing. Finally, beyond demonstrating that there are age differences in relational processing, the literature on support for relational processing at encoding and category cued recall also indicates that processing item-specific information in the context of a relational structure is most likely to reduce age differences in memory performance

DISTINCTIVE PROCESSING

This section will focus on studies that examine age differences in memory when variables that are thought to influence item-specific processing and relational processing are manipulated in the same study. First, three studies are reviewed that have applied techniques from Hunt and Einstein (1981) and Hunt and Seta (1984) to study adult age differences in memory. The section concludes by describing studies that have investigated potential age differences in the von Restorff effect, the modality effect in false memory, and the consistency effect, all of which have been discussed in terms of distinctive processing.

Extending Hunt and Seta (1984) and Hunt and Einstein (1981) to Older Adults

In this section I will discuss three studies that have employed orthogonal manipulations of item-specific and relational processing to examine age differences in memory performance. Hunt and Seta (1984) manipulated the type of processing engaged during an incidental learning task by asking participants to either sort words into the appropriate taxonomic category or to rate each word for pleasantness. Hunt and Seta also manipulated category size. The study list consisted of words from six categories and each category included 1, 2, 4, 8, 12, or 16 items. Larger categories are assumed to induce spontaneous relational processing. Free-recall performance was best when the combination of orienting task and category size encouraged both relational and item-specific processing. When categories were small, recall was better following the sorting task, which encouraged relational processing. For large categories, recall was best following the pleasantness-rating task, which encouraged item-specific processing. Processing item-specific information within a relational context produced the best memory.

The same basic paradigm was used by Guttentag (1988), Fisher and McDowd (1993), and Luszcz et al. (1990) to investigate memory performance in younger and older adults. In all cases the small categories were better remembered following the sorting task and large categories were better following the rating task. The effect of the orienting task on small categories was reduced for older adults in the Luszcz et al., but the same basic pattern was evident. Given that the findings of Hunt and Seta were replicated with older adults, this indicates that the combination of item-specific and relational processing is the best situation for memory performance for older adults as well as younger adults. It should be noted that the combination of relational and item-specific processing did not eliminate age differences in memory performance on the free-recall test. However, for words that were rated at encoding, the age difference was eliminated by providing category label cues to aid recall in both the Luszcz et al. and Fisher and McDowd experiments. In the Fisher and McDowd experiment, the age effect was also eliminated for words that had been sorted by providing the category label cues. (Guttentag, 1988, did not have a cued-recall condition).

Hunt and Einstein (1981) also manipulated orienting task and list structure. As in Hunt and Seta (1984), participants performed a rating task or a sorting task. Rather than using category-size variations to influence relational and item-specific processing, Hunt and Einstein used two different types of lists. The related list consisted of six words from each of six categories. The unrelated list consisted of six words from each of six more loosely defined ad hoc categories, such as liquid things. Performance was best when participants either rated the related list or sorted the unrelated list, or when participants performed both tasks on either list.

Fisher and McDowd (1993, Experiment 1) and Luszcz et al. (1990, Experiment 1) both also used the same manipulations with older adults (the former also included a young adult age group). The Luszcz et al. experiment included the condition in which both tasks are performed, the Fisher and McDowd experiment did not include this condition. The older adults in these experiments showed the same pattern of results as the young adults in Hunt and Einstein (1981). There was an effect of age in the Fisher and

McDowd experiment, but age did not interact with the other manipulations, indicating that the combined benefits of item-specific and relational processing are similar for younger and older adults.

In summary, when both item-specific and relational processing are manipulated in younger and older adults, the same pattern of effects emerges in free recall: both age groups benefit the most when the two types of processing are combined. The benefits of combined relational and item-specific processing only eliminated the age difference in memory performance when additional support was provided in the form of category label cues at the time of retrieval.

The Consistency Effect

The *consistency effect* refers to findings of better memory for items that are inconsistent with expectations than for items that are consistent with expectations. Mäntylä and Bäckman (1992) investigated the consistency effect in younger and older adults in a naturalistic setting. Participants briefly viewed a room arranged as a typical office. The office setting provided the relational context. The room contained objects that would be expected in an office setting (telephone) and objects that would not be expected in an office (hand mixer). After moving to a different room, participants' were given an old/new recognition test in which they designated items that had been in the office as old and other items as new. Following the recognition test, participants were taken back to the office and were given a token test. On the token test, participants were asked whether various objects in the office had been changed out with a slightly different object (e.g., replacing a black traditional telephone with a white modern telephone).

Both the younger and older adults showed equivalent consistency effects on the recognition test. Participants were better at recognizing items that were inconsistent with the office setting than they were at recognizing items that were consistent with the office setting. Thus, younger and older adults were equally sensitive to the distinctive nature of the inconsistent items. An age difference did emerge on the token test. Younger adults were better able to recognize changes in inconsistent items than changes in consistent items. There was no difference in change-detection abilities as a function of consistency for the older adults. The Mäntylä and Bäckman (1992) study shows that older adults can benefit from distinctiveness, when distinctiveness is defined as a difference in the context of similarity, but that the benefit may not be as large as that for younger adults.

The Modality Effect in False Recall

The failure on the part of older adults to encode sufficient item-specific information can lead to increased memory errors (e.g., Hess, 1984; Hess and Higgins, 1983). A paradigm for investigating memory errors that has recently received considerable attention is the Deese-Roediger-McDermott (DRM) paradigm (see Schacter & Wiseman, Chapter 5 this volume). In the DRM paradigm participants are presented with lists of words that are highly associated with critical nonpresented items. On subsequent memory tests, participants frequently report that the critical items had been presented. These false memories can reach very high levels, frequently as high as correct recall. However, Smith & Hunt (1998) discovered that when the highly associated items are presented visually, participants are much less likely to falsely remember the nonpresented critical items as having been presented than if the study list is presented auditorally. This is the modality effect in false memory.

In order to avoid false memories in the DRM paradigm, study-list items must be discriminated from highly associated critical lures. The overlap in relational information between the study items and the critical item could lead to the generation, or coming to mind, of the critical item at study or at test. Thus, externally perceived study-list items must be distinguished from critical items that the participant might have thought of but did not perceive. This discrimination must involve item-specific processing along some dimension that differentiates the study item from the critical item. Smith and Hunt argued that visually encoded items included perceptual information that is more helpful for making the discrimination between studied and related critical items. Thus, the modality effect arguably depends on distinctive processing (Smith & Hunt, 1998; Smith, Hunt, & Gallagher, 2005).

If older adults experience deficits in distinctive processing, then they may be less likely to show a modality effect in false memory. In two experiments, older adults failed to show a modality effect in false recall (Smith, Lozito, & Bayen, 2005). Smith, Payne, and Engle (2000) failed to find a modality effect in false recall in individuals with lower working-memory spans. Thus, reduced resources may account for the lack of a modality effect in false recall for older adults. Consistent with this idea is a study by Gallo and Roediger (2003), in which older adults do show a modality effect on false recognition. The recognition test provides more environmental support than the free-recall test. Furthermore, Gallo and Roediger focused participants' attention on particular aspects of the original encoding experience by asking participants to recall the modality of presentation for each item and to judge the quality of their memory for each item. Once again, older adults show deficits in distinctive processing that can be overcome if additional support is provided.

The von Restorff Effect

The von Restorff effect refers to better memory for an item that is isolated in a list of to-be-remembered items (Hunt, 1995). For instance, the isolate may be a number while all other items in the list are consonant strings. The von Restorff effect is a result of distinctive processing (Hunt, Chapter 1 this volume, 1995; Hunt & Lamb, 2001; Dunlosky, Hunt, & Clark, 2000). If older adults are less adroit at distinctive processing, then the von Restorff effect may be reduced for older adults.

Cimbalo and Brink (1982) investigated the von Restorff effect in younger and older adults. Participants viewed 12 study lists that each consisted of nine consonants shown one at a time. In half of the lists, the fifth consonant, which served as the isolate, was larger than the other consonants. The remaining lists were control lists in which all consonants were the same size. Following the intentional study task, participants tried to recall the lists in order of occurrence. The younger adults showed the von Restorff effect in that memory for the fifth item was better when in the isolation lists than in the control lists. The older adults did not show the isolation effect. There are some limitations to the study in terms of the control-list selection (see Hunt, 1995, for a discussion of appropriate control lists). Furthermore, the demand to recall the items in order may have influenced recall: Friedman (1966) found that when the requirement to recall items in order was dropped, age effects in a short-term memory task were eliminated. However, despite these potential problems, the study provides evidence once again that older adults experience a deficit in distinctive processing.

Distinctive Processing: Summary

The studies by Fisher and McDowd (1993), Guttentag (1988), and Luszcz et al. (1990) provide evidence that older adults benefit most when item-specific and relational processing are combined, replicating effects found with younger adults (Hunt & Einstein, 1981; Hunt & McDaniel, 1993; Hunt & Seta, 1984). Investigations of effects that can be explained by considering the processing of difference in the context of similarity show deficits for older adults, indicating age-related changes in distinctive processing. Furthermore, evidence suggests that age-related differences in distinctive processing may be attributable to age-related reductions in cognitive resource availability.

THREE POINTS CONCERNING DISTINCTIVENESS APPLIED TO MEMORY AND AGING

Hunt (Chapter 1 this volume) raised four points to consider when thinking about distinctiveness and memory. Three of these points, which are particularly relevant to the literature on distinctiveness and memory reviewed in this chapter, are discussed in this section.

Distinctiveness Is a Process, Not Inherent in Materials

Given that distinctiveness is not inherent in certain materials, but instead describes a way of processing information that can lead to good memory for that information, we might expect to find age differences in the benefits of distinctive processing, depending on the nature of those processes.

Younger adults do better than older adults on measures of working-memory span, indicating that older adults may have reduced resources relative to younger adults (Light, 1996; Verhaeghen et al., 1993; Zacks et al., 2000). If distinctive processes in a given situation are heavily dependent on our limited cognitive resources, older adults may be less inclined to spontaneously engage in those processes or they may be less able to engage in those processes as fully as are younger adults. Providing additional support can help to overcome these age differences (Craik, 1986). Providing support that facilitates either relational, item-specific, or preferably both kinds of processing may increase the chances that older adults will benefit fully from distinctive processing.

Several of the findings reviewed in this chapter concur with the proposal that distinctive processing may be more difficult for older adults owing to reduced resources. Luszcz et al. (1990) and Fisher and McDowd (1993) found that distinctive processing can eliminate age difference in recall as long as older adults are provided with adequate support at retrieval in the form of category label cues. In their study of the consistency effect, Mäntylä and Bäckman (1992) found that older adults did not show the consistency effect on a token test while younger adults did show improved performance for inconsistent items on the token test. When younger adults encoded the office scene while performing a secondary task they subsequently failed to show the consistency effect on the token test. This indicates that the age differences in distinctive processing are related to age differences in cognitive resources. Similarly, Smith et al. (2000) found the same pattern of results for younger adults with lower working-memory span scores as had been found with older adults in a false-memory study (Smith, Lozito, & Bayen, 2005). Neither the younger adults with lower working-memory capacity nor the older adults showed a reduction in false recall following visual-study presentation relative to auditory-study presentation. The lack of a modality effect in older adults could be due to reduced resources needed to engage in the appropriate distinctive processing.

Difference Alone Is Insufficient

The best illustration of this point is the heterogeneous control list used in the von Restorff paradigm (Hunt, Chapter 1 this volume, 1995). Unlike the isolation list in which all of the items except for the isolate are related (e.g., a number in a list of consonant string), in the heterogeneous list all items are different from each other (e.g., a number, a letter string, a color blotch, etc.). The number is better remembered in the isolation list than in the heterogeneous control list. There is no memorial advantage for the number in the heterogeneous control list, despite the fact that it is different from all the other items, because all of the items are different. Distinctiveness requires difference in the context of similarity, and the similarity is missing in the heterogeneous list. The one study with older adults in the von Restorff paradigm (Cimbalo & Brink, 1982) did not use a heterogeneous list so we cannot compare the effects of distinctiveness with the effects of difference only in that case. However, the research applying the methods of Hunt and Einstein (1981) and Hunt and Seta (1984) do allow this type of comparison.

In the Fisher and McDowd (1993), Guttentag (1988), and Luszcz et al. (1990) studies, there were cases in which item-specific processing alone was encouraged by the particular combination of orienting task and materials. Recall that in these studies participants performed either a sorting task or a pleasantness-rating task at encoding. The pleasantness-rating task focused participants on each item individually and therefore encouraged item-specific processing. A study list composed of small categories or unrelated items does not encourage processing of the relationships between the items. Thus, the small categories and unrelated list items would also encourage item-specific processing. When both the task and the materials focused on the particular items at the expense of relational processing, memory suffered. Thus, it appears that difference alone is insufficient to explain the benefits of distinctive processing for older adults as well as younger adults.

Distinctiveness Is Relative

Something can be distinctive only relative to something else. If distinctiveness is conceptualized as difference in contrast to similarity, this leads to the realization that trying to separately examine the contributions of the difference part and the similarity part will be misleading. By changing one, you are changing the other. Consideration of just organization, for instance, without attending to potential differences within that organization will likely produce confusion. This is exactly the case for the literature on memory and aging. Do older adults have a deficit in relational processing? The answer was not at all clear (Salthouse, 1991). The reanalysis of the memory and aging literature, from the perspective that difference and similarity interact, brings some order to the situation.

ACKNOWLEDGMENT

Preparation of this chapter was supported in part by a Gorden H. DeFriese Career Development Award from the Institute on Aging at the University of North Carolina at Chapel Hill.

REFERENCES

Amrhein, P. C., Bond, J. K., & Hamilton, D. K. (1999). Locus of control and the age difference in free recall from episodic memory. *The Journal of General Psychology, 126,* 149–159.

Anderson, N. D., & Craik, F. I. M. (2000). Memory and the aging brain. In E. Tulving & F. I. M. Craik (Eds.), *The Oxford handbook of memory* (pp. 411–425). New York: Oxford University Press.

Balota, D. A., Dolan, P. O., & Duchek, J. M. (2000). Memory changes in healthy older adults. In E. Tulving & F. I. M. Craik (Eds.), *The Oxford handbook of memory* (pp. 395–409). New York: Oxford University Press.

Basden, B. H., Basden, D. R., & Bartlett, K. (1993). Memory and organization in elderly subjects. *Experimental Aging Research, 19*, 29–38.

Brosseau, J., & Cohen, H. (1996). The representation of semantic categories in aging. *Experimental Aging Research, 22*, 381–391.

Burke, D. M., & Light, L. L. (1981). Memory and aging: The role of retrieval processes. *Psychological Bulletin, 90*, 513–546.

Burns, D. J., & Brown, C. A. (2000). The category access measure of relational processing. *Journal of Experimental Psychology: Learning, Memory, and Cogntion, 26*, 1057–1062.

Byrd, M. (1986). The use of organizational strategies to improve memory for prose passage. *International Journal of Aging and Human Development, 23*, 257–265.

Cherry, K. E., & Jones, M. W. (1999). Age-related differences in spatial memory: Effects of structural and organizational context. *The Journal of General Psychology, 126*, 53–73.

Cimbalo, R. S., & Brink, L. (1982). Aging and the von Restorff isolation effect in short/term memory. *The Journal of General Psychology, 106*, 69–76.

Craik, F. I. M. (1986). A functional account of age differences in memory. In F. Klix & H. Hagendorf (Eds.), *Human memory and cognitive capabilities* (pp. 409–422). Amsterdam: Elsevier.

Craik, F. I. M., & Byrd, M. (1982). Aging and cognitive deficits: The role of attentional resources. In F. I. M. Craik & S. E. Trehub (Eds.), *Aging and cognitive processes* (pp. 191–211). New York: Plenum Press.

Craik, F. I. M., Byrd, M., & Swanson, J. M. (1987). Patterns of memory loss in three elderly samples. *Psychology and Aging, 2*, 79–86.

Craik, F. I. M., & Jennings, J. M. (1992). Human memory. In F. I. M. Craik & T. A. Salthouse (Eds.), *The handbook of memory and aging* (pp. 51–110). Hillsdale, NJ: Lawrence Erlbaum Associates.

Craik, F. I. M., & Lockhart, R. S. (1972). Levels of processing: A framework for memory research. *Journal of Verbal Learning and Verbal Behavior, 11*, 671–684.

Craik, F. I. M., & Simon, E. (1980). Age difference in memory: The role of attention and depth of processing. In L. W. Poon, J. L. Fozard, L. S. Cermak, D. Arenberg, & L. W. Thompson (Eds.), *New directions in memory and aging* (pp. 95–112). Hillsdale, NJ: Laurence Erlbaum Associates.

Dunlosky, J., Hunt, R. R., & Clark, E. (2000). Is perceptual salience needed in explanations of the isolation effect? *Journal of Experimental Psychology: Learning, Memory, and Cognition, 26*, 649–657.

Erber, J. T. (1984). Age differences in the effect of encoding congruence on incidental free and cued recall. *Experimental Aging Research, 10*, 221–223.

Eysenck, M. W. (1974). Age differences in incidental learning. *Developmental Psychology, 10*, 936–941.

Fisher, L. M., & McDowd, J. M. (1993). Item and realtional processing in young and older adults. *Journal of Gerontology: Psychological Science, 48,* P62–P68.

Friedman, H. (1966). Memory organization in the aged. *Journal of Genetic Psychology, 109,* 3–8.

Frieske, D. A., & Park, D. C. (1993). Effects of organization and working memory on age differences in memory for scene information. *Experimental Aging Research, 19,* 321–332.

Gallo, D. A., & Roediger, H. L. III. (2003). The effects of associations and aging on illusory recollections. *Memory and Cognition, 31,* 1036–1044.

Guttentag, R. E. (1988). Processing relational and item-specific information: Effects of aging and division of attention. *Canadian Journal of Psychology, 42,* 414–423.

Guttentag, R. E., & Hunt R. R. (1988). Adult age differences in memory for imagined and performed actions. *Journal of gerontology: Psychology Sciences, 43,* 107–108.

Hay, J. F., & Jacoby, L. L. (1999). Separating habit and recollection in young and older adults: Effects of elaborative processing and distinctiveness. *Psychology and Aging, 14,* 122–134.

Hertzog, C., Dixon, R. A., & Hultsch, D. F. (1990). Relationships between metamemory, memory predictions, and memory task performance in adults. *Psychology and Aging, 5,* 215–227.

Hess, T. M. (1984). Effects of semantically related and unrelated contexts on recognition memory of different-aged adults. *Journal of Gerontology, 39,* 444–451.

Hess, T. M., & Arnould, D. (1986). Adult age differences in memory for explicit and implicit sentence information. *Journal of Gerontology, 41,* 191–194.

Hess, T. M., Flannagan, D. A., & Tate, C. S. (1993). Aging and memory for schematically vs. taxonomically organized verbal materials. *Journal of Gerontology, 48,* 37–44.

Hess, T. M., & Higgins, J. N. (1983). Context utilization in younger and old adults. *Journal of Gerontology, 38,* 65–71.

Howard, D. V., Mc Andrews, M. P., & Lasaga M. I. (1981). Semantic priming of lexical decision in young and old adults. *Journal of Gerontology, 36,* 707–714.

Hultsch, D. F. (1971). Organization and memory in adulthood. *Human Development, 14,* 16–29.

Hultsch, D. F. (1974). Learning to learn in adulthood. *Journal of Gerontology, 29,* 202–208.

Hultsch, D. F. (1975). Adult age differences in retrieval: Trace-dependent and cue-dependent forgetting. *Developmental Psychology, 11,* 197–201.

Hultsch, D. F., Hertzog, C., & Dixon, R. A. (1990). Ability correlates of memory performance in adulthood and aging. *Psychology and Aging, 5,* 356–368.

Hunt, R. R. (1995). The subtlety of distinctiveness: What von Restorff really did. *Psychonomic Bulletin & Review, 2*, 105–112.

Hunt, R. R., & Einstein, G. O. (1981) Relational and item-specific information in memory. *Journal of Verbal Learning and Verbal Behavior, 20*, 497–514.

Hunt, R. R., & Lamb, C. A. (2001). What causes the isolation effect? *Journal of Experimental Psychology: Learning, Memory, and Cognition, 27*, 1359–1366.

Hunt, R. R., & McDaniel, M. A. (1993). The enigma of organization and distinctiveness. *Journal of Memory and Language, 32*, 421–445.

Hunt, R. R., & Seta, C. E. (1984). Category size effects in recall: The roles of relational and individual item information. *Journal of Experimental Psychology: Learning, Memory, and Cognition, 10*, 454–464.

Hunt, R. R., & Smith, R. E. (1996). Accessing the particular from the general: The power of distinctiveness in the context of organization. *Memory and Cognition, 24*, 217–225.

Jackson, D. K., & Schneider, H. G. (1982). Age differences in organization and recall: An analysis of rehearsal processes. *Psychological Reports, 50*, 919–924.

Kausler, D. H. (1994). *Learning and memory in normal aging*. New York: Academic Press.

Laurence, M. W. (1966). Age differences in performance and subjective organization in the free-recall learning of pictorial material. *Canadian Journal of Psychology, 20*, 388–399.

Light, L. L. (1996). Memory and aging. In E. L. Bjork (Eds.), *Memory* (pp. 443–490). San Diego, CA: Academic Press.

Light, L. L., & Albertson, S. A. (1989). Direct and indirect test of memory for category exemplars in young and older adults. *Psychology and Aging, 4*, 487–492.

Luszcz, M. A., Roberts, T. H., & Mattiske, J. (1990). Use of relational and item-specific information in remebering by older and younger adults. *Psychology and Aging, 5*, 242–249.

Macht, M. L., & Buschke, H. (1983). Age differences in cognitive effort. *Journal of Gerontology, 38*, 695–700.

Mäntylä, T., & Bäckman, L. (1990). Encoding variability and age-related retrieval failures. *Psychology and Aging, 5*, 545–550.

Mäntylä, T., & Bäckman, L. (1992). Aging and memory for expected and unexpected objects in real-world settings. *Journal of Experimental Psychology: Learning, Memory, and Cognition, 18*, 1298–1309.

Mäntylä, T. & Craik, F. I. M. (1993). Context sensitivity and adult age differences in encoding variability. *European Journal of Cognitive Psychology, 5*, 319–336.

Mungas, D. Ehlers, C. L., & Blunden, D. (1991). Age differences in recall and information processing in verbal and spatial learning. *Canadian Journal on Aging, 10*, 320–332.

Murphy, M. D. (1979). Measurement and category clustering in free recall. In C. R. Puff (Ed.), *Memory organization and structure* (pp. 51–83). New York: Academic Press.

Norris, M. P., & West, R. L. (1993). Activity memory and aging: The role of motor retrieval and strategic processing. *Psychology and Aging, 8,* 81–86.

Park, D. C., Cherry, K. E., Smith, A. D., & Lafronza, V. N. (1990). Effects of distinctive context on memory for objects and their locations in young and older adults. *Psychology and Aging, 5,* 250–255.

Park, D. C., Smith, A. D., Dudley, W. N., & Lafronza, V. N. (1989). Effects of age and a divided attention task presented during encoding and retrieval on memory. *Journal of Experimental Psychology: Learning, Memory, and Cognition, 15,* 1185–1191.

Rabinowitz, J. C., Craik, F. I. M., & Ackerman, B. P. (1982). A processing resource account of age differences in recall. *Canadian Journal of Psychology, 36,* 325–344.

Rankin, J. L., & Collins, M. (1986). The effects of memory elaboration on adult age differences in incidental recall. *Experimental Aging Research, 12,* 231–234.

Rankin, J. L., & Firnhaber, S. (1986). Adult age differences in memory: Effects of distinctive and common encodings. *Experimental Aging Research, 12,* 141–146.

Rankin, J. L., & Hinrichs, J. V. (1983). Age, presentation rate, and the effectiveness of structural and semantic recall cues. *Journal of Gerontology, 38,* 593–596.

Rankin, J. L., Karol, R., & Tuten, C. (1984). Strategy use, recall, and recall organization in young, middle-aged, and elderly adults. *Experimental Aging Research, 10,* 193–196.

Riefer, D. M., & Batchelder, W. M. (1991). Age differences in storage and retrieval: A multinomial modeling analysis. *Bulletin of the Psychonomic Society, 29,* 415–418.

Rönnlund, M., Nyberg, L., Bäckman, L., & Nilsson, L.-G. (2003). Recall of subject-performed tasks, verbal tasks, and cognitive activities across the adult life span: Parallel age-related deficits. *Aging Neuropsychology and Cognition, 10,* 182–201.

Salthouse, T. A. (1991). *Theoretical perspectives on cognitive aging.* Hillsdale, NJ: Lawrence Erlbaum Associates.

Sanders, R. E., Murphy, M. D., Schmitt, F. A., & Walsh, K. K. (1980). Age differences in free recall rehearsal strategies. *Journal of Gerontology, 35,* 550–558.

Schacter, D. L., Kaszniak, Kihlstrom, J. F., & Valdiserri, M. (1991). The relation between source memory and aging. *Psychology and Aging, 6,* 559–568.

Sharps, M. J. (1991). Spatial memory in young and elderly adults: Category structure of stimulus sets. *Psychology and Aging, 6,* 309–312.

Shaw, R. J., & Craik F. I. M. (1989). Age differences in predictions and performance on a cued recall task. *Psychology and Aging, 4,* 131–135.

Smith, A. D. (1977). Adult age differences in cued recall. *Developmental Psychology, 13,* 326–331.

Smith, A. D. (1980). Age differences in encoding, storage, and retrieval. In L. W. Poon, J. L. Fozard, L. S. Cermak, D. Arenberg, & L. W. Thompson (Eds.) *New directions in memory and aging* (pp. 23–45). Hillsdale, NJ: Laurence Erlbaum Associates.

Smith, R. E., & Hunt, R. R. (1998). Presentation modality affects false memory. *Psychonomic Bulletin & Review, 5,* 710–715.

Smith, R. E., & Hunt, R. R. (2000a). The effects of distinctiveness require reinstatement of organization: The importance of intentional memory instructions. *Journal of Memory and Language, 43,* 431–446.

Smith, R. E., & Hunt, R. R. (2000b). The influence of distinctive processing on retrieval-induced forgetting. *Memory & Cognition, 28,* 503–508.

Smith, R. E., Hunt, R. R., & Dunlosky, J. (2005). *Aging, distinctive processing, and recall: An investigation using participant-generated cues.* Manuscript under review.

Smith, R. E., Hunt, R. R., & Gallagher, P. (2005). *The modality effect in false recall and false recognition.* Manuscript under review.

Smith, R. E., Lozito, J., & Bayen, U. J. (2005). Adult age differences in distinctive processing: The modality effect in false recall. *Psychology & Aging, 20,* 486–492.

Smith, R. E., Payne, T., & Engle, R. (2000). The modality effect on false recall as a function of working memory span. Poster presented at the annual meeting of the Psychonomic Society, New Orleans, LA, November, 2000.

Sternberg, R. J., & Tulving, E. (1977). The measurement of subjective organization in free recall. *Psychological Bulletin, 84,* 539–556.

Stuss, D. T., Craik, F. I. M., Sayer, L., Franchi, D. & Alexander, M. P. (1996). Comparisons of older people and patients with frontal lesions: Evidence form word list learning. *Psychology and Aging, 11,* 387–395.

Till, R. E., & Walsh, D. A. (1980). Encoding and retrieval factors in adult memory for implicational sentences. *Journal of Verbal Learning and Verbal Behavior, 19,* 1–16.

Tubi, N., & Calev, A. (1989). Verbal and visuospatial recall by younger and older subjects: Use of matched tasks. *Psychology and Aging, 4,* 493–495.

Tulving, E., & Pearlstone, Z. (1966). Availability versus accessibility of information in memory for words. *Journal of Verbal Learning and Verbal Behavior, 5,* 381–391.

Verhaeghen, P., Marcoen, A., & Goossens, L. (1993). Facts and fiction about memory aging: A quantitative integration of research findings. *Journals of Gerontology, 48,* 157–171.

Weinert, F. Schneider, W., & Knopf, M. (1988). Individual differences in memory development across the life-span. In P. B. Baltes, D. L. Featherman, & R. M. Learner (Eds.) *Life span development and behavior* (Vol. 9, pp. 39–85). Hillsdale, NJ: Lawrence Erlbaum Associates.

Weible, J. A., Nuest, B. D., Welty, J., Pate, W. E. II, & Turner, M. L. (2002). Demonstrating the effects of presentation rate on aging memory using the

California Verbal Learning Test (CVLT). *Aging Neuropsychology and Cognition, 9,* 38–47.

Wingard, J. A. (1980). Life-span developmental changes in mnemonic organization: A multimethod analysis. *International Journal of Behavioral Development, 3,* 467–487.

Witte, K. L., Freund, J. S., & Brown-Whistler, S. (1993). Adult age differences in free recall and category clustering. *Experimental Aging Research, 19,* 15–28.

Witte, K. L., Freund, J. S., & Sebby, R. A. (1990). Age differences in free recall and subjective organization. *Psychology and Aging, 5,* 307–309.

Worden, P. E., & Meggison D. L. (1984). Aging and the category-recall relationship. *Journal of Gerontology, 39,* 322–324.

Worden, P. E., & Sherman-Brown, S. (1983). A word-frequency cohort effect in young versus elderly adults' memory. *Developmental Psychology, 19,* 521–530.

Zacks, R. T., Hasher, L., & Li, K. Z. H. (2000). Human memory. In F. I. M. Craik & T. A. Salthouse (Eds.), *The handbook of aging and cognition* (pp. 293–358). Mahwah, NJ: Lawrence Erlbaum Associates.

Zivian, M. T., & Darjes, R. W. (1983). Free recall by in-school and out-of-school adults: Performance and metamemory. *Developmental Psychology, 19,* 513–520.

V

Distinctiveness in the Social Context

13

The Effects of Social Distinctiveness: The Phenomenology of Being in a Group

BRIAN MULLEN AND CARMEN PIZZUTO

"It's a poor sort of memory that only works backwards," the Queen remarked.
—Lewis Carroll (1885)
Through the Looking Glass

A central theme in social psychological research is the effect of the group on the individual. Stage fright, eyewitness identification, and hate speech are just a few of the phenomena studied by social psychologists that illustrate this broader concern for how the group affects the individual. The list of phenomena that illustrate the effect of the group on the individual coincides with the list of phenomena where the social context tends to be bifurcated into two subgroups.: "Speaker vs. audience," "suspect vs. witnesses," and "immigrant vs. natives" are specific examples of the pervasive tendency for people to respond to the social context in terms of "us vs. them." While these two subgroups will sometimes approximate moiety, it is often the case that one subgroup comprises a distinct numerical minority while the other comprises a larger majority. And, in many of these instances, memory processes operate to determine how the group affects the individual: The extent to which the audience remembers the speaker's performance (or the speaker remembers his or her lines), the extent to which the witnesses remember what the suspect looks like (or the suspect remembers his or her alibi), and the extent to which the natives remember unsavory attributes of the immigrant (or the immigrant remembers hostile acts of rejection) are specific examples of the operation of memory processes in the context of social groups of "us vs. them."

What is it like to be a part of a group? What do "We" have in common, and how do "We" differ from "Them"? How do our perceptions of and memories about the ingroup and the outgroup vary as a function of being in this group or that group? A central theme in the evidence described below is that the relative sizes of the ingroup and the outgroup will determine the distinctiveness of one group relative to another. In other words, guiding the research described in this chapter is the definition of *distinctiveness* as the increase in salience or attention afforded to a social group as a function of its relative numerical rarity: the smaller group is more distinctive (cf. Hunt, Chapter 1 this volume; Schmidt, 1991). The notion that relative group sizes may be a central structural or topographical determinant of group processes is not a new idea. Relative group size has figured prominently in the work of Diener (1980), Kanter (1977), McGuire (McGuire & McGuire, 1982), Mullen (1983, 1986, 1990, 1991, 2003), and Wicklund (1980, 1982), among many others. Historically, these ideas can be traced back to Koffka (1935), Simmel (1908/1950), and LeBon (1895).

Group Composition and Self-Focused Attention: "They're All Looking at Me"

Several social psychological researchers have invoked the gestalt *figure-ground principle* (Koffka, 1935) to explain the individual's attentional focus in the context of the group (e.g., Duval & Wicklund, 1972; Diener, 1980; Kanter, 1977; Mullen, 1983). This principle holds that perceptions are patterned into two aspects: figure, which stands out, appears distinct, closer, more thinglike, and is more easily remembered; and ground, which is indistinct, not clearly patterned or shaped, and appears further away (Kaufman, 1979; Koffka, 1935; Wertheimer, 1923). This is entirely consistent with considerations of the effect of the group on the individual's level of self-attention, or the state of taking one's self as the figural focus of attention (typically measured in terms of self-reports of self-consciousness or the use of first-person singular pronouns in spontaneous speech; see Cooley, 1908; Diener, 1980; Duval & Wicklund, 1972; Mullen, 1983; Royce, 1895; Wegner & Schaefer, 1978). It generally seems to be the case that the smaller stimulus is more likely to emerge as the distinct figure (Coren, Porac, & Ward, 1979). If the smaller stimulus emerges as the perceptual figure of attention, then the individuals in the smaller subgroup would tend to focus their attention on themselves and become more self-attentive. By the same token, the individuals in the larger subgroup would tend to focus their attention on those in the smaller subgroup and become less self-attentive.

Mullen (1990) reported the results of a meta-analytic integration of research examining this effect of group composition on self-focused attention. The results of 11 hypothesis tests, representing $\Sigma N = 1,927$ participant responses, revealed that there was a significant, $Z = 14.074$, $p = 6.29\text{E-}32$, strong, $r = .514$, tendency for the smaller subgroup to emerge as the figure of attentional focus. As depicted in Figure 13.1, the standardized degree of self-focused attention in conditions across studies varied as a linear function of the standardized relative size of the ingroup in conditions across studies. In other words, individuals in the smaller subgroup tended to focus their attention on themselves and become more self-

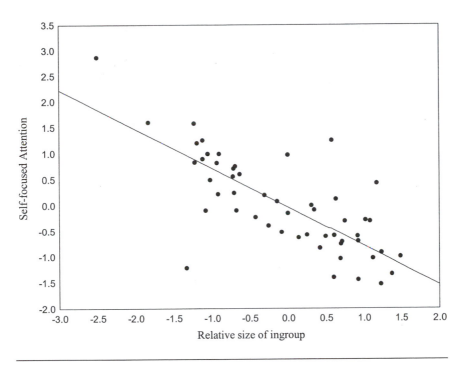

FIGURE 13.1 Prediction of self-focused attention as a function of relative in group size. Adapted from Mullen, 1990.

attentive. Note that the effect of relative group size on self-attention involves the measurement of an outcome (self-focused attention) that is not directly relevant to memory. However, this effect of relative group size on self-attention does provide a direct gauge of the extent to which relative group size determines the distinctiveness of social groups. Moreover, this effect of relative group size on self-attention also provides an important theoretical foundation for subsequent areas of research that more directly involve the measurement of memory outcomes (summarized below).

DISTINCTIVENESS AND PERCEPTIONS OF VARIABILITY: "THEY'RE ALL ALIKE"

Another aspect of the perception of groups that is significantly affected by the relative sizes of the ingroup and the outgroup is variability. Note that people have varying degrees of experience with ingroups and outgroups, and judgments of the variability of an ingroup relative to the outgroup apparently reflect differing reconstructions of these experiences with the groups. In other words, the effect of relative group size on judgments of variability involves the measurement of an outcome (variability judgments) that is at least indirectly relevant to memory. Goethals and Darley (1977) suggested that people will tend to perceive their own group as comprising a heterogeneous set of unique individuals, whereas an opposing group will be perceived as a homogeneous set of highly similar others. This type of pattern has been labeled the *magnification of diversity* (Goethals & Darley, 1977), the *outgroup homogeneity effect* (Jones, Wood, & Quattrone, 1981), or, more generally, the *relative heterogeneity effect* (Mullen & Hu, 1989).

The effect of relative ingroup size on relative heterogeneity was anticipated by Simmel (1908/1950): while the general tendency should be toward a perception of relative heterogeneity for the ingroup, this tendency should decrease as the size of the ingroup decreases, to the extent that small minorities actually evidence a relative homogeneity effect (perceiving the ingroup as less heterogeneous than the outgroup). This relative homogeneity effect could represent an information processing heuristic. For example, Tajfel (1969) and Tversky and Gati (1978, Study 4) described how the context may affect the perceived similarity of objects. Ingroup membership would be likely to acquire what Tversky and Gati called "diagnostic value" and may increase the perceived similarity of ingroup members through comparison with the outgroup. And the diagnosticity of ingroup membership, and the resultant perceived similarity of elements of the category (i.e., of members of the group), as discussed by Tversky and Gati (1978), would be likely to increase as the individual's ingroup emerges as the figural focus of attention.

Mullen and Hu (1989) reported the results of a meta-analytic integration of research examining this relative heterogeneity effect. The results of 63 hypothesis tests, representing $\Sigma N = 1,518$ participant responses, revealed that there was a significant, $Z = 12.186$, $p = 4.80\text{E}{-}27$, albeit rather weak, $r = .210$, tendency to perceive the ingroup as more heterogeneous than the outgroup. Moreover, as depicted in Figure 13.2, the relative heterogeneity effect increased as a function of the relative size of the ingroup, $r = .328$, $Z = 1.735$, $p = .04134$. In other words, the more distinctive the ingroup, the more homogeneous it is seen to be.

DISTINCTIVENESS AND PERCEIVED PREVALENCE: "EVERYONE AGREES WITH ME"

Social projection generally refers to the tendency to generate biased estimates of the prevalence of (or the consensus for) one's own ingroup (Allport, 1924). Note that people have varying degrees of experience with ingroups and outgroups, and judgments of the prevalence of an ingroup relative to the outgroup apparently reflect the ease with which these experiences are recalled. In other words, the effect of relative group size on

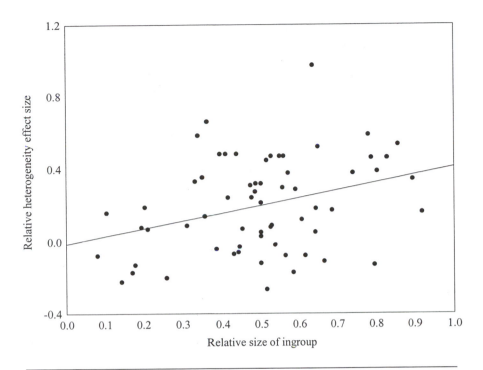

FIGURE 13.2 Prediction of the relative heterogeneity effect as a function of relative group size. Adapted from Mullen & Hu, 1989.

prevalence estimates involves the measurement of an outcome (prevalence estimates) that is directly relevant to memory. Studies have shown that when the wording of the estimation questionnaire focuses one's attention on the ingroup, the ingroup is perceived to be more prevalent (Mullen, Driskell, & Smith, 1989; Mullen & Hu, 1988). In the present context, this becomes relevant because increased perceived prevalence is one of the oldest and most common measures of cognitive availability (e.g., Hintzman, 1969; Tversky & Kahneman, 1974). Generally, the more available something is in memory, the more easily recallable that thing is (Asch & Ebenholtz, 1962; Tversky & Kahneman, 1974). Thus, if the relative sizes of groups influence their distinctiveness, and if the relative distinctiveness of groups influences their availability in memory, there should be an increase in the perceived prevalence for a group as a function of its relative rarity. In other words, people (both those in the minority and those in the majority) should tend to overremember the prevalence of the smaller minority to the extent that the smaller minority stands out and is distinctive.

Mullen and Hu (1988) reported the results of a meta-analytic integration of research examining these social projection effects. The results of 134 hypothesis tests, representing $\Sigma N = 8{,}550$ participant responses, revealed that there was a significant, $Z = 21.603$, $p = 9.77E-48$, moderate, $r = .332$, tendency for people in the majority to underestimate their consensus, coupled with a significant, $Z = 20.005$, $p = 8.39E-45$, strong, $r = .493$, tendency for people in the minority to overestimate their consensus. Moreover, as depicted in Figure 13.3, this social projection effect decreased as a function of the relative size of the ingroup, $r = -.765$, $Z = 29.343$, $p = 1.12E-59$. In other words, the smaller relative size of the minority makes it stand out, and thereby leads to an overestimation of the prevalence of the minority (both by the minority and by the majority). This pattern has subsequently been replicated at the primary level of analysis (Mullen & Smith, 1990). Thus, as its smaller relative size makes the minority stand out, people tend to overremember the prevalence for the smaller group.

DISTINCTIVENESS AND STEREOTYPING: "THEY ALL DO THAT"

Distinctiveness-based illusory correlations are erroneous judgments of the relation between two variables based on the co-occurrence of distinctive stimulus events. In the original demonstration of this phenomenon, Chap-

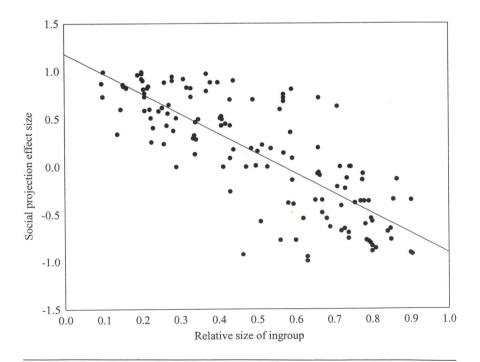

FIGURE 13.3 Prediction of the social projection effect as a function of relative group size. Adapted from Mullen & Hu, 1988.

man (1967) presented a list of word pairs to participants, each word being paired with others with equal frequency. Chapman observed that people consistently overestimated the frequency with which the two longest words in the list had been paired. In the context of a list of relatively short words, each long word was distinctive, and the pairing of these two distinctive long words was, apparently, particularly distinctive. It was this extreme distinctiveness, and the resultant increased availability in memory (Tversky & Kahneman, 1974), of the pairing of the two distinctive stimulus events that led subjects to overestimate the frequency of this particular word pair.

Hamilton and Gifford (1976) extended this information-processing phenomenon to the development of a paradigmatically new approach to the development of social stereotypes. In this paradigm, participants read a series of sentences describing members of one of two groups (the larger group A or the smaller broup B) engaging in one of two kinds of behaviors (frequent, positive behaviors or rare, negative behaviors). It was reasoned that overestimation of the co-occurrence of distinctive events could lead to an illusory correlation between relatively rare behaviors and the relatively smaller social group, leading to overremembering of the frequency of undesirable behaviors performed by minority group members. Note that people in this paradigm are exposed to a discrete series of events about members of the two groups engaging in the two types of behaviors, and estimates of the prevalence of a given type of group-behavior event apparently reflect the ease with which these events are recalled. In other words, the effect of relative group size on estimates of group-behavior events involves the measurement of an outcome (estimates of group-behavior events) that is clearly an indicator of memory. This extension of the distinctiveness-based illusory correlation paradigm provided a cognitive, nonmotivational foundation for the development of negative stereotypic beliefs about minority groups. Johnson and Mullen (1994) have confirmed the distinctiveness-based mechanism for this model of stereotype acquisition. For example, participants who had acquired a distinctiveness-based stereotype of the smaller group exhibited faster recognition latencies for smaller group–rarer behavior events, indicating that these distinctive events were in fact more accessible in memory.

Mullen and Johnson (1990) reported the results of a meta-analytic integration of research examining this distinctiveness-based illusory correlation effect. The results of 28 hypothesis tests, representing $\Sigma N = 1,401$ participant responses, revealed that there was a significant, $Z = 12.486$, $p = 7.55\text{E-}28$, moderate, $r = .344$, tendency for people to overestimate the co-occurrence of the smaller group's engaging in the rarer behavior. Moreover, as depicted in Figure 13.4, this distinctiveness-based illusory correlation effect increased as a function of the relative rarity of the smaller group–rarer behavior events, $r = -.343$, $Z = 2.335$, $p = .00977$. In other words, the paired-distinctiveness of the smaller group engaging in the rarer behavior leads people to overremember the co-occurrence of these two rare

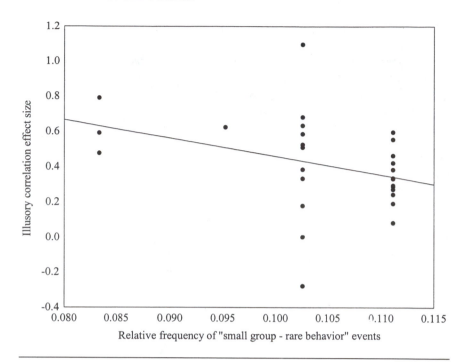

FIGURE 13.4 Prediction of the distinctiveness-based illusory correlation effect as a function of relative rarity of small group–rare behavior events. Adapted from Mullen & Johnson, 1990.

events, and this tendency gets stronger as the paired-distinctiveness of these two rare events increases.

DISTINCTIVENESS AND MEMORY FOR CROSS-RACE FACES: "THEY ALL LOOK THE SAME"

Another aspect of the perception of groups that is significantly affected by the relative sizes of the ingroup and the outgroup is the recognition of same- and other-race faces. Note that people are exposed to a series of faces of members of the ingroup and members of the outgroup, and sometimes later need to recognize those faces. In other words, the effect of relative group size on identification of ingroup and outgroup faces involves the measurement of an outcome (face recognition) that is clearly an indicator of memory.

The general tendency clearly seems to be for subjects to exhibit superior memory for faces belonging to members of their own racial group than for faces belonging to members of another group (e.g., Bothwell, Brigham, & Malpass, 1989). However, most reviews of this phenomenon are generally at a loss to provide a compelling theoretical account for this basic effect.

One possible account for the cross-racial facial identification effect derives from the possible correspondence between this effect and the relative heterogeneity effect described above. The relative heterogeneity effect refers to the tendency to think that members of the outgroup are similar. The cross-racial facial identification effect refers to the tendency to think that members of the outgroup look alike. Thus, both relative heterogeneity and cross-racial facial identification may be based on a failure to distinguish among individuals in the outgroup. If this is true, then the tendency for larger groups to exhibit greater relative heterogeneity should be matched by a corresponding tendency for larger groups to exhibit greater cross-racial facial identification. Given that in the United States white people are in a demographic majority, and black people are in a demographic minority, this leads to the prediction that the cross-racial facial identification effect should be stronger with white participants than with black participants.

Anthony, Copper, and Mullen (1992) reported the results of a meta-analytic integration of research examining this cross-racial facial identification effect. The results of 44 hypothesis tests, representing $\Sigma N = 1,725$ participant responses, revealed that there was a significant, $Z = 13.707$, $p = 5.21\text{E-}31$, and weak-to-moderate, $r = .284$, tendency for people to better remember ingroup faces. Moreover, as depicted in Figure 13.5, this cross-

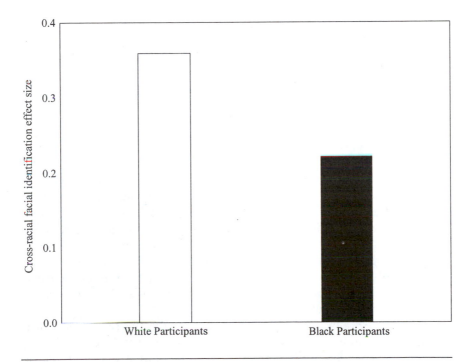

FIGURE 13.5 Prediction of the cross-racial facial identification effect as a function of relative group size. Adapted from Anthony et al., 1992.

racial facial identification effect was significant, $Z = 10.638$, $p = 9.27E-23$, and moderate, $r = .345$, for white participants, whereas this cross-racial facial identification effect was significant, $Z = 8.727$, $p = 3.12E-17$, but weak, $r = .218$, for black participants. Thus, the cross-racial facial identification effect appears to be stronger for the larger group (whites) and weaker for the smaller group (blacks).

DISTINCTIVENESS AND MEMORY FOR A TOKEN'S BEHAVIOR: "HE SAID, SHE SAID"

One specific area of research that has emphasized the impact of relative group size is the perception of the lone representative of a social category, typically referred to as a *token* (e.g., Biernat & Vescio, 1993, 1994; Kanter, 1977; Laws, 1975; Nesdale & Dharmalingham, 1986; Nesdale, Dharmalingham, & Kerr, 1987; Oakes, 1994; Taylor, Fiske, Etcoff, & Ruderman, 1978). Taylor et al. (1978, Study 3) initiated research into these effects of distinctiveness of people in mixed-gender groups. In the group-discussion paradigm introduced by this seminal study, participants viewed slide-and-tape portrayals of interacting small groups of varying gender composition and then responded to various questions about the discussion. Note that participants in these studies were exposed to a discrete series of events about members of two groups engaging in a discussion and were later asked to associate statements with the groups that made them. In other words, the effect of relative group size on the association between groups and statements involves the measurement of an outcome (statement identification) that is clearly an indicator of memory. The basic premise of this work is that the larger subgroup recedes as less distinctive and, therefore, statements by members of this larger group are less memorable. Conversely, the smaller subgroup emerges as more distinctive and therefore statements by members of this smaller group are more memorable.

However, narrative summaries of subsequent research in this paradigm have rendered conflicting conclusions. On the one hand, Lord and Saenz (1985) offered the sanguine observation that, "Because this bias of observers for perceptually distinctive stimuli has been the subject of considerable previous discussion . . . it requires little further comment" (p. 923). On the other hand, Oakes, Turner, & Haslam (1991) offered the more skeptical observation that "The empirical support for the distinctiveness hypothesis is equivocal" (p. 126). Clearly, the inconsistency deserves careful scrutiny and resolution.

Nichols, Abrams, and Mullen (2000) reported the results of a meta-analytic integration of research examining this mixed-gender discussion paradigm. The results of 44 hypothesis tests, representing $\Sigma N = 739$ participant responses, revealed that there was a significant, $Z = 10.522$, $p = 1.97E-22$, and small, $r = .166$, tendency for people to exhibit more extreme responses to members of the smaller group. However, when restricted to tests of better memory for statements by members of the smaller group, the results of 7 hypothesis tests, representing $\Sigma N = 477$ participant responses, revealed that there was a significant, $Z = 12.403$, $p = 1.26\text{E-}27$, and moderate, $r = .432$, tendency for people to exhibit better memory for statements by members of the smaller group. As depicted in Figure 13.6, the standardized degree of memory for statements by members of the smaller group in conditions across studies varied as a linear function of the standardized relative size of the smaller group in conditions across studies. This provides clear evidence for a significant effect of the relative size of the token's gender subgroup on the tendency to better remember statements by members of that smaller group.[1]

A MODEL OF THE PHENOMENOLOGY OF BEING IN A GROUP

Consider the following general summary of the patterns revealed above. On the one hand, as the size of a target group decreases, that group becomes more distinctive: People in that group become more self-focused;

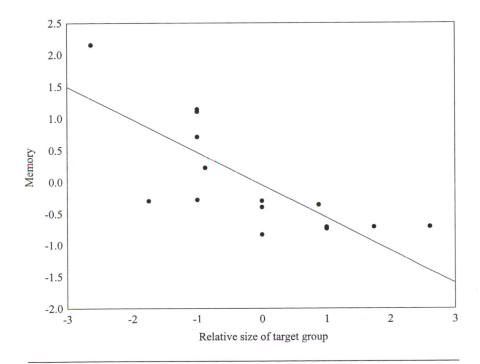

FIGURE 13.6 Prediction of prominence of the token in memory effect as a function of relative group size. Adapted from Nichols et al., 2000.

that group is seen as homogeneous; people overremember the prevalence of that group; people overremember the performance of rare, negative behaviors by members of that smaller group; the capacity to remember faces from that group is diminished; and statements made by members of that group are remembered better. On the other hand, as the size of a target group increases, that group becomes less distinctive: People in that group become less self-focused; that group is seen as heterogeneous; people underremember the prevalence of that group; people underremember the performance of rare, negative behaviors by members of that larger group; the capacity to remember faces from that group is enhanced; and statements made by members of that group are remembered less well.[2]

There is a remarkable consistency of results across these several and varied research domains (for similar patterns regarding the effects of relative group sizes on other social phenomena, see Mullen, 1983, 1986, 2001, 2003; Mullen, Brown, & Smith, 1992; Mullen, Chapman, & Peaugh, 1989; Mullen, Driskell, & Smith, 1989). Some of these effects of relative group sizes appear to operate on basic perceptual mechanisms, like the effects of relative group sizes on self-focused attention (Mullen, 1990). Some of these effects of relative group sizes appear to operate on indicators of semantic memory systems, like the effects of relative group sizes on estimates of prevalence for the ingroup (Mullen & Hu, 1988). Finally, some of these effects of relative group sizes appear to operate on indicators of episodic memory systems, like the effects of relative group sizes on recall of the group-behavior events in the distinctiveness-based illusory correlation paradigm (Mullen & Johnson, 1990), or the effects of relative group sizes on recognition of faces in the cross-racial facial identification paradigm (Anthony et al., 1992).

Evidence derived from research into other aspects of cognitive processes points to plausible mechanisms for the effects summarized above. These results converge on the basic effects of group composition on figure-ground effects and distinctiveness. In accord with the mechanisms specified above, the individual's self will emerge as the figural focus of attention as the relative size of the ingroup decreases; individuals will overestimate the prevalence of the rarer event when they estimate the consensus of the groups; individuals will overremember the co-occurrence of the smaller group's engaging in the rarer behavior; and individuals will overremember statements made by the distinctive token in a group discussion.

The distinctiveness of the group in turn seems to determine how individuals will represent the ingroup and the outgroup in memory. Two broad classes of cognitive representation have been identified: prototype representations and exemplar representations. According to prototype models of category representation (Posner & Keele, 1970; Reed, 1972), a category is represented by the prototype—some "average" or most typical category member. Instances are identified as category members if they are more similar to the category's prototype than they are to a prototype of another category. According to exemplar models of category representation (Brooks,

1978; Medin & Schaffer, 1978), a category is represented by an accumulation of information about known exemplars of that category. Instances are identified as category members if they are similar to the retrieved representations of known exemplars. Both prototype representations and exemplar representations can contribute to the handling of information about category members, for nonsocial information tasks (Homa, Sterling, & Trepel, 1981; Smith & Medin, 1981; Medin, Altom & Murphy, 1984) and for social information tasks (Linville, Fischer, & Salovey, 1989; Mullen et al., 1992; Park & Hastie, 1987; Rothbart & John, 1985; Smith & Zarate, 1990).

Previous research indicates an increase in the use of prototype representations when subjects were presented with the prototypes, compared to when subjects had to abstract the prototypes for themselves from exemplar information (e.g., Medin et al., 1984; Smith & Zarate, 1990). As discussed at length by Sherman and Corty (1984), studies that use poorly formed or unfamiliar prototypes often show superiority of exemplar representations, whereas studies that use well-defined and easily accessible prototypes often show superiority of prototype representations. These diverse effects converge on the tendency for people to use prototypes when those prototypes are primed or made easily accessible. In the present context, prototype representation for a particular group seems to be engaged or made more easily accessible when the relatively small size of that group enhances the distinctiveness of that group. Mullen, Johnson, and Anthony (1994) have confirmed this expectation in the context of the category-verification paradigm. Participants in a smaller social group exhibited a processing advantage for prototype-consistent ingroup members and for prototype-inconsistent outgroup members, whereas participants in a larger social group exhibited a processing advantage for prototype-inconsistent ingroup members and for prototype-consistent outgroup members.

Thus, information about the group that is more distinctive will be represented in memory in terms of prototypes, whereas information about the nondistinctive group will be will be represented in memory in terms of exemplars. This assumption simply makes explicit a paradoxical effect that has been implicit in previous research on minority groups (e.g., Crocker & McGraw, 1984; Hamilton & Gifford, 1976; Taylor et al., 1978): The group to which we pay the most attention, by virtue of its distinctiveness, is the group that will be cognitively represented with the simplest strategy. Thus, information about the minority group will be processed (both by members of the minority group and by members of the majority group) in terms of prototype representation, whereas information about the majority group will be processed (both by members of the minority and by members of the majority) in terms of exemplar representation.

The effect of distinctiveness on how individuals represent the ingroup and outgroup in memory can account for each of the remaining patterns revealed in the evidence presented above. For example, Park and Hastie (1987) reported that prototype representations yield judgments of smaller variability than do exemplar representations. This accounts for the effects of social distinctiveness on perceptions of relative heterogeneity: Both the minority and the majority employ a prototype representation of the minority, which in turn yields judgments of smaller variability for the minority. Similarly, this accounts for the effects of social distinctiveness on the cross-racial facial identification effect: both the minority and the majority employ a prototype representation of the minority, which in turn yields reduced accuracy in discriminating minority group faces.

Effects of Encouraging Exemplar Representation: "They Look Like People"

This model of the phenomenology of being in a group[3] can be summarized as follows: The relative sizes of the ingroup and the outgroup influence the distinctiveness of one group relative to another, with the smaller subgroup emerging as the figural focus of attention and the larger group receding into the perceptual ground. The distinctiveness of the group in turn seems to determine how individuals represent the ingroup and the outgroup in memory, with both the minority and the majority employing a prototype representation of the minority and an exemplar representation of the majority. If this model captures something of the fabric of social reality, it leads to a specific view of the development of, and possible interventions to address, intergroup hostility. That is, intergroup hostility may develop as a result of the majority's tendency to engage in prototype cognitive representations of the minority; and interventions might be designed to address intergroup hostility by encouraging members of the majority to engage in exemplar cognitive representations of the minority.

A number of studies have considered the role of complexity in the cognitive representations in intergroup perception. Several studies (e.g., Coffman, 1967; Koenig & King, 1964) have documented that people with low cognitive complexity respond to outgroups with more extreme negative evaluations. Moreover, children with more advanced classification skills are less likely to use rigid stereotypes than those with less advanced cognitive skills (e.g., Bigler & Liben, 1993; Leahy & Sherk, 1984). Overall, there seems to be a consistent tendency for more simplified cognitive representations to be associated with more extreme, negative, and stereotypic responses totarget groups.

The research summarized above suggests that if the prevailing mode of cognitive representation for the minority were shifted from prototype to exemplar, the outgroup would become subject to more complex and more positive perceptions. In an effort to examine this line of reasoning, Mullen, Pizzuto, and Foels (2002) performed a series of studies that attempted to encourage participants to represent a target group in memory in terms of exemplars and thereby encourage more complex and more positive perceptions of that target group. For example, Mullen et al. (2002, Experiment 3) had participants examine 11 drinking glasses that were identical in shape but varied in height and width. Participants examined the glasses under two instructional conditions. In *exemplar training*, participants were instructed to pay attention to the differences among glasses, to keep in mind what each glass looked like, and to think about each glass. Participants then compared each glass to a "comparison object"—a glass that corresponded to the arithmetic average of the 11 glasses. In *prototype training*, participants were instructed to pay attention to what the glasses had in common, to keep in mind what the average glass looked like, and to think about the typical glass; and the comparison object was a white ceramic coffee mug.

Participants in both conditions then viewed a booklet containing photographs of indigenous people, similar to the typical portrayals in the magazine *National Geographic*. These photographs portrayed a single indigenous person with some counterstereotypic cultural anomaly (e.g., a bare-breasted young black woman is posed against a background of thatch and mud huts, but she is wearing cassette headphones). After briefly viewing a photograph, the participants were signaled to turn to the next page in the booklet, where they were instructed to write about the person they just saw. After exemplar training, participants identified 69.7% of the cultural anomalies, whereas after prototype training participants identified 47.2% of the cultural anomalies ($F_{(1,21)} = 4.633$, $p = .0431$). In other words, participants in the exemplar-training condition were almost twice as likely to remember having seen the cultural anomalies. Moreover, after prototype training, participants were equally likely to characterize the indigenous people in descriptive terms like "tribal" or "native" (0.94%) and in deprecatory terms like "dirty" or "hungry" (0.76%), whereas after exemplar training, participants were more likely to use descriptive terms (2.26%) and less likely to use deprecatory terms (0.08%) ($F_{(1,21)} = 9.970$, $p = .00475$). In other words, participants in the exemplar training condition were nine times less likely to remember the indigenous people as appearing dirty or hungry. These results indicate that the (prototype vs. exemplar) training on nonsocial targets generalized to the cognitive representation of subsequent social targets: compared to prototype training, exemplar training led to a more enriched, and less deprecatory, cognitive representation of those subsequent social targets.

CONCLUSIONS

This approach, linking group composition, distinctiveness, and cognitive representations, provides an integrative account for a variety of social-cognition and group-processes phenomena. Social psychological researchers have long searched for "magic numbers" that could summarize the effects of the group on the individual. For example, Slater (1958) proposed that the optimum group size was approximately 5 persons. Old (1946) proposed that the optimum group size was approximately 0.7 persons. The present perspective encourages a consideration of relative group sizes as varying along a continuous, and pervasively influential, metric. The patterns reported in these integrations, based on hundreds of hypothesis tests and thousands of subject responses, provide a consistent picture of what it is like to belong to "We" instead of "them." The relative sizes of the ingroup and the outgroup will lead the smaller subgroup to emerge as the figural focus of attention and the larger group to recede into the perceptual ground. The distinctiveness of these groups in turn will lead both the minority and the majority to employ a prototype representation of the minority and an exemplar representation of the majority. And, despite how pervasive these tendencies may be, recent evidence seems to indicate that these tendencies can be modified through training to encourage more complex exemplar-based cognitive representations of social targets.

ACKNOWLEDGMENTS

Portions of this paper were presented at the 49th Annual Meeting of the Southwestern Psychological Association, New Orleans, LA, April 2003.

NOTES

1. It should be emphasized that studies included in this paradigm do not indicate an increased memory for which members of the smaller group said *what* thing; rather, the phenomenon measured by studies in this paradigm is simply an increased memory for things said by members of the smaller group (regardless of which members said what).
2. It should be emphasized that the effects of relative group sizes summarized above were derived from, and generalize to, a wide range of groups, including artificial hypothetical groups (e.g., group A vs. group B in the distinctiveness-based illusory correlation paradigm), small ad hoc groups created in the social psychological laboratory (e.g., the red group and the green group in the relative heterogeneity effect), and large-scale trans-historical ethnic categories (e.g., blacks and whites in the cross-racial facial-identification effect). Sometimes the smaller (sub)group is the lone individual (e.g., the self in front of an audience in the self-attention paradigm). Sometimes the smaller (sub)group is a group of similar individuals (e.g., blacks in the cross-racial facial-identification effect). As discussed at length by several scholars, these pervasive effects of relative group sizes are highly contextual: An adult male entering a setting otherwise populated by females will become focused on his distinctiveness defined in terms of his masculinity, whereas the same adult male entering a setting populated by children will become focused on his distinctiveness defined in terms of his adulthood (see Diener, 1980; Duval & Wicklund, 1972; Kanter, 1977; McGuire &

McGuire, 1982; Mullen, 1983, 1986, 1990, 1991, 2003; Turner, Hogg, Oakes, Reicher, & Wetherell, 1987; Wegner & Schaefer, 1978; Wicklund, 1980, 1982).

3. The source of this phrase is a passage in a popular *Star Trek* novel. Captain James Kirk's cognitive representation of Vulcans evidences an obvious shift from prototype to exemplar representation. In most of the *Star Trek* mythology, the lone Vulcan target of Human cognitive representations (Mr. Spock) embodies a rare minority of one, subject to extreme prototype representation. However, at one point, the Vulcan targets of Human cognitive representations are the vast majority: in a great hall on the planet Vulcan, Captain Kirk is one of approximately 1,000 non-Vulcans among approximately 14,000 Vulcans:

> Jim found himself suffering from the ridiculous feeling that he was being stared at. . . . As he chatted with them he was once again rather delighted that Vulcans were in fact different from one another. A lot of people had the idea that Vulcans were all tall, dark, and slender, men and women alike. But though a large percentage of them did indeed fit into those parameters, there were also short Vulcans, blond Vulcans, and even a redhead over by one of the tables. . . . "*They look like people,*" Jim thought, and then had to laugh at the idea. (Duane, 1988, p. 233; emphasis added)

REFERENCES

Allport, F. H. (1924). *Social psychology*, Cambridge, MA: Riverside Press.

Anthony, T., Copper, C., & Mullen, B. (1992). Cross-racial facial identification: A social cognitive integration. *Personality and Social Psychology Bulletin, 18*, 296–301.

Asch, S. E., & Ebenholtz, S. M. (1962). The principle of associative symmetry. *Proceedings of the American Philosophical Society, 106*, 135–163.

Biernat, M., & Vescio, T. K. (1993). Categorization and stereotyping: Effects of group context on memory and social judgement. *Journal of Experimental Social Psychology, 29*,166–202.

Biernat, M., & Vescio, T. K. (1994). Still another look at the effects of fit and novelty on the salience of social categories. *Journal of Experimental Social Psychology. 30*, 399–406.

Bigler, R. S., & Liben, L. S. (1993). A cognitive developmental approach to racial stereotyping and reconstructive memory in Euro-American children. *Child Development, 64*, 1507–1518.

Bothwell, R. K., Brigham, J. C., & Malpass, R. S. (1989). Cross-racial identification. *Personality and Social Psychology Bulletin, 15*, 19–25.

Brewer, M. B., Dull, V., & Lui, L. (1981). Perceptions of the elderly: Stereotypes as prototypes. *Journal of Personality and Social Psychology, 41*, 656–670.

Brooks, L. (1978). Nonanalytic concept formation and memory for instances. In E. Rosch & B. B. Lloyd (Eds.). *Cognition and categorization* (pp. 169–211). Hillsdale, NJ: Lawrence Erlbaum Associates.

Chapman, L. J. (1967). Illusory correlation in observational report. *Journal of Verbal Learning and Verbal Behavior, 6,* 151–155.

Coffman, T. L. (1967). *Personality structure, involvement, and the consequences of taking astand.* Unpublished Ph.D. dissertation, Princeton University.

Cooley, C. H. (1908). A study of the early use of self words by a child. *Psychological Review, 15,* 339–357.

Coren, S., Porac, C., & Ward, L. M. (1979). *Sensation and perception.* New York: Academic Press.

Crocker, J., & McGraw, K. M. (1984). What's good for the goose is not good for the gander: Solo status as an obstacle to occupational achievement for males and females. *American Behavioral Scientist, 27,* 357–370.

Diener, E. (1980). Deindividuation: The absence of self-awareness and self-regulation ingroup members. In P. B. Paulus (Ed.), *Psychology of group influence* (pp. 209–244). Hillsdale. NJ: Lawrence Erlbaum Associates.

Duane, D. (1988). *Spock's world.* New York: Pocket Books.

Duval, S., & Wicklund. R. A. (1972). *A theory of objective self-awareness.* New York: Academic Press.

Goethals, G. R., & Darley, J. M. (1977). Social comparison theory: An attribution approach. In J. Suls & R. L. Miller (Eds.), *Social comparison processes: Theoretical and empirical perspectives* (pp. 259–278). Washington, DC: Hemisphere.

Hamilton, D. L., & Gifford, R. K. (1976). Illusory correlation in interpersonal perception: A cognitive basis of stereolypic judgements. *Journal of Experimental Social Psychology, 12,* 392–407.

Hintzman, D. L. (1969). Apparent frequency as a function of frequency and spacing of repetitions. *Journal of Experimental Psychology, 80,* 139–145.

Homa, D., Sterling, S., & Trepel, L. (1981). Limitations of exemplar-based generalization and the abstraction of categorical information. *Journal of Experimental Psychology: Human Learning and Memory, 7,* 415–439.

Johnson, C., & Mullen, B. (1994). Evidence for the accessibility of paired distinctiveness indistinctiveness-based illusory correlation in stereotyping. *Personality and Social Psychology Bulletin, 20,* 65–70.

Jones, E. E., Wood, G. C, & Quattrone, G. A. (1981). Perceived variability of personal characteristics in ingroups and outgroups: The role of knowledge and evaluation. *Personality and Social Psychology Bulletin. 7,* 523–528.

Kanter, R. M. (1977). Some effects of proportions on group life: Skewed sex ratios and responses to token women. *American Journal of Sociology, 82,* 465–490.

Kaufman, I. (1979). *Perception: The world transformed.* New York: Oxford University Press.

Koffka, K. (1935). *Principles of gestalt psychology.* New York: Harcourt, Brace.

Koenig, F. W., & King, M. B. (1964). Cognitive simplicity and outgroup stereotype. *Social Forces, 42,* 324–327.

Laws, J. L. (1975). The psychology of tokenism: An analysis. *Sex Roles, 1,* 51–67.

Leahy, R. L., & Shirk, S. R. (1984). The development of classifactory skills and sex-trait stereotypes in children. *Sex Roles, 10,* 281–292.

LeBon, G. (1895). *The crowd.* New York: Viking Press.

Linville, P. (1982). Self-complexity as a cognitive buffer against stress-related illness and depression. *Journal of Personality and Social Psychology, 52,* 663–676.

Linville, P., Fischer, G. W., & Salovey, P. (1989). Perceived distributions of the characteristics of ingroup members and outgroup members. *Journal of Personality and Social Psychology 57,* 165–188.

Lord, C. G., & Saenz, D. S. (1985). Memory deficits and memory surfeits: Differential cognitive consequences of tokenism for tokens and observers. *Journal of Personality and Social Psychology. 49,* 918–926.

McGuire, W. J., & McGuire, C. V. (1982). Significant others in self-space: Sex differences in developmental trends in the self. In J. Suls (Ed.), *Social psychological perspectives on the self* (pp. 207–241). Hillsdale, NJ: Lawrence Erlbaum Associates.

Medin, D. L., Altom, M. W., & Murphy, T. D. (1984). Given versus induced category representations: Use of prototype and exemplar information in classification. *Journal of Experimental Psychology: Learning. Memory, and Cognition, 10,* 333–352.

Medin, D. L., & Schaffer, M. M. (1978). Context theory of classification learning. *Psychological Review, 85,* 207–238.

Mullen, B. (1983). Operationalizing the effect of the group on the individual: A self-attention perspective. *Journal of Experimental Social Psychology, 19,* 295–322.

Mullen, B. (1986). Atrocity as a function of lynch mob composition: A self-attention perspective. *Personality and Social Psychology Bulletin, 12,* 187–197.

Mullen. B. (1990). *Selves, others, salience, and phenomenology.* Paper presented at the annual meeting of Empire State Social Psychology, Blue Mountain Lake, NY.

Mullen, B. (1991). Group composition, salience, and cognitive representation: The phenomenology of being in a group. *Journal of Experimental Social Psychology, 27,* 297–323.

Mullen, B. (2001). Ethnophaulisms for ethnic immigrant groups. *Journal of Social Issues, Immigrants and Immigration, 57,* 457–475.

Mullen, B. (2003). The effects of social distinctiveness: The phenomenology of being in a group. In A. Guinote & Y. Trope (Chairs), The psychology of minorities: Basic mechanisms and social implications. Small group meeting sponsored by the European Association of Experimental Social Psychology, London, England.

Mullen, B., Brown, R., & Smith, C. (1992). Ingroup bias as a function of salience, relevance, and status: An integration. *European Journal of Social Psychology, 22,* 103–122.

Mullen, B., Chapman, J., & Peaugh, S. (1989). Focus of attention in groups: A self-attention perspective. *Journal of Social Psychology, 129,* 807–817.

Mullen, B., Driskell, J. E., & Smith, C. (1989). Availability and social projection: The effects of sequence of measurement and wording of question on estimates of consensus. *Personality and Social Psychology Bulletin, 15,* 84–90.

Mullen, B., & Hu, L. (1988). Social projection as a function of cognitive mechanisms: Two meta-analytic integrations. *British Journal of Social Psychology, 27,* 333–356.

Mullen, B., & Hu, L. (1989). Perceptions of ingroup and outgroup variability: A meta-analytic integration. *Basic and Applied Social Psychology, 10,* 233–252.

Mullen, B., & Johnson, C. (1990). Distinctiveness-based illusory correlation in stereotyping: A meta-analytic integration. *British Journal of Social Psychology, 29,* 11–28.

Mullen, B., & Johnson, C. (1993). Cognitive representation in ethnophaulisms as a function of group size: The phenomenology of being in a group. *Personality and Social Psychology Bulletin, 19,* 296–304.

Mullen, B., & Johnson, C. (1995). Cognitive representation in ethnophaulisms and illusory correlation in stereotyping. *Personality and Social Psychology Bulletin, 21,* 420–433.

Mullen, B., Johnson, C., & Anthony, T. (1994). Relative group size and cognitive representations of ingroup and outgroup: The phenomenology of being in a group. *Small Group Research, 25,* 250–266.

Mullen, B., Pizzuto, C., & Foels, R. (2002). Altering intergroup perceptions by altering prevailing mode of cognitive representation: "They look like people." *Journal of Personality and Social Psychology, 83,* 1333–1343.

Mullen, B., Salas, E., & Driskell, J. E. (1989). Salience, motivation, and artifact as contributions to the relation between participation rate and leadership. *Journal of Experimental Social Psychology, 25,* 545–559.

Mullen, B., & Smith, C. (1990). Social projection as a function of actual consensus. *Journal of Social Psychology, 130,* 501–506.

Nesdale, A. R., & Dharmalingham, S. (1986). Category salience, stereotyping, and person memory. *Australian Journal of Psychology, 38,* 145–151.

Nesdale, A. R., Dharmalingham, S., & Kerr, G. K. (1987). Effect of subgroup ratio on stereotyping. *European Journal of Social Psychology, 17,* 353–356.

Nichols, D. R., Abrams, D., & Mullen, B. (2000). Effects of gender composition in groups. I: An integration of the group discussion paradigm. Presented at the 1st annual meeting of SPSP, Nashville, TN.

Oakes, P. J. (1994). The effects of fit vs. novelty on the salience of social categories: A response to Biernat and Vescio (1993). *Journal of Experimental Social Psychology, 30,* 390–398.

Oakes, P. J., Turner, J. C., & Haslam, S. A. (1991). Perceiving people as group members: The role of fit in the salience of social categorizations. *British Journal of Social Psychology, 30,* 125–144.

Old, B. S. (1946). On the mathematics of committees, boards, and panels. *Scientific Monthly, 63,* 129–134.

Park, B., & Hastie, R. (1987). Perception of variability in category development: Instance versus abstraction-based stereotypes. *Journal of Personality and Social Psychology, 53*, 621–635.

Posner, M. I., & Keele, S. W. (1970). Retention of abstract ideas. *Journal of Experimental Psychology, 83*, 304–308.

Reed, S K. (1972). Pattern recognition and categorization. *Cognitive Psychology, 3*, 382–407.

Rothbart, M., & John, O.P. (1985). Social categorization and behavioral episodes: A cognitive analysis of the effects of intergroup contact. *Journal of Social Issues, 41*, 81–104.

Royce, J. (1895). Self-consciousness, social consciousness, and nature. *The Philosophical Review, 4*, 465–485; 577–602.

Schmidt, S. R. (1991). Can we have a distinctive theory of memory? *Memory & Cognition, 19*, 523–542.

Sherman, S. J., & Corty, E. (1984). Cognitive heuristics. In R. S. Wyer & T. K. Srull (Eds), *Handbook of social cognition* (pp. 153–180). Hillsdale, NJ: Lawrence Erlbaum Associates.

Simmel, G. (1908/1950). *The sociology of Georg Simmel*, K. Wolff, Trans. New York: Free Press.

Slater, P. E. (1958). Contrasting correlates of group size. *Sociemtry, 21*, 129–139.

Smith, E. E., & Medin, D. L. (1981). *Categories and concepts*. Cambridge, MA: Harvard University Press.

Smith, E. R., & Zarate, M. A. (1990). Exemplar and prototype use in social cognition. *Social Cognition, 8*, 243–262.

Tajfel, H. (1969). Cognitive aspects of prejudice. *Journal of Social Issues, 25*, 79–97.

Taylor, S. E., & Fiske, S. T. (1978). Salience, attention, and attribution: Top of the head phenomena. In I. Berkowitz (Ed.), *Advances in experimental social psychology* (Vol. 11, pp. 250–283). New York: Academic Press.

Taylor, S. I., Fiske, S. T., Etcoff, N. L., & Ruderman, A. J. (1978). Categorical bases of person memory and stereotyping. *Journal of Personality and Social Psychology, 36*, 778–793.

Turner, J. C., Hogg, M. A., Oakes, P. J., Reicher, S. D., & Wetherell, M. S. (1987). *Rediscovering the social group: A self-categorization theory*. Oxford: Basil Blackwell.

Tversky, A., & Gati, I. (1978). Studies of similarity. In E. Rosch & B. B. Lloyd (Eds.), *Cognition and categorization* (pp. 38–72). Hillsdale, NJ: Lawrence Erlbaum Associates.

Tversky, A., & Kahneman, D. (1974). Judgement under uncertainty: Heuristics and biases. *Science, 185*, 1124–1131.

Wegner, D. M., & Schaefer, D. (1978). The concentration of responsibility: An objective self-awareness analysis of group size effects in helping situations. *Journal of Personality and Social Psychology, 36*, 147–155.

Wertheimer, M. (1923). Untersuchengen zur lehre von der Gestalt: II. *Psychologische Forschung, 4*, 301–350.

Wicklund, R. A. (1980). Group contact and self-focused attention. In P. B. Paulus (Ed.), *Psychology of group influence*. Hillsdale, NJ: Lawrence Erlbaum Associates.

Wicklund, R. A. (1982). How society uses self-awareness. In J. Suls (Ed.), *Psychological perspectives on the self* (Vol. I). Hillsdale, NJ: Lawrence Erlbaum Associates.

14

Distinctiveness and Memory: A Comparison of the Social and Cognitive Literatures

Susan Coats and Eliot R. Smith

This chapter is concerned with the effects of distinctiveness on explicit memory in social psychology. We have several goals in writing this chapter. One is to draw comparisons between the social and cognitive literatures on the topic of distinctiveness and memory, with the aim of better understanding the extent to which the findings in each area may be applicable to the other. A second goal is to review several prominent lines of research in the social literature, each of which invokes the concept of distinctiveness to explain or describe memory phenomena. Lastly, the distinction between relational and item-specific processing is offered as a way to integrate these related but disparate areas of investigation and, by doing so, form links between the social and cognitive literatures.

The extent to which a stimulus is distinctive, of course, depends on its context. In both the social and cognitive literatures, distinctiveness has often been presented as the property of a stimulus in a particular situation (Schmidt, 1991; Higgins, 1996). Many researchers' usage of the term in the social domain is consistent with the following offered by Schmidt: "*distinctiveness* refers to stimuli that are incongruous with active conceptual frameworks or that contain salient features not present in active memory" (Schmidt, 1991, p. 537). For an example in the social domain, consider that a stimulus person who occupies a numerical minority position (e.g., a single male presented with many women in a stimulus display) is deemed distinctive (Taylor, Fiske, Etcoff, & Ruderman, 1978). Since we review distinctiveness phenomena in the social literature, we will frequently use the term in this manner in order to be consistent with this literature. In several cases, the critical stimuli may be "distinctive" owing to the prevailing context and in others the critical stimuli may be "distinctive" owing to incongruity with one's long-term experience (which corresponds to Schmidt's distinction between primary and secondary distinctiveness, respectively).

313

We also discuss the type of processing induced by that distinctiveness. Distinctiveness may be said to encourage specific types of processing of an item, which in turn enhances discrimination of that item at retrieval. Hunt (Hunt, Chapter 1 this volume; Hunt & McDaniel, 1993) maintains that combined processing of both similarity and differences yields enhanced discrimination of an item. The distinction between relational and item-specific processing is central to this discussion. *Relational processing* refers to processing of features common to all stimulus items. Such processing serves to interrelate items or organize them according to some scheme. Processing the interrelations among events helps participants form links that act as memory cues, so that retrieval of some items will cause people to remember others. In contrast, *item-specific processing* refers to the processing of properties of individual items not shared by other items. This processing serves to discriminate between items or events. The combination of relational and item-specific processing enhances memory because it specifies both the context defining an event and the unique properties of a particular item within the event. The concepts of item-specific and relational processing have been applied to a broad range of phenomena and have provided novel insights and predictions across many disparate areas (Hunt & McDaniel, 1993).

CONTRASTING DISTINCTIVENESS IN THE SOCIAL AND COGNITIVE LITERATURES

One of the primary aims of this volume is to extend the discoveries and insights of one domain to another. However, applying findings indiscriminately, without considering the differences among domains, may obscure and mislead rather than elucidate. In this next section we assess differences between the social and cognitive fields in the treatment of distinctiveness on memory.

Cognitive and social researchers often differ in terms of the objectives underlying the study of distinctiveness on memory. Making explicit these differences may facilitate exchange of ideas between the two areas. In the cognitive literature memory itself is the object of study, whereas in the social literature memory is most often a tool in service of social judgment, stereotyping, and impression formation, which themselves are the objects of study. Memory measures in the social literature are, therefore, usually included primarily to gain insight into other phenomena. As just one example, explicit memory has been assessed in order to better understand why perceivers make relatively extreme evaluations of individuals who are salient owing to their group's relative small size in a stimulus array (e.g., Nichols, Abrams, & Mullen, 2000; Lord & Saenz, 1985; Taylor et al., 1978).

This dual focus on social judgments and memory has led to a number of important discoveries about the relationship between judgments and memory (Hastie & Kumar, 1979; Hastie & Park, 1986). Although one might reasonably expect that a participant's trait ratings and evaluations about a target are related to the information that he or she recalls about that target, the two are quite often not related (Hastie & Kumar, 1979; Hastie & Park, 1986). Notably, this dissociation is particularly likely to occur in certain situations involving distinctive information—for instance, information that is incongruent with expectations (Hastie & Kumar 1979; Stangor & McMillon, 1992). Although a thorough discussion of this topic is beyond the scope of this chapter, we briefly note that such dissociations are common when perceivers make judgments about a target during stimulus presentation (Hastie & Park, 1986). Such judgments are commonly said to be formed "online." In contrast, "memory-based" judgments are formed at the time of test and depend on retrieval of stimulus items.

The dual interest in memory and judgment within social psychology has also had methodological consequences. Stimulus displays and memory measures presented in the social domain have tended to be more circumscribed than those in the cognitive domain. For instance, studies often use only a single measure of explicit memory, and entire paradigms frequently rely heavily on a single memory measure. And not surprisingly, the prototype stimulus is a description of a person or group. This is in contrast to the cognitive literature, in which the stimulus items are of many types and are associated in many different ways (e.g., the stimuli may comprise lists of categories, unrelated items from various categories, words with varying orthographic features). Most of the research that examines distinctive memory phenomena in the social realm involves presenting participants with information (typically traits or behaviors) about one or two individuals or one or two groups. Information is constructed so that some aspects of the stimuli are distinctive and then memory is assessed. That the stimuli comprise information ascribed to individual or group targets has important consequences for information processing. First, the stimuli are related by virtue of their ascription to a group or individual. According to Hunt and Einstein (1981), items that are related or belong to the same category encourage relational processing. There is considerable evidence suggesting that perceivers often expect some degree of coherence and unity in such stimuli and will often engage in organizational processing, such as integrating the information about the target and resolving inconsistencies (Hastie & Kumar, 1979; Wyer & Srull, 1989). This is especially true when the target is an individual, as perceivers typically expect an especially high degree of coherency in such a target (McConnell, Sherman, & Hamilton, 1994a; 1997). Indeed, as we discuss below, the degree of coherence that the participant expects in a target (often referred to as *entitativity* in the literature) has been found to be of critical importance to numerous social memory phenomena.

Second, the typical stimulus items in social psychological research are sentences describing some behaviors (or less common, traits) that are ascribed to a particular person or group. In contrast, much of the research examining the effects of distinctiveness on memory in the cognitive literature rely on lists of single word items, such as in studies on the von Restorff effect (e.g., Dunlosky, Hunt, & Clark, 2000; Hunt & Einstein, 1981; Schmidt, 1991). The stimuli in social studies often involve the encoding, organization, and retrieval of associated information. For instance, in paradigms offering information about two-person targets, one common explicit measure is a cued-recall task in which participants are presented at test with stimulus items (e.g., behavioral statements) that were ascribed to one of the targets during the study phase. The participant is asked to indicate which target was paired with the behavior. Performance on this task is contingent on the memory for the associative relation between the behavior and the target.

This cued-recall task has been most frequently used in paradigms comparing memory for stimuli ascribed to two groups (e.g., the illusory correlation and the recognition confusion paradigms). In the study phase of such paradigms, participants are exposed to group members who belong to one of two groups, and each member is associated with a behavior. The cued memory task that follows comes in two flavors. In one variation, the participant is asked to indicate whether the person who performed the behavior belongs to "group A" or "group B." In another variation, the participant is presented with pictures of all the group members (pictures are presented during the study phase along with the behavioral information) and asked to identify which *individual* performed the behavior. Performance on either version of the task depends heavily on relational information. Pertinent to this discussion is a conceptual distinction made by Worthen and Loveland (2003; Worthen, Chapter 7 this volume) between inter-item relational and intra-item relational processing (see also Hunt, Chapter 1 this volume, for a discussion of event-based and item-based processing). Inter-item relational information concerns the relations between the items (separate person-behavior pairs in this paradigm), and intra-item relational processing taps relations between the behavior and the person associated with that behavior. In variations in which the participant is asked to identify which *group* was associated with the target, both types of relational processing likely contribute to accurate performance. This is because accurate performance on this cued-recall task may be accomplished by retrieving information about which particular individual performed the behavior (i.e., intra-item relational information) or by retrieving information about which group was associated with the behavior (i.e., inter-item relational information). However, when the participant is asked to identify which *individual* was associated with the target, accurate performance depends more heavily on intra-item relational processing. We return to this topic later in the chapter.

The following sections of the chapter will review several widely documented findings in the social literature involving distinctiveness and memory. This is not intended to be an exhaustive review. We primarily limit our review to explicit memory. Mullen (Chapter 13 this volume) nicely captures many of the effects of distinctiveness on evaluation, stereotyping, and other such phenomena, much of which may be considered a form of implicit memory.

After a brief review of each finding, we analyze the finding within the framework of item-specific and relational processing. Our contribution is to discuss both of these *types* of processing as they are enhanced by stimulus distinctiveness. In contrast, existing social-psychological models of these effects tend to rely on assumptions about different *amounts* of a single type of processing (e.g., an assumption that distinctive items receive "more attention" and "better encoding"). The intent here is not to replace any formal models in the areas reviewed. In fact, we believe the constructs of item-specific and relational processing are compatible with a variety of formal models (e.g., Garcia-Marques & Hamilton, 1996; Hastie, 1980; Srull & Wyer, 1989). Rather, the purpose is to bring distinct areas under a common umbrella and to highlight previously unrecognized parallels.

THE INCONGRUENCY EFFECT

One of the more active research questions to emerge over the last 20 years in social cognition is whether an expectation about a social target will affect a perceiver's memory for information as a function of its relevance to the expectation (Hastie & Kumar, 1979; Rojahn & Pettigrew, 1992; Stangor & McMillan, 1992; Srull, 1981). This question has sparked a large volume of research, in part because early work appeared to arrive at discrepant answers. Hastie and Kumar's (1979) seminal research is the most frequently cited in this area. Hastie and Kumar presented participants with a trait expectation of a target, followed by behaviors attributed to the target that varied in whether they were consistent with, inconsistent with, or irrelevant to the trait expectation. Then participants were asked to recall the behaviors. Participants' memory for inconsistent behaviors was better than their memory for consistent behaviors, and memory for expectation-irrelevant behaviors was worst of all. Of the many studies that followed, some were consistent with the Hastie and Kumar finding while some were not. Both Stangor and McMillan (1992) and Rojahn and Pettigrew (1992) published extensive meta-analyses of the existing research on memory for expectancy-congruent and expectancy-incongruent information. Their analyses indicate that although there is generally a recall advantage for inconsistent information, this tendency is modified by a number of important variables.

Factors That Qualify the Incongruency Effect

One of the most critical factors in the relationship between incongruity and recall is whether the target is an individual or a group. Incongruent effects occur for individual targets but typically do not occur when the target is a group. Hamilton & Sherman (1996) argue that differences between groups and individuals in terms of entitativity largely underlie this finding. *Entitativity* refers to the perception that a social aggregate is perceived as possessing unity and coherence. Although both individuals and groups can exhibit varying levels of entitativity, perceivers hold different expectations about the amount of entitativity in individual and group social targets (Hamilton & Sherman, 1996; McConnell et al., 1997). Perceivers typically expect unity and coherence in the traits of individuals. These strong expectations of unity lead perceivers to search for consistencies in target behaviors, to form coherent and stable impressions of individuals. In contrast, individual members of a group are not expected to behave in consistent ways. Because of this expectation of variability, perceivers will typically be less motivated to form an integrated impression of group targets or to reconcile behavioral inconsistencies as they encounter target-relevant information. But what if a particular group is perceived as being high in entitativity? McConnell et al. (1997) tested the prediction that participants exposed to groups high in entitativity would preferentially recall incongruent behavior. Their results were in accord with the prediction.

Explicit processing instructions also moderate the incongruity effect. Differences between memory-processing goals and impression-formation goals have typically been tested. Impression instructions direct the participant to form a coherent impression of the target. Memory instructions direct the participant to try to memorize the statements. Impression instructions typically yield an incongruity effect, whereas memory instruction sets often do not (except in some studies where the target was an individual).

The manner by which incongruency is established is another moderator. The recall advantage for incongruent information is stronger and more reliable when incongruency is manipulated in the immediate context than when based on preexisting stereotypes (Stangor & McMillan, 1992). Further, the magnitude of the incongruency effect is inversely related to the proportion of incongruent items in the stimulus set (Stangor & McMillan, 1992). Participants with limited cognitive capacity or who are exposed to complex processing tasks (e.g., large number of targets, large number of traits, less exposure time) recall consistent information at least as well as inconsistent information (Stangor & McMillan, 1992).

Current Explanations for the Incongruency Effect

The prevailing explanation for the incongruency effect is that the recall advantage of the incongruent information results from special processing devoted to incongruent information to reconcile it with the prevailing expectation, typically in an attempt to form a coherent impression of the target (Stangor & McMillan, 1992). It is maintained that because inconsistent information violates an expectancy, it is surprising, draws people's attention, and initiates attempts to explain the inconsistency. Such information is extensively processed in relation to the target and to other information about the target. The various moderators of the incongruency effect identified by the meta-analyses are consistent with this explanation. In general, the meta-analyses demonstrate that any variable expected to decrease such incongruency-resolution processes will attenuate recall of inconsistent information, in some cases leading to recall advantages for consistent information. Thus, individual targets result in the incongruency effect and group targets do not because it is only in the former case that perceivers expect a high amount of unity and coherence in the target. This expectation of unity motivates perceivers to form an integrated impression and thus to reconcile behavioral inconsistencies. Similarly, impression-formation goals, which typically yield an incongruity effect, also motivate the perceiver to form a coherent impression of the target and thus to resolve any inconsistencies. Differences in the strength of the effect based on whether the expectancy is formed during the experimental session or based on previously established stereotypes are explained by maintaining that such trait expectancies are stronger than those based on stereotypes. Trait expectancies are stronger because they are based on information that applies specifically to the target rather than being based on attributes that are known to apply to members of the same class as the target (Srull, Lichtenstein, & Rothbart, 1985). Lastly, the incongruency effect is weakened under conditions that strain cognitive functioning because participants are unable to engage in inconsistency resolution.

Recognition

Thus far we have discussed the effects of incongruity on free recall. In large part this is because most studies in this area have relied exclusively on free recall to measure explicit memory. But, of course, use of different memory measures yields important information about the processes that underlie the effect. Recognition measures have been used occasionally to examine the incongruity effect. In general, recognition measures that have been corrected for response bias show an overall advantage for expectancy-incongruent information (Stangor & McMillan, 1992). However, a number of the moderator variables discussed earlier tend to produce opposite effects on free recall and recognition sensitivity. Whereas memory set instructions (relative to impression-formation instructions) and complex processing conditions attenuate the incongruity effect on free-recall measures, these same factors increase the incongruity effect on recognition measures. However, the type of target (group vs. individual) has the same effect on free recall and recognition measures, such that both show an advantage for incongruent material with individual targets.

The Incongruency Effect Explained by Item-Specific and Relational Processing

Examining the incongruency effect within the framework of item-specific and relational processing serves two purposes. First, such an analysis may ultimately provide new insights into the effect, as it has with many memory phenomena in the cognitive literature. In addition, such an analysis should serve to bring the incongruency effect under a common umbrella with similar effects in both the social and cognitive literatures and thus aid us in drawing parallels between these two domains. In this analysis, we focus specifically on how each moderator variable of the incongruency effect impacts the contribution of item-specific and relational processing, and how such a framework may explain differences on the recall and recognition measures.

First, it is important to consider differences between the two memory measures: free recall and recognition. These measures differ in the extent to which item-specific and relational information contribute to performance. Free recall is thought to depend on both item-specific and relational information (Hunt & McDaniel, 1993). This is because relational information aids in generating information and item-specific information aids in making discriminations within a class of events. In contrast, recognition depends primarily on item-specific information, as the task is largely one of discrimination. Understanding the cause of the effect also requires consideration of the nature of the stimuli and especially the relationship between the congruent and incongruent items in the paradigms. In the incongruency paradigm, all the items relate to one another by virtue of their ascription to a single target. In addition, the incongruent items typically indicate a trait that is in *opposition* to information provided by other information (e.g., unfriendly vs. friendly). The critical and control items are thus related by way of contradiction. In other paradigms invoking the distinctiveness effect on memory, the critical items are often unrelated to the control items. We elaborate on this point in a later section, where we compare the incongruency effect to other memory phenomena.

With this as background, we review the findings.

Recall

The effect of incongruency on recall occurs most strongly with individual targets and/or with impression instructions. These findings can be interpreted as the result of differences in item-specific and relational processing during encoding and at test. Individual targets and impression instructions both encourage the encoding of relational information. Such processing serves to interrelate and organize the information. And in these circumstances, the incongruent items receive a disproportionate amount of relational processing as the perceiver seeks to reconcile that item with the prevailing configuration. Because the incongruent information is at odds with the preponderance of information about the individual, such items will receive somewhat greater item-specific processing as well. With relatively high levels of both types of processing, incongruent items will be well recalled.

In contrast, when perceivers operate under memory instructions, relational processing is diminished. The incongruent items may receive a disproportionate amount of item-specific processing, but in the absence of extensive relational processing the advantage of these items in recall will be lessened or negated.

We maintain that group targets diminish relational processing as well, but primarily only for the incongruent items. Here, the standard impression-formation instructions encourage relational processing of the congruent items. However, because perceivers expect less consistency within group targets than for individual targets, the incongruent items relating to groups do not require particular elaboration or resolution to form an impression of the target (as is the case with individual targets). As a consequence, the incongruent items receive relatively little relational processing. Thus the advantage of these items in recall will, once again, be diminished.

Recognition

The incongruency effect on recognition, although examined in many fewer studies, occurs most strongly with memory instructions (compared to impression instructions). This, we suggest, is because memory instructions encourage item-specific processing (and impression-formation relational processing), as just argued. Under these conditions, the incongruent items receive an especially high degree of item-specific processing (though less relational processing) relative to the other items because the incongruent items are inconsistent with the preponderance of information about the target. In the absence of impression instructions, the perceiver lacks motivation to reconcile the incongruent items. Such items are better recognized because item-specific processing is more likely to aid later recognition memory.

Lastly, the incongruency effect on recognition is stronger for individual targets than for group targets. With standard impression instructions, the critical difference between these two target types is that the incongruent information receives a relatively high degree of relational processing when the target is an individual, but little when it is a group (which serves to negate the effect for group targets on recall). The congruent items receive high levels of relational processing regardless of target type. Group targets, however, should not diminish the enhanced processing of item-specific information for the incongruent information. Therefore, when the target is a group, incongruent items enhance recognition performance, but not recall.

The Incongruency Effect, the Isolation Effect, and the Issue of Salience

In the cognitive literature, the isolation paradigm has been the prototype paradigm for examining the effect of distinctiveness on memory (Hunt, Chapter 1 this volume). This paradigm entails presenting participants with material, a small proportion of which differs on some dimension from the majority of the material. Participants operating under memory instructions consistently show better recall for the isolates. Why is it that the isolation effect occurs with intentional memory instructions, but the incongruency effect on recall does not?[1] We suggest this is because the two effects occur for very different reasons. Hunt and Lamb (2001) explain that the isolation effect under standard memory conditions occurs because of a failure to process differences among the homogeneous controls. Consistent with this explanation, Hunt and Lamb (2001) conducted a study of the isolation effect by comparing the effect of those operating under intentional memory instructions and those operating under a difference judgment between the current word and the previous word. Only in the former condition was an isolation effect found. The reason for this pattern becomes clear once one considers the stimuli that are typically used in the paradigm. In the standard isolation paradigm, the items on the list are single words reporting exemplars from categories. The isolated item is that which belongs to a different category from the other items on the list, which themselves are exemplars of a single category. Thus, the control items are both highly similar to one another and very dissimilar from the isolate. As a consequence the control items receive little item-specific processing under normal memory instructions.

The stimuli used in the incongruency paradigm differ from that of the isolation paradigm in several important ways. Most significantly, the critical and control items in the incongruity paradigm are considerably more "similar" than are the corresponding items in the isolation paradigm. In the isolation paradigm, the only obvious relationship between the critical and control items is their appearance on the same list. In the incongruency paradigm, all the items relate to one another by virtue of their ascription to a single target. In addition, the incongruent items typically indicate a trait that *opposes* information provided by the other items. This is far different from being unrelated. As stated previously, the incongruency effect occurs under impression instructions primarily because under these conditions the incongruent items are subject to a particularly high degree of relational processing. The incongruent items become highly relevant to the other items when the perceiver operates under the goal of integrating these items with congruent items. When participants process the information in the absence of such a goal (i.e., memory instructions), such items receive relatively little relational processing and the advantage of the items in recall is diminished. The finding that the instruction set has opposite effects on incongruency depending on the type of memory measure is consistent with this view. Under impression-formation instructions, incongruent items are not better recognized, which makes sense if the recall advantage under these conditions were due primarily to greater relational processing of the incongruent items.

The incongruency and isolation effects are similar in some ways. Both have been explained as resulting from additional attention directed to the isolate or uncharacteristic items at encoding (Hastie, 1980; Schmidt, 1991; Stangor & McMillon, 1992; Srull & Wyer, 1989). Such items, it is argued, are subjectively experienced as salient and surprising, receive enhanced encoding, and as result are remembered better. Recently however, Hunt and McDaniel (1993) have demonstrated that the isolation effect does not depend on the salience of the item at encoding. The effect occurs even when the critical item appears early in the list where the isolated item is not perceived as unusual to the participant. This finding calls into question the prevailing view in social psychology about the cause of the incongruency effect, or at least the contention that the critical items are recalled better because of differential processing owing to their salience.

There are, however, reasons to suspect that the role that salience plays in the production of these two effects may differ. Again, consider the important differences between the two paradigms. As discussed earlier, in the standard isolation paradigm, the items on the list are single words reporting exemplars from categories. The isolated item is set for spontaneous categorical and item-specific processing (Hunt & Lamb, 2001). In the incongruency paradigm, the items are typically behaviors that imply some trait. The semantic meaning of the items and the relations among items in the congruency paradigm are likely not spontaneously realized. Furthermore, as we discussed earlier, the two effects have different causes. Whereas the isolation effect occurs because of a failure to process differences among the homogeneous controls (Hunt & Lamb, 2001), the incongruency effect occurs primarily because the incongruent items are subject to a particularly high degree of relational processing. The incongruent and congruent items, rather than being unrelated, are, in some ways, especially related owing to the fact that they are contradictory. Because of differences such as these, it is not unreasonable to suspect that salience and subsequent attention directed to such items may be necessary for the type of reconciliation or relational processing that underlies the effect. Several studies have demonstrated that incongruent items receive extensive processing when initially encountered (Bargh & Thein, 1985). And perhaps more telling, a study by Sherman and Hamilton (1994) demonstrated that incongruent information, more so than congruent information, involves the reactivation of previously encountered information about the person in question. This finding supports the notion that incongruent information encourages efforts to reconcile the item with the overall impression during encoding.

Of course, empirically separating salience from such incongruency should be quite easily accomplished in the incongruency paradigm by varying the placement of the incongruent items.[2] Such a study should answer the question of whether salience is necessary for the incongruency effect to occur. If the effect were to occur in cases in which the incongruent items appeared early on the list, an amended version of the prevalent explanation for the effect may be retained by positing that the reconciliation process can occur subsequent to exposure.

THE ILLUSORY CORRELATION EFFECT

The illusory correlation is generally defined as the erroneous perception of the co-occurrence of rare characteristics (Chapman, 1967; Hamilton & Gifford, 1976). In social psychology usage, this effect is typically concerned with the perceived linkage between minority group membership and rare (usually undesirable) behaviors. An influential study by Hamilton & Gifford (1976) stimulated a great deal of social psychological interest in this phenomenon, in large part because of its potential role in the formation of stereotypes. Hamilton and Gifford presented participants with a number of statements each describing a member of one of two groups (group A or group B), performing either a desirable or an undesirable behavior. There were twice as many descriptions of group A than of group B (24 and 12, respectively) and more of the behaviors were desirable than undesirable (24 and 12, respectively). Although the frequency of sentences for the two groups was unequal, the ratio of desirable to undesirable behaviors was the same for both groups. After reading the sentences, participants completed three measures to assess their perceptions of the two groups. Participants were presented with the original behaviors and asked which group was associated with each statement (the group assignment task). Participants also estimated the frequency of undesirable behaviors performed by the members of each group. Finally, ratings were made of each group on a set of desirable and undesirable traits. Phi coefficients, a measure of perceived correlation, were computed from the group assignments and frequency estimates. Of these three measures, only the assignment task is clearly an explicit measure of memory (and is essentially a cued-recall task). And even that task, like the other two, could be driven more by a participant's overall evaluative impression of each group than by specific memory for the group associated with each behavior.

Across all three measures, participants' responses indicated an erroneous perception of an association between the smaller group B and the performance of undesirable behaviors. Participants' responses in the group-assignment task may reveal some insight regarding the nature of this bias. Participants tended to correctly attribute the rare (undesirable) behaviors to the minority group, and they tended to incorrectly attribute a subset of the rare (undesirable) behaviors performed by the majority group to the minority group. This served to further augment estimates of the minority group's rare (undesirable) behaviors. Hamilton and Gifford's basic findings have been replicated many times (Mullen & Johnson, 1990).

Only very rarely have more standard measures of memory, such as recall or recognition, been used in the illusory correlation paradigm. Two studies that included recall measures in the study of illusory correlation found greater recall for the co-occurring infrequent items (i.e., the minority group's negative behaviors) than of the other categories of items (Hamilton, Dugan & Trolier, 1985; Stroessner, Meiland, & Cook, 1999, as cited in Stroessner & Plaks, 2001). However, McConnell, Sherman, & Hamilton (1994b) report a recall advantage for the infrequent items, but not a particular advantage for the co-occurring infrequent items. Stroessner, Hamilton, and Mackie (1992) found no effect of category type on recall. However, their recall task was performed after participants had completed a number of other dependent measures, which may have contaminated performance on the task.

Current Explanations for the Illusory Correlation Effect

Hamilton and Gifford (1976) explained the illusory correlation effect as being due to the distinctiveness of the co-occurrence of infrequent stimulus information (those items describing a member of the smaller group performing an infrequently occurring type of behavior). According to this account, such co-occurrences are noticed and receive differential processing. As a consequence, these items become well represented in memory and are easily retrievable when judgments are subsequently called for. Hence, to the extent that subjects apply the availability heuristic (Tversky & Kahneman, 1973), those items have differential impact on those judgments.

Recent research, however, indicates that distinctiveness at the time of encoding is not a necessary precondition for the formation of bias. Following the work of Hunt and McDaniel (1993) cited earlier, McConnell and his colleagues (McConnell et al., 1994b) altered the presentation order of stimuli so that the co-occurring infrequent stimuli were not distinctive at the time that participants encountered them. Still the illusory correlation emerged. This finding shows that distinctiveness at the time of encoding is not a necessary precondition for the formation of bias. These results are problematic for the original distinctiveness-based account, in which distinctive stimuli were assumed to receive greater attention at encoding. The results seem to require postulating processes that operate after original encoding that could alter the processing given an item (Hunt & McDaniel, 1993; Hunt, Chapter 1 this volume).

Several alternative explanations for the illusory correlation effect have been proposed, which do not posit any special processing of the infrequently occurring items. Smith (1991) argued that participants may be sensitive to the *difference* between the number of positive and negative items recalled, and not to the proportionate differences between positive group A and group B behaviors. Thus, because the difference between positive and negative behaviors is greater for group A than group B, the majority group (A) is seen as more positive than the minority group (B). By means of a computer simulation, Smith demonstrated that illusory correlations might result from the memory processes modeled by Hintzman's (1986) exemplar memory model. Fiedler and his colleagues have also critiqued the distinctiveness-based account (Fiedler, 1991; Fiedler & Armbruster, 1994; Fiedler, Russer, & Gramm, 1993). The central theme in Fiedler's argument is that the illusory correlation is a consequence of information loss that produces regression in the subject's estimates of those frequencies. A number of studies conducted by Fielder and his colleagues (cited above) demonstrate quite clearly that illusory correlations can arise in certain situations without any differential processing of the infrequent information.

However, other evidence is quite consistent with the distinctiveness interpretation proposed by Hamilton and Gifford (1976). Data show that the co-occurring infrequent items in the illusory correlation paradigm receive differential processing and are more accessible than other item types. Among this evidence is the finding that the distinctive items receive greater processing times than the other three item types when they are distinctive at the time of presentation (Stoessner et al., 1992). Further, these processing differences predict the magnitude of the bias. In addition, several studies have demonstrated that participants respond most quickly to the undesirable behaviors performed by the smaller group (suggesting heightened accessibility), and these latencies were predictive of the magnitude of the bias (Johnson & Mullen, 1994; McConnell et al., 1994b). The alternative accounts presented above would need to be extended to explain these findings. Thus, it appears that the distinctiveness interpretation proposed by Hamilton and Gifford (1976) is one explanation for the illusory correlation effect, but mechanisms other than differential processing of distinctive items likely also contribute to the formation of illusory correlations or are able to account for the bias under some circumstances.

Factors that Qualify the Illusory Correlation Effect

Although the illusory correlation has proved highly reliable, a number of variables have been shown to moderate the effect. Interestingly, some of these variables are ones that were shown to moderate the incongruity effect presented earlier. Type of target (group vs. individual) is one such moderator. In the standard illusory correlation study, the participants are presented with information regarding two groups (group A and group B). Several studies manipulated the type of target and found a typical illusory correlation bias for group targets but no such bias for individual targets (Hamilton & Sherman, 1996; McConnell et al., 1997; McConnell et al., 1994a; Schaller & Maass, 1989, Experiment 2). Thus, type of target has the opposite effect on the two phenomena. The incongruity effect primarily occurs when the target is an individual, whereas the illusory correlation effect typically occurs when the target is a group.

Type of instruction is another factor that moderates both the incongruency effect and the illusory correlation. Ordinarily in the illusory correlation paradigm, participants operate under memory-set instructions. Participants are asked to listen carefully to the items and are told that their memory for the information will be tested afterwards. Studies that have manipulated instruction set by including an impression formation condition find that the effect occurs for participants in the memory-set instruction condition only (McConnell et al., 1994a; Pryor, 1986; McConnell et al., 1997). Once again, an important moderator (type of instruction) has an opposite impact on the incongruity effect and the illusory correlation.

In their meta-analysis, Mullen and Johnson (1990) found an increase in the illusory correlation effect as a function of the number of exemplars present (however, the effect of the number of exemplars did not reach significance for the group-assignment measure). The number of items in the stimulus set was also found to moderate the incongruency effect (but in that case, the item number served to attenuate the effect). The results of studies examining the moderating effect of other factors assumed to impinge on cognitive capacity have been mixed. Positive mood (e.g., Bodenhausen, Kramer, & Susser, 1994; Sinclair & Mark, 1995; Stroessner & Mackie, 1992), and sometimes negative mood (Cohen, Weingartner, Smallberg, Pickar, & Murphy, 1982), can decrease the thoroughness with which available information is processed. Stroessner et al. (1992) assessed participants' processing latencies as a means of investigating differential attention to the co-occurring infrequent items. Only participants in a neutral mood differentially attended to the minority group's infrequent behavior, and only these participants formed illusory correlations. In a study by Fiedler, Russer and Gramm (1993), distraction served to minimize the illusory correlation among the usual group targets. However, when participants were presented with individual targets, distraction was found to enhance the effect. Spears & Haslam (1997) maintain that illusory correlations form when experimental participants have moderate available capacity but do not when capacity is either higher or lower.

Studies seeking to examine the generalizability of the effect have revealed additional moderators. Does the effect occur when the infrequent behaviors are positive rather than negative? The answer is yes, but the effect is significantly weaker (Mullen & Johnson, 1990). This finding makes sense in light of the fact that undesirable behaviors are more unusual and unexpected in general (as well as in the local stimulus set). Other studies illustrate that directly involving the self often has a strong impact on the effect (Berndsen, Spears, & van der Plight, 1996; Spears, van der Plight & Eiser, 1985). For instance, Spears and his colleagues (1985) used as stimulus items attitude statements that purportedly expressed the opinions of people from two different towns (thus pro or con attitude statements replaced negative and positive behaviors). Although an illusory correlation effect was found on the group-assignment task and frequency judgments for participants whose attitude position was congruent with the minority-attitude position, the effect was almost nonexistent for subjects whose own positions were congruent with the majority position. The authors explain this finding by suggesting that attitude-congruent positions appear more salient than others owing to their self-relevance, thereby resulting in an elimination of the illusory correlation among the majority-congruent attitude holders (cf. Schmidt, Chapter 3 this volume). Several studies show that membership in one of the target groups affects formation of the illusory correlation. Schaller and Maass (1989, Experiment 2) led participants to believe that they were members of either the majority group, the minority group, or neither group. Those assigned to a group made frequency estimates, group assignments, and evaluative judgments that favored the ingroup (Schaller & Maass, 1989; Schaller, 1991).

The Illusory Correlation Effect Explained by Item-Specific and Relational Processing

A number of important variables moderate both the incongruity effect and the illusory correlation effect, but curiously they seem to have opposite effects. Most notably, the incongruity effect on recall occurs with individual targets and /or with impression-set instructions, whereas the illusory correlation occurs for group targets and/or when memory instructions are used. In this section we apply the concepts of item-specific and relational processing to the illusory correlation effect. We believe this conceptual framework provides a common foundation from which to understand the impact of these moderator variables on the two effects reviewed in this chapter.

First, it is important to consider differences among the various memory tasks the paradigms typically employ. The incongruency effect is typically demonstrated on free-recall measures, and the illusory correlation effect with the group-assignment task, frequency estimates, and evaluation task. The illusory correlation effect on recall, which has only rarely been examined, has been less consistent (Hamilton, Dugan, & Trolier, 1985; McConnell et al., 1994b). For reasons stated earlier, the group-assignment task depends primarily on relational information (for which both intra-item and inter-item information benefits performance). In contrast, the retrieval process that underlies frequency estimations are assumed to be rather quick, effortless, and not dependent on extensive retrieval of instances (Hintzman, 1986, 1988; Garcia-Marques & Hamilton, 1996). Rather, they are assumed to be heuristic in nature and to abide by the availability heuristic (Tversky & Kahneman, 1973). Lastly, the illusory correlation effect is also typically demonstrated on evaluative judgments.

The specific characteristics of the two paradigms, such as the number and configuration of targets and the nature of the items, are also critical to understanding when and why the effect occurs. In the standard illusory correlation paradigm, participants are provided information about individuals belonging to *two* groups (compared with information about one person in the standard incongruency paradigm). The distinction we made previously between intra-item and inter-item processing is relevant here. In the standard incongruency paradigm, all items pertain to a single target. In contrast, in the standard illusory correlation paradigm, each item (usually a behavior) is ascribed to one individual who belongs to one of two groups. Thus, in the later case, relational processing may occur at several levels—

at the individual level (intra-item relational) and/or at the group level (inter-item relational). The relationship between the critical and control items in the illusory correlation paradigm is also pertinent. The uniqueness of the co-occurring items in the illusory correlation paradigm is based on obvious categorical membership (group A vs. B) and behaviors that are either good or bad. The good and bad behaviors are not directly in opposition to one another to the same extent as the corresponding items in the incongruency paradigm (for example, "honest" and "clumsy" are evaluatively opposite, but not directly inconsistent like "honest" and "dishonest"). Thus, in some ways, the items in the illusory correlation paradigm are more analogous to items used in the isolation paradigm than in the incongruency paradigm.

Together these differences (in memory measures, number of targets, and items) can account for the finding that the illusory correlation occurs with memory instructions and group targets, whereas the incongruity effect occurs with impression instructions and individual targets. As discussed previously, we believe the incongruity effect occurs primarily because impression instructions and individual targets enhance relational processing of the incongruent items, thereby aiding recall. More specifically, impression and individual target enhance inter-item relational processing of the incongruent items, as the perceiver seeks to reconcile that item with the prevailing configuration on the target.

In contrast, the illusory correlation effect typically does not occur with impression instructions and individual targets, but rather with memory instructions and group targets. It is important to note that the illusory correlation effect depends on the perceiver's ability to recognize that some group/behavior *combinations* occur less frequently than others. As stated earlier, under conditions of impression instruction or with individual targets, relational processing is encouraged. Such processing encourages the formation of target impressions based on the combined information retained about each target. As a consequence, all items receive considerable inter-item relational processing. Although the undesirable behaviors may receive greater inter-item relational processing than the desirable behaviors, there are a proportionate number of undesirable actions per group. Thus, the consequence of such processing should not result in differential associations between desirability of behaviors and target. Group assignments, frequency estimates, and evaluation under such circumstances should therefore show little if any advantage for the co-occurring infrequent items.

Group targets and memory instructions especially, however, diminish the encoding of inter-item relational information (as people are less motivated to form coherent impressions of the targets). In such cases, the co-occurring infrequent items receive a disproportionate amount of item-specific processing owing to their infrequency. This is analogous to the enhanced item-specific processing of the isolates in the isolation paradigm in the cognitive domain. In addition, these items will receive considerable intra-item processing because it is the combination of the infrequent target and infrequent behavior that renders these particular items unusual. As a consequence, accuracy should be high for the co-occurring infrequent items in the group-assignment task (which benefits from both intra-item and inter-item relational processing) but poor for the other item types. For these other types of items, responses will be based largely on guessing that is biased by retrieval of the co-occurring infrequent items, resulting in an overall overestimation of the infrequent behaviors to the infrequent group. Participants' responses to evaluation judgments and frequency estimation will be based on the ease of retrieval of instances, which will largely be skewed to the co-occurring infrequent items.

CONCLUSION

In this chapter we have assessed the contributions of both relational and item-specific processing to several areas of investigation involving distinctiveness and memory prominent in the social literature. We believe application of this conceptual framework provides a level of integration among diverse findings in the literature and may provide novel insights or new extensions within each area. As a last example, we believe that applying the framework of item-specific and relational processing may help to clarify findings and unify disparate viewpoints among research examining the effects of relative group size on memory and judgment. This area is concerned with whether individuals presented as members of a relatively small group are remembered or judged differently from members of a balanced or large group (Taylor et al., 1978; Klauer, Wegener, & Ehrenberg, 2002; Oakes & Turner, 1986). The current dispute concerns whether such individuals are particularly likely to be subject to categorization (which roughly corresponds to relational processing) or individualization (which roughly corresponds to item-specific processing). Much existing social psychological theory views these two states as endpoints of a single continuum (see Smith & DeCoster, 2000, for an exception). When viewed in terms of item-specific and relational processing, it becomes clear that infrequent or minority members may receive (depending on the context) both increased individuation *and* increased categorization, and that different memory and judgment measures may tap information that is encoded by these different processes.

We began this chapter by reviewing differences between social and cognitive psychology in the treatment of distinctiveness and memory. We suspect many of these differences can be understood and explained by identifying how each impacts item-specific and relational processing. For instance, self-categorization may produce many of its effects through strategic shifts in the way the material is processed (e.g., information about ingroup members who behave well may encourage relational processing whereas information about ingroup members who behave poorly may encourage item-specific processing). If so, many areas in the social domain may benefit from consideration of how item-specific and relational processing contribute to phenomena. Likewise, the social literature may serve as a rich resource for those in the cognitive field who are interested in understanding how factors such as affect, motivation, associated stimuli, and self involvement impact item-specific and relational processing.

ACKNOWLEDGMENTS

Portions of this paper were presented at the 49th Annual Meeting of the Southwestern Psychological Association, New Orleans, LA, April 2003.

NOTES

1. One complication that arises in drawing parallels between the two paradigms is that the incongruency paradigm is itself quite varied, and often confounds several factors that may contribute to the effect. For instance, many studies reporting the incongruency effect use an approach similar to that of the isolation paradigm in the cognitive literature. That is, the incongruent items are defined relative to the immediate context. In other studies, however, the incongruency effect is examined by varying the typicality of the material in the stimulus set. In these studies, the incongruent items are those that are incongruent with previously established stereotypes or with trait expectations created before receiving the list of information. The ratio of congruent to incongruent items is held constant. The former constitutes what Schmidt (1991) refers to as primary distinctiveness and the later as secondary distinctiveness. The incongruency effect tends to be stronger in the latter case (Stangor & McMillan, 1992). Yet a third variant are studies in which the "distinctive" items are both rare in the immediate context and incongruent with previous experience. With these complications in mind we proceed.

2. However, incongruency effects have been found in studies in which incongruency was based on preexisting stereotypes or on trait expectancies describing the target prior to receiving the list of behaviors and in which the frequency of incongruent to congruent items in the stimulus set was the same (Dutta, Kanungo, & Friebergs, 1972; Kanungo & Das, 1960, Stangor & Ruble, 1989). In such cases, the incongruent items are different only with respect to a preexisting expectation. In such cases, it would seem difficult to empirically separate salience from difference.

REFERENCES

Bargh, J. A., & Thein, R. D. (1985). Individual construct accessibility, person memory, and the recall-judgment link: The case of information overload. *Journal of Personality and Social Psychology, 49,* 1129–1146.

Berndsen, M., Spears, R., & van der Plight, J. (1996). Illusory correlation and attitude-based vested interest. *European Journal of Social Psychology, 26,* 247–264.

Beirut, M., & Vescio, T. K. (1993). Categorization and stereotyping: Effects of group context on memory and social judgment. *Journal of Experimental Social Psychology, 29,* 166–202.

Bodenhausen, G. V., Kramer, G. P., & Susser, K. (1994) Happiness and stereotypic thinking in social judgment. *Journal of Personality and Social Psychology, 66,* 621–632.

Chapman, L. J. (1967). Illusory correlation in observational report. *Journal of Verbal Learning and Verbal Behavior, 6,* 151–144.

Cohen, R. M., Weingartner, H., Smallberg, S. A., Pickar, D., & Murphy, D. L. (1982). Effort and cognition in depression. Archives of General Psychiatry, 39, 593–597.

Dunlosky, J., Hunt, R. R., & Clark, E. (2000). Is perceptual salience needed in explanations of the isolation effect? *Journal of Experimental Psychology: Learning, Memory, and Cognition, 26,* 649–657.

Dutta, S., Kanungo, R. N., & Friebergs, V. (1972). Retention of affective material: Effects of affect on retrieval. *Journal of Personality and Social Psychology, 23,* 64–80.

Fiedler, K. (1991). The tricky nature of skewed frequency tables: An information loss account of distinctiveness-based illusory correlations. *Journal of Personality and Social Psychology, 60,* 24–36.

Fiedler, K., & Armbruster, T. (1994). Two halfs may be more than one whole: Category split effects on frequency illusions. *Journal of Personality and Social Psychology, 66,* 633–645.

Fiedler, K., Russer, S., & Gramm, K. (1993). Illusory correlations and memory performance. *Journal of Experimental Social Psychology, 29,* 111–136.

Fiske, S. T., Lin, M., & Neuberg, S. L. (1999). The continuum model, then years later. In S. Chaiken & Y. Trope (Eds.), *Dual process theories in social psychology* (pp. 231–254). New York: Guilford Press.

Garcia-Marques, L., & Hamilton, D. L., (1996). Resolving the apparent discrepancy between the incongruency effect and the expectancy based illusory correlation effect: The TRAP model. *Journal of Personality and Social Psychology, 71,* 845–860.

Garcia-Marques, L, Maddox, K. B., & Hamilton, D. L., (2002). Exhaustive and heuristic retrieval processes in person cognition: Further tests of the TRAP model. *Journal of Personality and Social Psychology, 82,* 193–207.

Hamilton, D. L. (1981). Illusory correlation as a basis for stereotyping. In D. L. Hamilton (Ed.), *Cognitive processes in stereotyping and intergroup behavior* (pp. 115–144). Hillsdale, NJ: Lawrence Erlbaum Associates.

Hamilton, D., Dugan, D., & Trolier, P. (1985). The formation of stereotypic beliefs: Further evidence for distinctiveness-based illusory correlations. *Journal of Personality and Social Psychology, 48,* 5–17.

Hamilton, D. L., & Gifford, R. K. (1976). Illusory correlation in interpersonal perception: A cognitive basis of stereotypic judgments. *Journal of Experimental Social Psychology, 12,* 392–407.

Hamilton, D. L., & Sherman, S. J. (1996). Perceiving persons and groups. *Psychological Review, 103,* 336–355.

Hastie, R. (1980). Memory for behavioral information that confirms or contradicts a personality impression. In R. Hastie, T. M. Ostrom, E. B. Ebbesen, R. S. Wyer, D. L. Hamilton, & D. E. Carlston (Eds.), *Person memory: The cognitive basis of social perception* (pp. 155–177). Hillsdale, NJ: Lawrence Erlbaum Associates.

Hastie, R. (1984). Causes and effects of causal attribution. *Journal of Personality and Social Psychology, 46,* 44–56.

Hastie, R., & Kumar, P. (1979). Person memory: Personality traits as organizing principles in memory for behaviors. *Journal of Personality and Social Psychology, 37,* 25–38.

Hastie, R., & Park, B. (1986). The relationship between memory and judgment depends on whether the judgment task is memory-based or on-line. *Psychological Review, 93,* 258–268

Higgins, E. T. (1996). Knowledge activation: accessibility, applicability, and salience. In E. T. Higgins & A. W. Kruglanski (Eds.), *Social psychology: Handbook of basic principles* (pp. 133–168). New York: Guilford Press.

Hintzman, D. L. (1986). "Schema abstraction" in a multiple-trace memory model. *Psychological Review, 93,* 411–28.

Hintzman, D. (1988). Judgments of frequency and recognition memory in a multiple-trace memory model. *Psychological Review, 95,* 528–551.

Hunt, R. R., & Einstein, G. O. (1981). Relational and item-specific information in memory. *Journal of Verbal Learning and Verbal Behavior, 20,* 497–514.

Hunt, R. R., & Lamb, C. A. (2001). What causes the isolation effect? *Journal of Experimental Psychology; Learning, Memory, and Cognition, 27,* 1359–1366.

Hunt, R. R., & McDaniel, M. A. (1993). Enigma of organization and distinctiveness. *Journal of Memory and Language, 32,* 421–445.

Johnson, C., & Mullen, B. (1994). Evidence for the accessibility of paired distinctiveness in distinctiveness-based illusory correlation in stereotyping. *Personality and Social Psychology Bulletin, 20,* 65–70.

Kanungo, R. N., & Das, J. P. (1960). Differential learning and forgetting as a function of the social frame of reference. *Journal of Abnormal and Social Psychology, 61,* 82–86.

Klauer, K. C., Wegener, I., & Ehrenberg, K. (2002). Perceiving minority members as individuals: Te effects of relative group size in social categorization. *European Journal of Social Psychology, 32,* 223–245.

Lord, C. G., & Saenz, D. S. (1985). Memory deficits and memory surfeits: Differential cognitive consequences of tokenism for tokens and observers. *Journal of Personality and Social Psychology. 49,* 918–926.

McConnell, A. R., Leibold, J., & Sherman, S. J. (1997). Within-target illusory correlations and the formation of context-dependent attitudes. *Journal of Personality and Social Psychology, 73,* 675–686.

McConnell, A. R., Sherman, S. J., & Hamilton, D. L. (1994a). On-line and memory based aspects of individual and group target judgments. *Journal of Personality and Social Psychology, 67,* 173–185.

McConnell, A. R., Sherman, S. J., & Hamilton, D. L. (1994b). Illusory correlation in the perception of groups: An extension of the distinctiveness-based account. *Journal of Personality and Social Psychology, 67,* 414–429.

McConnell, A. R., Sherman, S. J., & Hamilton, D. L. (1997). Target entitativity: Implications for information processing about individual and group targets. *Journal of Personality and Social Psychology, 72,* 750–762.

Mullen, B. (1991). Group composition, salience, and cognitive representations: The phenomenology of being in a group. *Journal of Experimental Social Psychology, 27,* 297–323.

Mullen, B., Brown, R., & Smith, C. (1992). Ingroup bias as a function of salience, relevance, and status: An integration. *European Journal of Social Psychology, 22,* 103–122.

Mullen, B., & Johnson, C. (1990). Distinctiveness based illusory correlations and stereotyping: A metaanalytic integration. *British Journal of Social Psychology, 29,* 11–28.

Nichols, D. R., Abrams, D., & Mullen, B. (2000). *Effects of gender composition in groups. I: An integration of the group discussion paradigm.* Presented at the 1st annual meeting of SPSP, Nashville, TN.

Oakes, P. J., & Turner, C. (1986). Distinctiveness and the salience of social category memberships: Is there a perceptual bias towards novelty? *European Journal of Social Psychology, 16,* 325–344.

Pryor, J. (1986). The influence of differential encoding sets upon the formation of illusory correlations and group impressions. *Personality and Social Psychology Bulletin, 12,* 216–226.

Rojahn, L., & Pettigrew, T. F. (1992). Memory for schema-relevant information: A meta-analytic resolution. *British Journal of Social Psychology, 31,* 81–110.

Sanbonmatsu, D. M., Sherman, S. J., & Hamilton, D. L. (1987). Illusory correlation in the perception of individuals and groups. *Social Cognition, 5,* 1–25.

Schmidt, S. R. (1991). Can we have a distinctiveness theory of memory? *Memory and Cognition, 19,* 523–542.

Shaller, M. (1991). Social categorization and the formation of group stereotypes: Further evidence for biased information processing in the perception of group-behavior correlations. *European Journal of Social Psychology, 21,* 25–35.

Shaller, M., & Maass, A. (1989). Illusory correlation and social categorization: toward an integration of motivational and cognitive factors in stereotype formation. *Journal of Personality and Social Psychology, 56,* 709–721.

Sherman, J. W., & Hamilton, D. L. (1994). On the formation of inter-item associative links in person memory. *Journal of Experimental Social Psychology, 30*, 203–217.

Sinclair, R. C., & Mark, M. M. (1995). The effects of mood state on judgmental accuracy: Processing strategy as a mechanism. *Cognition and Emotion, 9*, 417–438.

Smith, E. R. (1991). Illusory correlation in a simulated exemplar-based memory. *Journal of Experimental Social Psychology, 27*, 107–123.

Smith, E. R., & DeCoster, J. (2000). Dual-process models in social and cognitive psychology: Conceptual integration and links to underlying memory systems. *Personality and Social Psychological Review, 4*, 108–131.

Spears, R., & Haslam, S. A. (1997). Stereotyping and the burden of cognitive load. In R. Spears, P. J. Oakes, N. Ellemers, & S. A. Haslam (Eds.), *The social psychology of stereotyping and group life* (pp. 171–207). Oxford, UK: Blackwell.

Spears, R., van der Plight, J., & Eiser, J. R. (1985). Illusory correlation in the perception of group attitudes. *Journal of Personality and Social Psychology, 48*, 863–875.

Srull, T. K. (1981). Person memory: Some tests of associative storage and retrieval models. *Journal of Experimental Psychology: Human Learning and Memory, 7*, 440–463.

Srull, T. K., Lichtenstein, M., & Rothbart, M. (1985). Associative storage and retrieval processes in person memory. *Journal of Experimental Psychology: Learning Memory and Cognition, 11*, 316–345.

Srull, T. K., & Wyer, R. S. (1989). Person memory and judgment. *Psychological Review, 96*, 58–83.

Stangor, C., & McMillan, D. (1992). Memory for expectancy-congruent and expectancy incongruent information. A review of the social and developmental literatures. *Psychological Bulletin, 111*, 42–61.

Stangor, C., & Ruble, D. N. (1989). Differntial effects of gender schemas and gender constancy on children's information processing and behavior. *Social Cognition, 7*, 353–372.

Stroessner, S., & Plaks, J. (2001). Illusory correlation and stereotype formation: Tracing the area of research over a quarter century. In G. Moskowitz (Ed.), *Cognitive Social Psychology: The Princeton symposium on the legacy and future of social cognition* (pp. 247–259). Mahwah, NJ: Lawrence Erlbaum.

Stroessner, S, J., Hamilton, D. L., & Mackie, D. M. (1992). Affect and stereotyping: The effect of induced mood on distinctiveness-based illusory correlations. *Journal of Personality and Social Psychology, 62*, 564–576.

Stroessner, S. J., & Mackie, D. M. (1992). The impact of induced affect on the perception of variability in social groups. *Personality and Social Psychology Bulletin, 18*, 546–554.

Taylor, S. E., Fiske, S. T., Etcoff, N. L., & Ruderman, A. (1978). Categorical bases of person memory and stereotyping. *Journal of Personality and Social Psychology, 36*, 778–793.

Tversky, A., & Kahneman, D. (1973). Availability: A heuristic for judging frequency and probability. *Cognitive Psychology, 5*, 207–232.

Worthen, J. B., & Loveland, J. M. (2003). Disruptive effects of bizarreness in free and cued recall for self-performed and other-performed acts: The costs of item-specific processing. In S. P. Shohov (Ed.), *Advances in psychology research* (Vol. 24, pp. 3–16). Hauppauge, NY: Nova Science Publishers.

Wyer. R. S., & Srull, T. K. (1989). *Memory and cognition in its social context*. Hillsdale, NJ: Lawrence Erlbaum Associates.

VI

THE NEUROSCIENCE OF DISTINCTIVENESS AND MEMORY

15

Multiple Electrophysiological
Indices of Distinctiveness

Monica Fabiani

Several types of distinctiveness are typically identified in the literature (Schmidt, 1991). Among them, *primary distinctiveness* refers to the fact that some events come to stand out by virtue of the context in which they are embedded, whereas *secondary distinctiveness* refers to events that violate our expectancies based on our general world knowledge, rather than on their immediate context. In either case, distinctiveness is not necessarily an attribute that the event possesses, but the result of processes that allow for the event to be differentiated from its immediate or more general context (see also Hunt, Chapter 1 this volume, for a similar approach). Within this framework, I will refer to an additional concept—that of *subjective distinctiveness* (Donchin & Fabiani, 1991). By and large, experimental manipulations of the context in which stimuli are embedded are effective in making them stand out in the eyes of the participants. However, there will be variability in this phenomenon across subjects and across trials for any given subject. These variations could be explained, at least in part, by variability in the "comparator" processes that take place, which depend on each individual subject's previous experience and current brain state, as well as on the specific environmental conditions in which particular data are collected. In other words, distinctiveness may be conceived as the result of the interaction between the stimulus (within its context) and the subject's processing.

In this chapter I will review data from event-related brain potential studies (ERPs; Fabiani, Gratton, & Coles, 2000). These data are based largely on paradigms manipulating primary distinctiveness, and are sometimes collected for the explicit purpose of assessing the memory consequences of this manipulation (and their relationship to the underlying brain activity). More often, however, distinctiveness manipulations are used for the purpose of investigating how the brain responds to events that stand out. From these data, inferences are made about various aspects of cognition, including sensory and working memory, whereas the explicit longer term memory consequences of these manipulations are not tested (and are often not easily testable).

This review is not meant to be exhaustive, but is intended to illustrate how, at the neural level, the processing of distinctive events is underlined by multiple phenomena, each of which may contribute, directly or indirectly, to the enhanced memory performance that often accompanies distinctive events. In other words, it is important to remember that the relationship between a broad and multiply defined psychological construct, such as distinctiveness, and a particular aspect of brain activity is unlikely to be completely characterized by a one-to-one mapping.

For reasons of space and focus, I am restricting this review to studies in which ERPs are recorded during encoding (when events are first presented or studied) within paradigms in which distinctiveness (most often primary distinctiveness) is manipulated. It is clear, however, that some of the processes that may in the end contribute to enhanced memory performance may occur during the rehearsal or retrieval of the events.[1]

Sensory Brain Responses to Events That "Stand Out"

The human central nervous system is tuned to process differences rather than regularities, starting with the earliest stages of sensory processing. This is reflected in the occurrence of inhibitory processes that enhance our perception of borders and edges (Gilbert, Hirsch, & Wiesel, 1990) and by the rapid habituation of neurons to repeated stimulation, which may be at the basis of many perceptual priming effects (Reber, Gitelman, Parrish, & Mesulam, 2003; Reber, Stark, & Squire, 1998). This processing bias may have an inherent ecological validity, as changes in the environment may signal potentially dangerous situations and should therefore be processed.

In psychophysiology, research on components of the orienting reflex (OR; Sokolov, 1963; Sokolov & Vinogradova, 1975; Donchin, Fabiani, Packer, & Siddle, 1991; Siddle & Packer, 1991) has intersected since the 1970s with cognitive research on the consequences of processing rare, novel, or distinctive information (Donchin & Fabiani, 1991; Donchin, 1981; Donchin & Coles, 1988a, 1988b). Two short-latency ERP components provide examples of this early processing level, the N1 (or N100; e.g., Hillyard, Vogel, & Luck, 1998) and the mismatch negativity (MMN; Ritter, Deacon, Gomes, Javitt, & Vaughan, 1995).

The auditory N100 is elicited by any stimulus that reaches the auditory threshold of the individual; it is negative in polarity and peaks approximately 100 milliseconds from stimulus onset (hence its name; Näätänen, 1988; Näätänen & Picton, 1987; Woods, 1995). Dipole analyses of ERP (e.g., Scherg, Vajsar, & Picton, 1989) and magnetoencephalographic data (e.g., McEvoy, Levanen & Loveless, 1997), as well as optical data (Rinne et al., 1999), indicate that it originates, at least in part, in the auditory cortex. The amplitude of this component is modulated by selective attention, as the auditory N100 is larger for attended than for unattended channels (Hillyard, Hink, Schwent, & Picton, 1973). Similarly, the N100/P150 complex in the visual domain is generated in visual cortex (Di Russo, Martinez, Sereno, Pitzalis, & Hillyard, 2002; Martinez et al., 1999; Shigeto, Tobimatsu, Yamamoto, Kobayashi, & Kato, 1998) and its amplitude is also modulated by attention. Although both of these brain responses are by and large elicited in an "obligatory" fashion (i.e., whenever sensory information is processed by the appropriate cortical sensory system), some of the factors that affect them are relevant to the present discussion on brain markers of distinctiveness.

First, the auditory N100 does diminish in amplitude with repetition (Woods & Elmasian, 1986; Budd, Barry, Gordon, Rennie, & Michie, 1998; see also Näätänen, 1992). This decrease has specific temporal properties, in that it is maximal when the interval between stimuli is 400 milliseconds. Recent research from our laboratory (Sable et al., 2004) indicates that this decrease is not due to neuronal refractoriness after stimulation, but to other, possibly inhibitory, mechanisms that take approximately 400 milliseconds to reach their full capacity. Changes in the stimulus being presented appear to cause immediate recovery of the N100 amplitude (e.g., Woods & Elmasian, 1986; for a review see Näätänen, 1992, chapter 4), suggesting that distinctive items (i.e., items that are different and occur rarely within the context) will trigger the release from the underlying inhibitory mechanisms.[2] Although the relationship between the auditory N100 and subsequent memory has not been explicitly tested, some additional pieces of evidence suggest that a relationship—albeit indirect—may exist. In fact, whereas in young adults the N100 quickly attenuates with repeated stimulations, in normal older adults it does so only to a smaller extent, suggesting that the normally occurring inhibitory mechanisms may not be working as efficiently with age (Golob, Miranda, Johnson, & Starr, 2001; Fabiani, Low, Wee, Sable & Gratton, 2005). This, in turn, suggests that, with aging, processing may be devoted to repeated information that should instead be ignored, presumably at the expenses of other more relevant processing that could be taking place instead. It is interesting to note that Cimbalo and Brink (1982) reported that the elderly do not show a von Restorff effect (i.e., a memory advantage for distinctive items; von Restorff, 1933) in a task in which young adults do.

Second, work recently completed in our laboratory (Brumback, Low, Gratton & Fabiani, 2004) indicates that young adults selected as having either high or low working-memory span based on the Operation-Span task (O-Span; Kane & Engle, 2000) show clear individual differences in their N100/P150 responses to simple auditory and visual stimuli. High-span subjects have larger N100/P150 amplitudes than low-span subjects, and measures of these components correctly classify individuals based on both span and fluid intelligence. These results suggest that these ERP components may index some elements of distinctiveness that are involved in early attention control. Further, they also suggests that early and seemingly sensory brain responses may have a profound influence on much more complex processes such as those involved in distinctiveness, working memory and fluid intelligence.

Another ERP component that may be relevant to this overview of the possible neural bases of distinctiveness is the MMN. The MMN is an auditory component (although seemingly analogous responses have been reported for the visual system; Fu, Fan, & Chen, 2003; Pazo-Alvarez, Cadaveira, & Amenedo, 2003; Gratton, Fabiani, Goodman-Wood, & De-Soto, 1998), with at least one generator in auditory cortex (see Alho, 1995; Ritter et al., 1995; Rinne et al., 1999). It is elicited by deviant and rare stimuli occurring within a series of repeated (standard) stimuli (*oddball paradigm*). In fact, the MMN component is obtained by subtracting the standard waveform from the deviant waveform. Unlike longer latency ERP components such as the P300[3] (see also the section on P300 and memory), the MMN can be elicited by any perceivable stimulus change even in the absence of attention (e.g., while the subject is passively listening to a sound series while engaged in some other task).

The MMN is considered an index of sensory memory, as its peak latency (approximately 200 milliseconds after stimulus onset) and other timing properties match reasonably well those estimated for echoic memory in the behavioral literature (see Cowan, 1984, 1987). To the extent that the MMN is elicited by potentially salient events that may have to be "transferred" into working memory for further processing, this component may index one of the shortest-latency steps in the processing stream following distinctive events. It is also interesting to note that the MMN is sensitive to both 'sensory" aspects of distinctiveness, such as those generated by any audible deviation in a stream of tones, and to "learned/experienced-based" aspects of distinctiveness. In fact, Näätänen et al. (1997) reported a study in which rare/deviant phonemes elicited enhanced MMN responses in the auditory cortex of the left hemisphere when they were prototypical to the subject's own language, with respect to when they were typical of another language.

SEMANTIC INCONGRUITY AND THE N400

An extensive review of the literature on incongruity, including a review of the N400, is provided in another chapter in this book (Michelon & Snyder, Chapter 16 this volume), so only a few key concepts will be reviewed here. The N400 (first described by Kutas & Hillyard, 1980; for reviews see Kutas & VanPetten, 1994; Fabiani et al., 2000) is elicited by words and pronounceable pseudowords (but not by nonwords that violate the rules of the language) presented in isolation, as well as within lists, sentences, and discourses. When unrelated words are presented within a list, the amplitudes of the N400s they elicit are inversely related to the words' frequencies in the language (Van Petten & Kutas, 1990; see also Van Petten & Kutas, 1991). The amplitude of N400 diminishes with word repetition and once a sentence context is established. When a sentence context is violated (e.g., such as in the sentence "I drink tea with cream and *socks*"), a large N400 is reinstated whose amplitude is inversely related to the subject's expectancy for the terminal word (*cloze probability*).

From this discussion, it appears that the N400, albeit occurring in response to linguistic stimuli, is governed by mechanisms similar to those modulating the sensory components described earlier, decreasing in amplitude as the eliciting stimuli become more regular and predictable within their context. According to this framework the N400 may in fact reflect some aspects of the processing of the "distinctiveness" of linguistic stimuli, as its decrease or absence may signal predictability. However, this may also indicate that the N400 is a better index of what is (not) *currently* in memory, rather than of what is likely to be in memory at a later time.

A few studies have investigated the relationship between the amplitude of the N400 elicited by words at encoding and subsequent memory performance (e.g., Neville, Kutas, Chesney, & Schmidt, 1986; Fabiani, & Donchin, 1995). The Neville et al. (1986) study (which used category-related sentences priming congruous and incongruous endings as stimuli) showed that the memory for semantically incongruous words was generally poor and was not predicted by the amplitude of the N400 when the words were first encoded. A study by Fabiani and Donchin (1995) used a von Restorff (or isolation) paradigm in which subjects were given lists of words to memorize. Within each list, all but one of the words (the semantic isolate) were members of the same semantic category. Semantic isolates were remembered better than the same words presented within a homogeneous context, but only when subjects performed a lexical decision task. These words also elicited a large N400, but the amplitude of this component did not distinguish between later recalled and not recalled words, whereas a P300, also elicited by the semantic isolates, did (see section on P300 and memory). Similar findings were obtained by Bartholow, Fabiani, Gratton, and Bettencourt (2001), who tested memory for incongruous words at the end of sentences with a cued-recall procedure and found that memory performance was close to zero for this group of words (see also section on violation of expectancies).

In summary, it appears that words that elicit a large N400 at encoding are often poorly recalled at test (but not always; see Fabiani & Donchin. 1995), thus suggesting an inverse relationship between N400 amplitude and subsequent memory performance. However, the *trial-by-trial* variability in N400 amplitude is not associated with later recall; rather, the presence of a large N400 may on average signal poor recall of the *group* of words that elicited it. In experiments in which memory enhancements to semantically incongruous words are found (e.g., Fabiani & Donchin, 1995), it is the amplitude of P300, rather than that of the N400, that predicts subsequent memory performance. This may suggest that it is not semantic distinctiveness per se that predicts recall, but rather some type of task- or context-dependent processing that may be associated with (or a consequence of) semantic distinctiveness.

These findings appear in contrast with behavioral research indicating better memory for bizarre sentences (e.g., McDaniel, Einstein, DeLosh, May, & Brady, 1995). However, other research indicates that both significance (e.g., Schmidt, 2002; Chapter 3 this volume) and bizarreness (Worthen & Wood, 2001; Worthen, Chapter 7 this volume) can have both facilitative and disruptive effects on memory. In addition, experiments in which N400s are recorded to incongruous words in sentences differ in many ways from apparently similar behavioral research, including the relative frequency of occurrence of the bizarre stimuli within the experimental context and the specific instructions given to the subjects. It is also possible that the examination of other memory indices, such as response bias and detail confusion, could help clarify the relationship between the N400, bizarreness, and memory.

VIOLATION OF EXPECTANCIES IN PERSON PERCEPTION AND RELATED MEMORY EFFECTS

An ERP paradigm that bears some similarities with those used to study semantic incongruity effects has been used in studies of person perception (Bartholow et al., 2001). In this paradigm, the subjects read paragraphs, each describing fictitious characters possessing a given trait, and then were presented with sentences describing behaviors of that person that were either consistent or inconsistent with that trait. For example, a fictitious woman named Efrin could be described as kind. In the sentences following the descriptive paragraph some of her behaviors were consistent with those exhibited by a kind person (e.g., "She gave her daughter a kiss"). Others were neutral (e.g., "She gave the conductor her ticket"), and a few were inconsistent (e.g., "She gave her dog a kick"). Finally, a few sentences were also semantically incongruous (e.g., "She brought home the moon"). Several interesting findings were obtained using this paradigm. First, behaviors that violated the subjects' expectancies about the fictitious person elicited a larger P300 than those conforming to expectations. Second, these same behaviors (and especially those that were negative) were remembered better than consistent behaviors in a follow up cued-recall test. This is consistent with the idea that out-of-character behaviors may be more distinctive than those that are expected. They also confirm previous research showing a negative bias under these conditions (*misanthropic memory effect*; Trafimow & Finlay, 2001; Ybarra, Schaberg, & Keiper, 1999; Ybarra & Stephan, 1996). In contrast, semantically incongruent endings, which elicited large N400s, were hardly recalled at all, also confirming results of previous research (Neville et al., 1986).

In a follow-up study using this paradigm (Bartholow, Pearson, Gratton, & Fabiani, 2003) it was hypothesized that alcohol intoxication might change the dynamics of person perception, including memorability. It was found that, just as in the Bartholow et al. (2001) study, behaviors that were inconsistent with the character presented earlier were recalled better. Under placebo conditions, inconsistent negative behaviors were recalled better than inconsistent positive behaviors, replicating the findings of Bartholow et al. (2001) and of previous research on the misanthropic memory effect. However, under alcohol intoxication, the reverse was true and participants remembered better inconsistent but positive behaviors.

From these studies, it appears that mood and social context may affect which type of distinctive information is processed and how, and that drugs such as alcohol may change these relationships. Further, it is useful to note that incongruous information within a person-perception context elicits a larger P300-like response (rather than reinstating a large N400). It could be hypothesized that this may reflect the fact that the context is set by the paragraph preceding each group of sentences, rather than by general knowledge. However, even violations of long-held stereotypes appear to elicit P300-like responses (Osterhout, Bersick, & McLaughlin, 1997; but see recent work on sentences relying on context set by the previous discourse: van Berkum, Zwitserlood, Hagoort, & Brown, 2003).

P300 AND MEMORY: STUDIES USING THE ISOLATION OR VON RESTORFF PARADIGM

The P300 (also called P3 or P3b) is an ERP component first described by Sutton, Braren, Zubin, and John (1965; for a review see Fabiani et al., 2000). It has a positive polarity and a peak latency of at least 300 milliseconds (hence its name). In experiments using words as stimuli, its peak latency often exceeds 600 milliseconds (thus peaking *after* the N400 in experiments where both components are elicited), and may even occur after a response choice is made (e.g., Kutas, McCarthy, & Donchin, 1977). The amplitude of P300 is inversely proportional to the probability of occurrence of a rare stimulus within a series of homogeneous stimuli (Duncan-Johnson & Donchin, 1977), and it is further modulated by local changes in the sequence when stimuli are equiprobable (Squires, Wickens, Squires, & Donchin, 1976; Brumback, 2005). For a P300 to be elicited, it is required that the stimuli be attended by the subject (unlike the MMN described earlier), and noticeable and attended changes within otherwise regular series (regardless of sensory modality) will all elicit a P300. Thus, oddball tasks in which a P300 is elicited typically require that subjects count or respond to the rare stimuli (or give a choice response to both classes of stimuli).

Donchin (1981; see also Donchin & Coles, 1988a, 1988b) proposed that the P300 may index a process of "context updating" whereby working memory is updated because of changes occurring in the environment, with the purpose of modifying behavior on future trials. For example, the amplitude of the P300 on trials in which an error occurs predicts reaction time slowing in subsequent trials (Donchin, Gratton, Dupree, & Coles, 1988).

From this brief overview, it is easy to note the similarity between the stimuli (and related paradigms) typically eliciting large P300s, and those used to study the effects of primary distinctiveness on memory. For example, in the isolation (or von Restorff) paradigm stimuli are usually rendered distinctive by making them rare within their context. Within this framework, it can be expected that the amplitude of P300 will clearly distinguish between isolated stimuli (distinctive and rare, therefore eliciting large P300s) and nonisolated stimuli (homogeneous and frequent, therefore eliciting small P300s). Further, and more interestingly, it can be hypothesized that the *trial-by-trial* variability of the P300 elicited by the *isolates* at *encoding* would predict *subsequent* recall. In other words, within a group of stimuli eliciting large P300s, it can be predicted that those that were later recalled would have elicited, at encoding, larger P300s than those that were not.[4] We tested these and other hypotheses in a series of studies in which P300 was elicited in the context of a von Restorff paradigm (Fabiani, Gratton, Chiarenza, & Donchin, 1990; Fabiani, Karis, & Donchin, 1986, 1990; Fabiani, & Donchin, 1995; Karis, Fabiani, & Donchin, 1984).

Karis et al. (1984) recorded ERPs to unrelated words grouped in lists of 15. Most of the lists contained a word, presented in one of the five middle-serial positions, which was written in either a smaller or larger font than the other words (isolate). A free recall followed each list, and at the end of the experiment subjects were debriefed about which strategies they had used to memorize the words. Several interesting findings came out of this study. First, a memory advantage for distinctive words was evident (as compared to nonisolated words in the same serial positions; the von Restorff, or isolation, effect), but only for subjects who had used rote mnemonic strategies to memorize the words. Subjects who used elaborative strategies (based on making up stories involving several words in each list) did not show any recall advantage for the isolated words. Accordingly, only for subjects who used rote strategies and had a memory advantage for the distinctive words did the amplitude of the encoding P300 predict subsequent recall. For those subjects who used elaborative strategies and recalled isolates and nonisolates equally well, the amplitude of P300 at encoding did not predict subsequent memory, but the amplitude of a longer latency frontal slow wave did.

These results suggest two critical points. First, the amplitude of the encoding P300 does not simply index individual differences in the amount of "attention" or "extra-processing" devoted to the distinctive items, which, in turn, will determine the subsequent memory outcome. In fact, subjects using rote and elaborative strategies had equally large P300s to the isolates, indicating that all of them processed the distinctive feature. However, the rehearsal processes following the P300 (some of which may be indexed by the slow-wave activity observed in the elaborators) determined whether or not the variance in P300 amplitude was predictive of subsequent memory.

Three additional follow-up studies were conducted to further corroborate these initial findings, and in particular the role of strategies in the P300/memory relationship, and in the memory for distinctive information. First, we considered that, when memory is tested incidentally, subjects are not likely to engage in elaboration in order to improve their memory performance. Therefore, under these conditions, differences in subjects' strategy should disappear, and the P300 elicited by distinctive items at encoding should predict subsequent memory in all subjects. To test this prediction, we (Fabiani et al., 1986) ran subjects in an "oddball" paradigm in which unique male and female names were used as stimuli. Names of one gender occurred rarely (20%) and subjects were asked to count either the rare or frequent names to ensure that they were processing the stimuli. At the end of the experiment subjects were unexpectedly administered a free-recall task and asked to remember as many names as they could. As predicted, under these conditions the encoding P300 was larger for recalled than not recalled names, and individual differences were not apparent.

Cimbalo, Nowak, and Soderstrom (1981) had reported that children had very large isolation effects. We hypothesized that this may be due to the fact that, spontaneously, children rely solely on rote rehearsal strategies (Bjorklund & Muir, 1987). Thus, as for the incidental memory study described above, the correlation between the amplitude of the P300 elicited by isolated items at encoding and their subsequent recall should be particularly evident in children. This is exactly what we found in a study in which ERPs were recorded in 10-year-old children in a von Restorff paradigm (Fabiani et al., 1990). Children spontaneously used only rote memorization strategies, and large memory advantages for isolated words, as well as a P300/memory relationship, were found in all subjects.

In a third study we tested more directly the hypothesis that the use of rote mnemonic strategies is critical for the occurrence of a von Restorff effect and a relationship between the encoding P300 and subsequent memory (Fabiani et al., 1990). In this study we directly manipulated strategy instructions *within* subjects and examined whether this manipulation was successful in inducing or eliminating a memory advantage for distinctive items and the P300/memory relationship. Subjects were run in an isolation paradigm identical to that used by Karis et al. (1984). However, in different sessions, they were given either rote or elaborative rehearsal strategy instructions. As predicted, this manipulation was effective in changing the memory outcome, as well as the relationship between the encoding processes indexed by the P300 and subsequent recall. Under rote rehearsal instructions, distinctive items were recalled better than other items, and the P300 they elicited predicted recall. In contrast, under elaborative rehearsal instructions, distinctive items were not recalled better than other items, and the P300 they elicited was not correlated with subsequent memory.

In a fourth study (Fabiani & Donchin, 1995), we examined whether the relationship between isolation, encoding P300, and recall was restricted to items isolated by means of changing some of their physical features (e.g., font size), or whether it extended to semantic distinctiveness (i.e., to items rendered distinctive by embedding them among other items from a different semantic category, such as the word *car* in the midst of flower names). Specifically, isolation was achieved by means of both physical (font size) and semantic (category membership) features; we also used two types of orienting tasks (lexical decision and physical decision). We found that people engaged in lexical decision had memory advantages for both types of distinctive items, whereas people engaged in the physical (shallow) task had only advantages for items made distinctive by changing their font size. The P300 (but not the N400) elicited at encoding predicted subsequent recall for both types of isolated items.

Taken together with the rest of the literature previously reviewed, these findings suggest that semantic isolation may in fact facilitate recall, but only under specific task (and perhaps context) conditions. Orienting tasks that facilitate item-specific processing may help memorization of semantically distinctive items because distinctiveness can be used as a cue for recall. However, when the orienting tasks facilitate relational processing, semantic distinctiveness may be deleterious for recall because subjects may rely heavily on the item-to-item relationships to aid retrieval. In other words, under conditions stressing relational processes, semantically distinctive items may be harder to integrate with other items because of their isolation. Note that, in the Fabiani and Donchin (1995) study, the encoding operations (which included an enhanced P300) facilitating the recall of semantically and physically distinctive items appeared to be similar, and largely based on item-specific processing. In this same study, Fabiani and Donchin also examined the positions in which isolates were written down during free recall. The results indicated that the isolated items were reported more often either at the beginning or at the end of the list of recalled words, suggesting the existence of organizational processes taking place either at retrieval or earlier (see Bruce & Gaines, 1976).

A study conducted by Otten and Donchin (2000) further investigated whether the P300/memory relationship is affected by the manner in which primary distinctiveness is induced. They manipulated the integrality between the stimuli to be memorized and the attributes that make them distinctive. Words were isolated either by varying their font size or by surrounding them with a frame at close or far distance. All isolated words, regardless of attribute, were recalled better than comparable nonisolated words. Further, words with distinctive font sizes (integral cues) elicited large P300s, whose amplitudes were predictive of subsequent recall. The frame attributes (nonintegral cues) elicited smaller P300s whose amplitudes were not correlated with subsequent recall. In these groups of words, however, recall was predicted by a longer latency slow-wave component.

In all the studies reviewed in this section it is apparent that whether or not the amplitude of P300 at encoding predicts subsequent recall depends on the interactions between the encoding processes indexed by the P300 and the rehearsal and retrieval conditions that follow. A large number of additional studies have found relationships between increased positive ERP responses elicited at encoding and subsequent memory (e.g., Otten & Rugg, 2001; Paller, McCarthy, & Wood, 1988; for reviews see Rugg, 1995; Paller, 2000). Most of these studies use paradigms that do not create primary distinctiveness conditions, and in which the ERP effects are usually interpreted as positivities, distinct from the P300 but partially overlapping with it (in cases where a P300 is elicited). Whether or not these ERP/memory effects are partly due to the processing of specific stimulus properties that may contribute to the trace distinctiveness of the stimuli (and thus to their likelihood of being later remembered) is unclear.

Brain Responses to Novel Stimuli and Their Effects on Memory

In the previous section I have reviewed studies in which distinctiveness was manipulated by making a task-relevant item stand out with respect to its context (e.g., the oddball and von Restorff paradigms). A variant of the oddball paradigm (the novelty oddball) introduces a third element into this picture. In this paradigm, in addition to standard (frequent) and rare (deviant) stimuli, some additional, rare, unexpected, and novel stimuli are introduced in the series. No instructions are associated with these stimuli, and subjects are reminded to ignore them and perform the regular oddball task (e.g., respond to rare target stimuli). In the auditory version of this paradigm (Knight, 1984, 1987), nontonal sounds (e.g., a dog bark) are randomly introduced into an oddball series of high- and low-pitched pure tones (see also Courchesne, Hillyard, & Galambos, 1975, for a visual version of the same task).

It is important to emphasize here that the tonal stimuli—even those that are infrequent—are repeated many times (sometime hundreds of times) in the course of an oddball study. The novel stimuli are typically not repeated and differ from each other in a number of ways, including pitch, easiness with which they can be named, and so on (Fabiani, Kazmerski, Cycowicz, & Friedman, 1996). Thus, as such, they are unpredictable and really stand out within the homogeneous context created by the tonal stimuli.

The novel and unexpected stimuli introduced in the series are hypothesized to induce an orienting response and grab the subjects' attention. With respect to the distinctiveness discussion relevant for this chapter, these stimuli also stand out with respect to the context created in the experiment and are therefore distinctive. In fact, as they differ from the rare but repeated target stimuli on a number of dimensions, they may be more salient and distinctive than the stimuli normally eliciting a P300. However, since they are not task relevant or associated with a response (just like the frequent stimuli), they may be processed to a lesser extent than the rare target stimuli. This generates a relatively unique situation with respect to primary distinctiveness paradigms, as task relevance and frequency of occurrence are dissociated.

Just like the rare items in a regular oddball paradigm, the novel items elicit a P300-like response, which, however, differs in various ways from that elicited by the rare/target stimuli. First, the latency of this component (often called P3a or novelty P3) is slightly shorter than that of the target-elicited P300. Second, the novelty P3 is larger at frontal electrodes, whereas the target P300 has a posterior maximum, which indicates that the neural generators of these two brain responses are at least partially different (for reviews see Friedman, Cycowicz, & Gaeta, 2001; Friedman, Kazmerski, & Fabiani, 1997; see also Comerchero & Polich, 1999; Goldstein, Spencer, & Donchin, 2002; Polich & Comerchero, 2003). Knight (1984) reported that the P3a/novelty P3 is eliminated in patients with frontal lobe lesions, whereas the posterior target P300 is maintained. These data suggest that the frontal lobes are likely to be an essential part of the neural circuitry underlying this component. Several investigators have proposed that the novelty P3 is a response to the attention-catching properties of novel stimuli and may be part of the orienting response.

Because frontal lobe function (as well as frontal lobe anatomy) is often affected by normal aging, recent research has focused on changes in the novelty P3 response in older adults (e.g., Fabiani & Friedman, 1995; Fabiani, Friedman, & Cheng, 1998; Friedman & Simpson, 1994; Friedman, Simpson, & Hamberger, 1993; Knight, 1987). A number of findings from these studies are relevant to the current discussion on the neural substrate of distinctiveness. First, older adults maintain a frontal P3a response to the novel stimuli much longer than young adults, in which this response habituates over time (Friedman & Simpson, 1994). This suggests that older adults may be more distracted by attention-grabbing but task-irrelevant information than young adults. Further, Fabiani and Friedman (1995) found that, in older adults, the P300 response to *target* (i.e., rare but repeated) stimuli had a frontal scalp distribution similar to the novelty P3a elicited by novel stimuli. In addition, older adults who exhibited a more pronounced frontal response to repeated *targets* were more impaired in tests of frontal lobe function, suggesting that the persistence of this response may be an index of frontal dysfunction (Fabiani et al., 1998).

These data have implications for the dynamics of distinctiveness-related processes over the life span, suggesting that older adults may devote additional processes to events that young adults can cease to orient to after a few repetitions. Fabiani and Friedman (1995) hypothesized that this lack of specificity of the frontal P3a response in aging may have consequences for the memory for the novel items. Consistent with this hypothesis, they found that older adults' performance in a recognition task following the oddball tasks was lower than for younger adults. However, this age-related recognition performance decrement could also be mediated by differences between younger and older adults in their sound naming abilities (Fabiani et al., 1996). In fact, when asked to name the novel sounds, young adults used specific names whenever feasible (e.g., *chicken*), whereas older adults often used more generic names (e.g., *bird*). This, in turn, could make individual items more confusable in a recognition test in which distractors from the same categories are used.

DISCUSSION

The data reported here are consistent with a model of the effects of distinctiveness on memory that stresses the interaction of at least three processing levels in determining the probability of successful memory (recall or recognition) of distinctive items: (1) encoding processes, (2) rehearsal strategies (when allowed), and (3) retrieval conditions. The use of ERP measures, and in particular of ERP components sensitive to primary distinctiveness, enables us to track encoding processes in some details. Specifically, the data indicate that, in conditions in which distinctiveness is manipulated by making stimuli stand out within their context, the P300 (or according to other authors, a less well defined positivity) is predictive of subsequent recall. Distinctiveness can be achieved through either physical, semantic, or, in principle, other forms of differentiation. However, the P300 is an "optional" ERP response, which may reflect the encoding of different stimulus dimensions, depending on task conditions. From the Fabiani and Donchin (1995) study, it appears that the relationship between P300 and subsequent recall for semantically deviant items holds only for conditions in which the orienting task involves semantic processing. Presumably this is because only under these conditions does the P300 reflect the encoding of semantic information.

As we have seen, other ERP components are sensitive to the items' distinctiveness. These include the N100 and MMN (for auditory stimuli), the N400 (for verbal stimuli) and the frontal P3/P3a. There is currently no evidence that trial-by-trial variability in the amplitude of these components predicts subsequent memory, at least directly. For the N400 there are a few studies indicating on average a reverse relationship, so that stimuli eliciting large N400s are, as a group, associated with low probability of recall. However, this overall effect is not reflected by a correlation with amplitude changes on a trial-by-trial basis. Indirect memory effects, possibly mediated by IQ or comprehension abilities, are of course possible, as the amplitude of N400 has been shown to be modulated by these factors in studies investigating brain activity in response to jokes (Coulson & Kutas, 2001) and metaphor processing (Kazmerski, Blasko, & Dessalegn, 2003).

There appears to be a substantial logical difference between components such as the N100 and the MMN and the target P300 in the context of processing distinctive information. Whereas the early sensory components (and possibly the N400) appear to be domain-specific, relatively automatic responses, the P300 is a more general and flexible brain response across different domains, so that it can reflect very different forms of stimulus dimensions. In this sense, P300 may reflect brain events that are more closely related to the concept of subjective distinctiveness. However, it is also the case that the paradigms, rehearsal, and retrieval conditions used in the studies reviewed above may be particularly appropriate for demonstrating a P300/memory relationship. By the same token, paradigms could be designed that could make the role of other ERP indices of distinctiveness more relevant to subsequent memory.

The studies reviewed in this chapter also highlight the role of rehearsal strategies in mediating the relationship between P300 and subsequent recall. This emphasizes the idea that successful and, in fact enhanced, recall may be achieved through multiple routes. For instance, an item may be retrieved more easily because its encoding conditions made it very distinctive. However, an item may also be easily retrieved because it is associated to many other items, making it more likely to be recalled if any of its associates is also recalled. Thus, under elaborative rehearsal conditions (i.e., conditions in which many relational connections are set up), the link between initial encoding distinctiveness (as indexed by the P300) and subsequent recall may become irrelevant. Interestingly, under these conditions, another ERP component (a frontal positive slow-wave) predicts recall. It could be hypothesized that this component represents an early index of the occurrence of elaborative rehearsal operations. An open—and perhaps difficult to address—question is whether the elaborative processes signaled by the frontal positive slow-wave may also be considered as yet another form of distinctiveness—namely, a trace distinctiveness resulting from being subjected to further and further processing.

In conclusion, studies of ERPs and distinctiveness indicate that this theoretical construct is central to the way our brain processes information and is represented by multiple indices. The data also highlight the fact that distinctiveness-related processes may occur at different levels, starting with short-latency sensory phenomena that are largely modality specific. These early processes, indexed by ERP components such as the N100 and the MMN, may signal that a given subsystem has processed a potentially relevant "change" either at a pre-attentive or early attentional level. Next, more general systems may intervene in the processing, such as those indexed by the N400, that may evaluate "change" at more symbolic/meaning-related levels. Finally, the system may use the relevant "changes" to alter goals and future behaviors, and some of these latter processes may be reflected by the P300 and its relationship to subsequent memory and possibly by some of the long-latency positivities and slow-wave components.

The relationship between a particular level of distinctiveness processing and subsequent memory may be greatly affected by the encoding, rehearsal and retrieval conditions, and by their interactions. This relationship, however, follows predictable patterns, which are largely determined by the degree of overlap that occurs between the distinctiveness dimensions generated at encoding and those emphasized during rehearsal and retrieval.

ACKNOWLEDGMENTS

I wish to acknowledge the support of NIA grant AG21887. I am also grateful to Kara Federmeier, Gabriele Gratton and Jeff Sable for their comments on an earlier draft of this chapter.

NOTES

1. An example of post-encoding processing is provided by the seminal work of Hedwig von Restorff (1933), from whom the von Restorff, or isolation, effect (the enhanced memory for events that stand out) takes its name. As a member of the Gestalt school, she was interested in demonstrating that figure-ground contrast could be obtained not only perceptually, but also at the "trace" (i.e., memory) level. To separate these two levels, in some of her experiments she presented distinctive ('isolated") events early on in a series. Thus, the item was encoded *before* any context against which the item could stand out was even established (e.g., compare the series A B C D E F G H I J with the "isolated" series A B A A A A A A A A). The enhanced recall of item B in the second list must be due to processes that occur after B itself is presented, for example when the subject categorizes and organizes the items in his/her mind.

2. Given the overlap between the N100 and the MMN, there is a possibility that the enhancement of the N100 seen after a stimulus change may be due in part to the occurrence of a MMN, rather than purely to a reinstatement of the N100.

3. As explained in more detail in the section on P300 and memory, the P300 is an ERP component commonly elicited by attended and task relevant stimuli. Its amplitude is inversely proportional to the stimulus probability within the context, hence its relevance to the concept of distinctiveness. Further, the amplitude of P300 at encoding is related to the subsequent memory for the eliciting item.

4. These analyses are done by tagging the waveform elicited by each individual word (recorded during study) on the basis on the outcome of the subsequent memory test. These subsequent-memory-tagged waveforms are then averaged into recalled and not-recalled bins, respectively. An alternative analysis is to sort the tagged encoding waveforms into quartiles, based

on the amplitude of the P300, and then calculate the percent recall associated with each quartile.

REFERENCES

Alho, K. (1995). Cerebral generators of the mismatch negativity (MMN) and its magnetic counterpart (MMNm) elicited by sound changes. *Ear and Hearing, 16,* 38–51

Bartholow, B., Fabiani, M., Gratton, G., & Bettencourt, A. (2001). A psychophysiological analysis of the processing time course of social expectancy violations. *Psychological Science, 12*(3), 197–204.

Bartholow, B. D., Pearson, M., Gratton, G. & Fabiani, M. (2003). Effects of alcohol on social information processing: A social cognitive neuroscience approach. *Journal of Personality and Social Psychology, 85*(4), 627–638.

Bjorklund, D. F., & Muir, J. E. (1987). Children's development of free recall memory: remembering on their own. In R. Vasta (Ed.), *Annals of Child Development* (Vol. 5, pp. 79–123) Greenwich, CT: JAI Press.

Brumback, C. R., Low, K. A., Gratton, G. & Fabiani, M. (2004). Sensory brain responses predict individual differences in working memory span and fluid intelligence. *NeuroReport, 15*(2), 373–376.

Brumback, C. R., Low, K., Gratton, G., & Fabiani, M. (2005). Putting things into perspective: Differences in working memory span and the integration of information. *Experimental Psychology, 52*(1), 21–30.

Bruce, D., & Gaines, M. T. (1976). Tests of an organizational hypothesis of isolation effects in free recall. *Journal of Verbal Learning and Verbal Behavior, 15,* 59–72.

Budd, T. W., Barry, R. J., Gordon, E., Rennie, C., Michie, P. T. (1998). Decrement of the N1 auditory event-related potential with stimulus repetition: Habituation vs. refractoriness. *International Journal of Psychophysiology, 31,* 51–68.

Cimbalo, R. S., & Brink, L. (1982). Aging and the von Restorff isolation effect in short/term memory. *The Journal of General Psychology, 106,* 69–76.

Cimbalo, R. S., Nowak, B. I., & Soderstrom, J. A. (1981). The isolation effect in children's short term memory. *Journal of General Psychology, 105,* 215–223.

Comerchero, M. D., & Polich J. (1999). P3a and P3b from typical auditory and visual stimuli. *Clinical Neurophysiology, 110*(1), 24–30.

Coulson, S., & Kutas, M. (2001). Getting it: human event-related brain response to jokes in good and poor comprehenders. *Neuroscience Letters, 316*(2), 71–74.

Courchesne, E., Hillyard, S.A., & Galambos, R. (1975). Stimulus novelty, task relevance, and the visual evoked potential in man. *Electroencephalography and clinical Neurophysiology, 39,* 131–143.

Cowan, N. (1984). On short and long auditory stores. *Psychological Bulletin, 96,* 341–370.

Cowan, N. (1987). Auditory sensory storage in relation to the growth of sensation and acoustic information extraction. *Journal of Experimental Psychology: Human Perception and Performance, 13,* 204–215.

Di Russo, F., Martinez, A., Sereno, M. I., Pitzalis, S., & Hillyard, S. A. (2002). Cortical sources of the early components of the visual evoked potential. *Human Brain Mapping, 15,* 95–111.

Donchin, E. (1981). Surprise! . . . Surprise? *Psychophysiology, 18,* 493–513.

Donchin, E., & Coles, M. G. H. (1988a). Is the P300 component a manifestation of context updating? *Behavioral and Brain Sciences, 11,* 355–372.

Donchin, E., & Coles, M. G. H. (1988b). On the conceptual foundations of cognitive psychophysiology: A reply to comments. *Behavioral and Brain Sciences, 11,* 406–417.

Donchin, E., & Fabiani, M. (1991). The use of event-related brain potentials in the study of memory: Is P300 a measure of event distinctiveness? In J. R. Jennings & M. G. H. Coles (Eds.), *Handbook of cognitive psychophysiology: Central and autonomic nervous system approaches* (pp.471–498). Chichester, UK: Wiley.

Donchin, E., Fabiani, M., Packer, J. S., & Siddle, D. A. T. (1991). Orienting, P300 and memory: Commentary. In J. R. Jennings & M. G. H. Coles (Eds.), *Handbook of cognitive psychophysiology: Central and autonomic nervous system approaches* (pp. 499–510). Chichester, UK: Wiley.

Donchin, E., Gratton, G., Dupree, D., & Coles, M. G. H. (1988). After a rash action: Latency and amplitude of the P300 following fast guesses. In G. Galbraith, M. Klietzman, & E. Donchin (Eds.), *Neurophysiology and psychophysiology: Experimental and clinical applications* (pp. 173–188). Hillsdale, NJ: Lawrence Erlbaum Associates.

Duncan-Johnson, C. C., & Donchin, E. (1977). On quantifying surprise: The variation of event-related potentials with subjective probability. *Psychophysiology, 14,* 456–467.

Fabiani, M., & Donchin, E. (1995). Encoding processes and memory organization: A model of the von Restorff effect. *Journal of Experimental Psychology: Learning, Memory and Cognition, 21*(1), 224–240.

Fabiani, M., & Friedman, D. (1995). Changes in brain activity patterns in aging: The novelty oddball. *Psychophysiology, 32,* 579–594.

Fabiani, M., Friedman, D., & Cheng, J. C. (1998). Individual differences in P3 scalp distribution in older adults, and their relationship to frontal lobe function. *Psychophysiology, 35,* 698–708.

Fabiani, M., Gratton, G., & Coles, M. G. H. (2000). Event-related brain potentials: Methods, theory and applications. In J. Cacioppo, L. Tassinary, & G. Berntson (Eds.), *Handbook of psychophysiology* (pp. 53–84). New York: Cambridge University Press.

Fabiani, M., Gratton, G., Chiarenza, G. A., & Donchin, E. (1990). A psychophysiological investigation of the von Restorff paradigm in children. *Journal of Psychophysiology, 4,* 15–24.

Fabiani, M., Gratton, G., Karis, D., & Donchin, E. (1987). The definition, identification, and reliability of measurement of the P300 component of the event related brain potential. In P. K. Ackles, J. R. Jennings, & M. G. H. Coles (Eds.), *Advances in psychophysiology* (pp. 1–78). Greenwich, CT: JAI Press.

Fabiani, M., Karis, D., & Donchin, E. (1986). P300 and recall in an incidental memory paradigm. *Psychophysiology, 23,* 298–308.

Fabiani, M., Karis, D., & Donchin, E. (1990). Effects of strategy manipulation in a von Restorff paradigm. *Electroencephalography and Clinical Neurophysiology, 75,* 22–35.

Fabiani, M., Kazmerski, V. A., Cycowicz, Y., & Friedman, D. (1996). Naming norms for brief environmental sounds: Effects of age and dementia. *Psychophysiology, 33,* 462–475.

Fabiani, M., Low, K. A., Wee, E., Sable, J. J., & Gratton, G. (revision submitted). Reduced suppression or labile memory? Mechanisms of inefficient filtering of irrelevant information in older adults. *Manuscript submitted for publication.*

Friedman D., Cycowicz, Y. M., & Gaeta, H. (2001). The novelty P3: an event-related brain potential (ERP) sign of the brain's evaluation of novelty. *Neuroscience Biobehavioral Reviews, 25*(4), 355–373.

Friedman, D., Kazmerski, V., & Fabiani, M. (1997). An overview of age-related changes in the scalp distribution of P3b. *Electroencephalography and Clinical Neurophysiology, 104,* 498–513.

Friedman, D., & Simpson, G. (1994). ERP Amplitude and scalp distribution to target and novel events: Effects of temporal order in young, middle-aged and older adults. *Cognitive Brain Research, 2,* 49–63.

Friedman, D., Simpson, G., & Hamberger, M. (1993). Age-related changes in scalp topography to novel and target stimuli. *Psychophysiology, 30,* 383–396.

Fu, S., Fan, S., & Chen, L. (2003). Event-related potentials reveal involuntary processing of orientation changes in the visual modality. *Psychophysiology, 40,* 770–775.

Gilbert, C. D., Hirsch, J. A., & Wiesel, T. N. (1990). Lateral interactions in visual cortex, *Cold Spring Harbor Symposia on Quantitative Biology, 55,* 663–677.

Goldstein, A., Spencer, K. M., & Donchin, E. (2002). The influence of stimulus deviance and novelty on the P300 and novelty P3. *Psychophysiology, 39*(6), 781–790.

Golob, E. J., Miranda, G. G., Johnson, J. K., & Starr, A. (2001). Sensory cortical interactions in aging, mild cognitive impairment, and Alzheimer's disease. *Neurobiology of Aging, 22,* 755–763.

Gratton, G., Fabiani, M., Goodman-Wood, M. R., & DeSoto, M. C. (1998). Memory-driven processing in human medial occipital cortex: An event-related optical signal (EROS) study. *Psychophysiology, 35,* 348–351.

Hillyard, S. A., Hink, R. F., Schwent, V. L., & Picton, T. W. (1973). Electrical signs of selective attention in the human brain. *Science, 182,* 177–180.

Hillyard, S. A., Vogel, E. K., & Luck, S. J. (1998). Sensory gain control (amplification) as a mechanism of selective attention: electrophysiological and neuroimaging evidence. *Philosophical Transactions of the Royal Society of London: Biology, 353*, 1257–1270.

Kane, M., & Engle. (2000). Working memory capacity, proactive interference, and divided attention: Limits on long-term memory retrieval. *Journal of Experimental Psychology: Learning, Memory, and Cognition, 26*(2), 336–358.

Karis, D., Fabiani, M., & Donchin, E. (1984). "P300" and memory: Individual differences in the von Restorff effect. *Cognitive Psychology, 16*, 177–216.

Kazmerski, V. A., Blasko, D. G., & Dessalegn, B. G. (2003). ERP and behavioral evidence of individual differences in metaphor comprehension. *Memory & Cognition, 31*(5), 673–689.

Knight, R. T. (1984). Decreased response to novel stimuli after prefrontal lesions in man. *Electroencephalography and Clinical Neurophysiology, 59*, 9–20.

Knight, R. T. (1987). Aging decreases auditory event-related potentials to unexpected stimuli in humans. *Neurobiology of Aging, 8*, 109–113.

Kutas, M., & Hillyard, S. A. (1980). Reading senseless sentences: Brain potentials reflect semantic incongruity. *Science, 207*, 203–205.

Kutas, M., McCarthy, G., & Donchin, E. (1977). Augmenting mental chronometry: The P300 as a measure of stimulus evaluation time. *Science, 197*, 792–795.

Kutas, M., & VanPetten, C. (1994). Psycholinguistics electrified: event-related brain potential investigations. In M. A. Gernsbacher (Ed.), *Handbook of psycholinguistics* (pp. 83–143). San Diego: Academic Press.

Lattner, S., & Friederici, A. D. (2003). Talker's voice and gender stereotype in human auditory sentence processing—evidence from event-related brain potentials. *Neuroscience Letters, 27, 339*(3), 191–194.

Martinez, A., Anllo-Vento, L., Sereno, M. I, Frank, L. R., Buxton, R. B., Dubowitz, D. J., Wong, E. C., Hinrichs, H., Heinze, H. J., & Hillyard, S. A. (1999). Involvement of striate and extrastriate visual cortical areas in spatial attention. *Nature Neuroscience, 2*, 364–369.

McDaniel, M. A., Einstein, G. O., DeLosh, E. L., May, C. P., & Brady, P. (1995). The bizarreness effect: It's not surprising, it's complex. *Journal of Experimental Psychology: Learning, Memory, and Cognition, 21*, 422–435.

McEvoy, L., Levanen, S., & Loveless, N. (1997). Temporal characteristics of auditory sensory memory: neuromagnetic evidence. *Psychophysiology, 34*, 308–316.

Näätänen, R. (1988). Implications of ERP data for psychological theories of attention. *Biological Psychology, 26*(1-3), 117–163.

Näätänen, R. (1992). *Attention and brain function.* Hillsdale, NJ: Lawrence Erlbaum Associates.

Näätänen, R., Lehtokoski, A., Lennes, M., Cheour, M., Huotilainen, M., Iivonen, A., Vainio, M., Alku, P., Ilmoniemi, R. J., Luuk, A., Allik, J., Sinkkonen, J., & Alho, K. (1997). Language-specific phoneme representations revealed by electric and magnetic brain responses. *Nature, 385(6615)*, 432–434.

Näätänen, R., & Picton, T. (1987). The N1 wave of the human electric and magnetic response to sound: A review and an analysis of the component structure. *Psychophysiology, 24, 375–425.*

Neville, H. J., Kutas, M., Chesney, G., & Schmidt, A. L. (1986). Event-related brain potentials during initial encoding and recognition memory of congruous and incongruous words. *Journal of Memory and Language, 25,* 75–92.

Osterhout, L., Bersick, M., & McLaughlin, J. (1997) Brain potentials reflect violations of gender stereotypes. *Memory & Cognition. 25(3),* 273–285.

Otten, L. J., & Donchin E. (2000). Relationship between P300 amplitude and subsequent recall for distinctive events: dependence on type of distinctiveness attribute. *Psychophysiology, 37(5),* 644–661.

Otten, L. J., & Rugg, M. D. (2001). Electrophysiological correlates of memory encoding are task-dependent. *Cognitive Brain Research, 12(1),* 11–18.

Paller, K. A. (2000). Neural measures of conscious and unconscious memory. *Behavioral Neurology, 12(3),* 127–141.

Paller, K. A., McCarthy G., & Wood, C. C. (1988). ERPs predictive of subsequent recall and recognition performance. *Biological Psychology, 26(1-3),* 269–276.

Pazo-Alvarez, P., Cadaveira, F, & Amenedo, E. (2003). MMN in the visual modality: a review. *Biological Psychology, 63(3),* 199–236.

Polich, J., & Comerchero, M. D. (2003). P3a from visual stimuli: typicality, task, and topography. *Brain Topography, 15(3),* 141–152.

Reber, P. J., Gitelman, D. R., Parrish, T. B., & Mesulam, M. M. (2003). Dissociating explicit and implicit category knowledge with fMRI. *Journal of Cognitive Neuroscience, 15(4),* 574–583.

Reber, P. J., Stark, C. E., & Squire, L. R. (1998). Contrasting cortical activity associated with category memory and recognition memory. *Learning & Memory, 5(6),* 420–428.

Rinne, T., Gratton, G., Fabiani, M., Cowan, N., Maclin, E., Stinard, A., Sinkkonen, J., Alho, K., & Näätänen, R. (1999). Scalp-recorded optical signals make sound processing from the auditory cortex visible. *NeuroImage, 10,* 620–624.

Ritter, W., Deacon, D., Gomes, H., Javitt, D. C., & Vaughan, H. G., Jr. (1995). The mismatch negativity of event-related potentials as a probe of transient auditory memory: A review. *Ear and Hearing, 16,* 52–67.

Rugg, M. D. (1995). ERP studies of memory. In M. D. Rugg & M. G. H. Coles (Eds.), *Electrophysiology of mind* (pp. 132–170). Oxford, UK: Oxford University Press.

Sable, J. J., Low, K. A., Maclin, E. L., Fabiani, M., & Gratton, G. (2004). Latent inhibition mediates N1 attenuation to repeating sounds. *Psychophysiology, 41*, 636–642.

Scherg, M., Vajsar, J., & Picton, T. W. (1989). A source analysis of the human auditory evoked potential *Journal of Cognitive Neuroscience, 1*, 336–355.

Schmidt, S. R. (1991). Can we have a distinctive theory of memory? *Memory & Cognition, 19*(6), 523–542.

Schmidt, S. R. (2002). Outstanding memories: The positive and negative effects of nudes on memory. *Journal of Experimental Psychology: Learning, Memory, & Cognition, 28*(2), 353–361.

Siddle, D. A. T., & Packer, J. S. (1991). Memory and autonomic activity: The role of the orienting response. In J. R. Jennings, & M. G. H. Coles (Eds.), *Handbook of cognitive psychophysiology: Central and autonomic nervous system approaches*. Chichester, UK: Wiley.

Shigeto, H., Tobimatsu, S., Yamamoto, T., Kobayashi, T., & Kato, M. J. (1998). Visual evoked cortical magnetic responses to checkerboard pattern reversal stimulation: a study on the neural generators of N75, P100 and N145. *Neurol. Sci., 156*, 186–194.

Sokolov, E. N. (1963). *Perception and the conditioned reflex*. New York: Macmillan.

Sokolov, E. N., & Vinogradova, O. S. (1975). *Neuronal mechanisms of the orienting reflex*. Hillsdale, NJ: Lawrence Erlbaum Associates.

Squires, K. C., Wickens, C., Squires, N. K., & Donchin, E. (1976). The effect of stimulus sequence on the waveform of the cortical event-related potential. *Science, 193*, 1142–1146.

Sutton, S., Braren, M., Zubin, J., & John, E. R. (1965). Evoked potential correlates of stimulus uncertainty. *Science, 150*, 1187–1188.

Trafimow, D., & Finlay, K. A. (2001). An investigation of three models of multitrait representations. *Personality and Social Psychology Bulletin, 27*, 226–241.

van Berkum, J. J., Zwitserlood, P., Hagoort, P., & Brown, C. M. (2003). When and how do listeners relate a sentence to the wider discourse? Evidence from the N400 effect. *Cognitive Brain Research, 17*(3), 701–718.

Van Petten, C., & Kutas, M. (1990). Interactions between sentence context and word frequency in event-related brain potentials. *Memory & Cognition, 18*(4), 380–393.

Van Petten, C., & Kutas, M. (1991). Influences of semantic and syntactic context on open- and closed-class words. *Memory & Cognition, 19*(1), 95–112.

Von Restorff, H. (1933). Uber die Wirkung von Bereichsbildungen im Spurenfeld. *Psychologische Forschung, 18*, 299–342.

Woods, D. L. (1995). The component structure of the N1 wave of the human auditory evoked potential. *Electroencephalography and Clinical Neurophysiology, 44*(Suppl.), 102–109.

Woods, D. L., & Elmasian, R. (1986). The habituation of event-related potentials to speech sounds and tones. *Electroencephalography & Clinical Neurophysiology, 65*(6), 447–459.

Ybarra, O., Schaberg, L., & Keiper, S. (1999). Favorable and unfavorable target expectancies and social information processing. *Journal of Personality and Social Psychology, 77,* 698–709.

Ybarra, O., & Stephan, W. G. (1996). Misanthropic person memory. *Journal of Personality and Social Psychology, 70,* 691–700.

Worthen, J. B, & Wood, V. V. (2001). A disruptive effect of bizarreness on memory for relational and contextual details of self-performed and other-performed acts. *American Journal of Psychology, 114*(4), 535–546.

16

Neural Correlates of Incongruity

PASCALE MICHELON AND ABRAHAM Z. SNYDER

Most of the objects in our environment are familiar and expected in a given situation. When you go to the gas station you usually see cars, gas pumps, and people, all these being very well known, contextually expected entities. Sometimes, however, you may notice a vehicle because of some specific property: it happens that one is orange while all the other cars are white. Or you may notice a customer because of his behavior: a man is trying to put quarters into the gas pump. It is likely that you will remember both the orange car and the man's odd behavior. A mnemonic advantage can be attributed to the distinctiveness of perceived events.

Two types of distinctiveness can be distinguished: primary and secondary distinctiveness (Schmidt, 1991). Primary distinctiveness is due to item contrast with respect to the surroundings. In our example, the orange car is distinct because all other cars are white. The likelihood that an item will be remembered increases as the number of properties shared with its contextual neighbors decreases (Hunt, 1995; Schmidt, 1991). If the orange car were among other orange cars or simply among other colored cars it would lose distinctiveness. Secondary distinctiveness is generated by violation of expectations about the world. In our example, the man's behavior is distinct because one knows that quarters are used in meters but not in gas pumps. In this chapter we will focus on secondary distinctiveness, which we suggest underlies the subjective percept of bizarreness or incongruity. The neural correlates of the encoding of incongruous information will be explored in an attempt to understand why it is better remembered.

INCONGRUITY: EFFECTS ON MEMORY

Multiple behavioral studies have shown a memory advantage for incongruous versus ordinary material. This result is commonly known as the *bizarreness effect*. Previous work has established that semantically incongruous sentences (e.g., "The soldier licked the kittens") are better recalled than ordinary sentences (e.g., "The man read a book"; Cornoldi, Cavedon, De Beni, & Pra Baldi, 1988; Engelkamp, Zimmer,& Biegelmann, 1993; Hirshman, Whelley, & Palij, 1989; McDaniel & Einstein, 1986; Nicolas & Marchal, 1996; Riefer & Rouder, 1992; Worthen & Marshall, 1996). Incongruity in these studies typically is induced by violating semantic consistency—for example, by attributing human actions to animals and artifacts or vice versa. Subjects typically are asked to read incongruous and ordinary sentences with attention to semantic content. A memory advantage on subsequent testing for incongruous material has so far been reliably demonstrated, mostly with recall tasks (more rarely with recognition tasks) and with mixed (including incongruous and ordinary items) rather than pure lists.

INCONGRUITY AND MEMORY: EXPLANATIONS

Three interpretations of the bizarreness effect will be considered here. One possibility is that incongruous stimuli elicit extra (more elaborated) processing because they are more difficult to understand in the context of expected properties and semantic norms (the *attentional* or *processing time* hypothesis; Merry, 1980; Wollen & Cox, 1981). According to this view, the extra elaboration given to incongruous items strengthens their memory trace much as deep, semantically elaborated tasks encourage memorization in standard memory paradigms (e.g., Craik & Lockhart, 1972; Craik & Tulving, 1975).

Another possibility is that primary distinctiveness plays a role in the bizarreness effect. This *distinctiveness* hypothesis, proposed by McDaniel & Eistein (1986), is based on the finding that bizarreness effects appear primarily with mixed lists (containing both ordinary and incongruous material). According to this view, incongruous material is well remembered because it is contextually distinctive. Worthen & Marshall (1996) indeed demonstrated that a mnemonic advantage can be observed for any type of material (ordinary or incongruous) as long as this material is isolated at study in the larger context of another type of material.

Another possibility is that incongruous stimuli elicit a surprise response owing to the violation of expectations, which enhances contextual cues available for later recall (the *surprise* or *expectation violation* hypothesis; Hirshman, 1988; Hirshman et al., 1989). According to this view, failure to understand the relation between incongruous items and their context can improve memory. Such failures occur because unexpected or novel combinations lead to a semantic "blind-alley" search resulting in better memory representation. Later, the blind-alley search cue mediates retrieval of the incongruous information on which the blind-alley search was committed.

The above-mentioned explanations of the bizarreness effect are not mutually exclusive. Indeed, it is possible that incongruous items receive extra processing *and* elicit a surprise response. At the same time, such extra processing may serve memory only in the context of primary distinctiveness.

Another avenue of inquiry distinguishes between encoding and retrieval. The attentional hypothesis postulates that the encoding of incongruous items is crucial in producing the memory advantage. In contrast, the distinctiveness and the surprise hypotheses propose that the memory advantage for incongruous items is mediated by processes occurring at the time of access. This claim is mostly based on the finding that the bizarreness effect occurs mostly for free recall and less so for recognition or cued recall, tasks that presumably lessen the role of retrieval processes (see Riefer & Rouder, 1992; Riefer & LaMay, 1998). McDaniel, DeLosh, and Merritt (2000) recently demonstrated that the bizarreness effect is eliminated when alternative retrieval strategies are encouraged, which was taken as evidence that the bizarreness effect occurs at retrieval rather than at encoding.

INCONGRUITY: NEURAL CORRELATES

We consider below two types of physiological data that may help in adjudicating between alternative explanations of how incongruity leads to better memory. First, we review some event-related potential (ERP) experiments that shed light on the electrophysiological correlates of encoding success. As well, such data may distinguish item features that lead to better memory. Second, we discuss functional neuroimaging experiments based on positron emission tomography (PET) and functional magnetic resonance imaging (fMRI). Functional neuroimaging has been used to localize the anatomical representation of processes associated with encoding success. Correlation of such data against other functional neuroimaging results may be used to draw inferences regarding which cognitive operations (e.g., working memory, spatial attention) contribute most to subsequent memory.

In principle, electrophysiology and functional neuroimaging both could be used to distinguish between encoding and retrieval hypotheses, provided that data are recorded at both stages of the entire memorization process. However, previous examinations of the neural correlates of incongruity have been focused mainly on encoding. Consequently, only indirect conclusions can be drawn regarding the contributions of encoding vs. retrieval processes to the bizarreness effect.

Neural Correlates of Primary Distinctiveness

The P300

One event-related potential that can be related to primary distinctiveness is the P300 (also known as P3). The P300 manifests as a scalp positivity peaking about 300 milliseconds after infrequent (oddball) stimuli (Johnson, 1986, 1993; Matt, Leuthold, & Sommer, 1992). Such stimuli are distinct only in the context of the task at hand. The P300 is the electrophysiological phenomenon most associated with orienting, a complex of processes including arousal, capture of attention, and memory formation (Sokolov, 1963).

Tasks eliciting the P300 response include the isolation paradigm (von Restorff, 1933) and target detection. In both type of tasks, one type of stimulus (oddball) is isolated—that is, infrequently presented. For example, oddball visual words may be presented in uppercase in the context of background words presented in lowercase. Oddball sounds may be assigned a different pitch. Subjects either detect the oddballs or perform an unrelated task. In detection tasks, three types of stimuli are used: a standard, high-probability stimulus requiring no overt response; a low-probability target to which subjects are asked to respond; and equally improbable, unexpected novel events (oddball stimuli). Detection paradigms give rise to two distinguishable electrophysiological responses: the P3a, which is elicited by the infrequent *and* unexpected stimuli (oddballs); and the P3b, which is elicited by task-relevant targets. The P3b response is strongly modulated by task relevance and does not habituate. The P3a exhibits a somewhat earlier latency, a more anterior scalp distribution and habituates rapidly (Courchesne, Hillyard, & Galambos, 1975; Knight & Nakada, 1998; Knight & Scabini, 1998).

Auditory oddball stimuli also elicit an electrophysiological response known as mismatch negativity (MMN; Naatanen, 1992). MMN occurs relatively early (110–140 milliseconds after deviant tone pips) and appears to be specific to auditory stimuli. Its likely generators are in auditory cortex (Liebenthal et al., 2003). As MMN seems to be related more to sensory than to cognitive processes, it will not be further discussed here.

The P300 and memory

As an extensive review of the relationship between the P300 and memory is provided in another chapter of this book (Fabiani, Chapter 15 this volume) only a few key results will be mentioned here. The electrophysiological phenomenon most consistently associated with better subsequent memory is late (350–800 milliseconds latency) scalp positivity (e.g., Paller, 1990; Rugg, Schloerscheidt, & Doyle, 1996). This response is often classified as belonging to the P300 family and can be experimentally manipulated in parallel with subsequent recall by varying the primary distinctiveness of presented items (Fabiani, Karis, & Donchin, 1986; Johnson, Pfefferbaum, & Kopell, 1985; Karis, Fabiani, & Donchin, 1984; Otten & Donchin, 2000). For instance, Fabiani et al. (1986) used an incidental memory paradigm in which subjects were asked to count either male or female names that were either rare or frequent. Memory for the names was later tested using a free-recall task. At encoding, rare names evoked larger P300 responses than frequent names. At test, rare names were better recalled than frequent names. Using back-sorting, it was determined that P300 responses evoked at study were larger for names that were later remembered, supporting the existence of a relationship between the amplitude of the P300 and subsequent recall.

Neural correlates of the P300

Correlative studies of patients with brain lesions suggest that the P300 is dependent on a widespread network of brain regions. A consistent finding is that the temporal-parietal junction as well as the posterior hippocampus lesions disrupt generation of the P300 (Knight, 1996; Knight & Scabini, 1988). Patients with posterior hippocampal lesions not only show dramatic reduction of the P3a (Knight, 1996) but also do not produce phasic skin conductance responses to novel events, which is a signature of the orienting response (see Williams et al., 2000). Patients with unilateral lesions of the dorsolateral prefrontal cortex also show reduced P3a (Knight, 1984). Lesions in the vicinity of the temporal-parietal junction affect both the P3a and the P3b (Knight, Scabini, Woods, & Clayworth, 1989).

In the neuroimaging domain, several fMRI correlates of the P3a have recently been reported suggesting that the hippocampus as well as the temporal, prefrontal, and parietal cortices contribute to the generation of this potential (Kirino, Belger, Goldman-Rakic, & McCarthy, 2000; McCarthy, Luby, Gore, & Goldman-Rakic, 1997; Strange, Henson, Friston, & Dolan, 2000). McCarthy and colleagues used a paradigm in which subjects were asked to respond to rare target stimuli (strings of Xs) presented among standard stimuli (strings of Os; McCarthy et al., 1997). Results showed that the middle frontal gyri and the inferior parietal lobules, which are usually involved in working-memory tasks, were activated by infrequent targets.

In a recent study using the isolation paradigm, Strange et al. (2000) showed that semantic, emotional, and perceptual oddball effects could be dissociated based on their neural correlates. Subjects viewed serially presented nouns including semantic (unrelated word meaning), perceptual (different type), and emotional (affectively charged) oddballs. Two regions were activated irrespective of the attribute conferring distinctiveness: a right prefrontal region and the inferior parietal lobule. Perceptual oddballs also evoked specific activity bilaterally in posterior fusiform regions. Emotional oddballs evoked specific activity in the left amygdala, a structure widely believed to be involved in emotional processing (Adolphs, 2002; Cardinal, Parkinson, Hall, & Everitt, 2002; Hamann, 2003; LeDoux, 2000). Finally, semantic oddballs evoked specific activity in the left prefrontal cortex, a region frequently associated with semantic processing (Cabeza & Nyberg, 2000). Strange et al. (2000) propose that two types of networks are activated when a stimulus embodying primary distinctiveness is presented: (1) a system detecting "generic deviance" that involves right prefrontal and fusiform cortices, and (2) regions that usually deal with the aspects of the stimulus that presently bear the deviance.

In sum, detection of primary distinctiveness seems to engage a widespread network of brain regions involving the hippocampus, temporal-parietal, and frontal cortices. The frontal regions may monitor discrepancies between expectations and experience while more posterior regions may play a role in working memory and attentional processes. The hippocampal formation may be generally activated by novel stimuli as a correlate of the process of creating new associations (Eichenbaum, 2001; Jacobs & Schenk, 2003; Small, 2002).

It has been proposed that primary distinctiveness may play a role in the bizarreness memory effect (McDaniel & Eistein, 1986). The neural data described above suggests that primary distinctiveness leads to enhanced working memory, discrepancy monitoring, and memory formation, which may relate to the memory advantage observed for incongruous information. However, as mentioned earlier, the mnemonic advantage of primary distinctiveness seems to apply to any kind of stimulus. Indeed, Worthen and Marshall (1996) showed that isolated items show a mnemonic advantage independently of their nature (incongruous or ordinary). So, the next question is: what is the role of incongruity itself in the memory effect? And what are the neural correlates of incongruity, independent of primary distinctiveness?

Neural Correlates of Secondary Distinctiveness

The N400

The ERP that can be directly related to secondary distinctiveness as defined earlier is the N400. The N400 potential is central-parietal scalp negativity that peaks 400 milliseconds after the presentation of (1) semantically incongruous words in the context of sentences (see Kutas & Hillyard, 1983) or (2) semantically unrelated pairs of words or pictures (see Hagoort, 2003; Holcomb, 1988; McPherson & Holcomb, 1999). In paradigms using incongruous sentence endings such as, "The man was reading a hotel," the amplitude of the N400 following the last word of a sentence is inversely related to its contextual likelihood. In paradigms using single stimuli, the amplitude of the N400 is larger in response to a word preceded by an unrelated word (e.g., *nurse* preceded by *dog*) than in response to a word preceded by a related word (e.g., *nurse* preceded by *doctor*). The N400 phenomenon is thought to be a correlate of the semantic conflict arising when perceived information is different from information expected based on context.

The N400 and memory

Although the relation between late scalp positivity and subsequent memory performance is clear, available data do not indicate a clear relationship between the N400 and subsequent memory. Only a few previous studies bear on this issue (e.g., Bartholow, Fabiani, Gratton, & Bettencourt, 2001;

Neville, Kutas, Chesney, & Schmidt, 1986). In the Neville et al. (1986) study, subjects made yes/no responses to propositions such as "A type of bird: robin," and "A type of insect: sun." Memory for the single words was later tested using a recognition task. Results showed that at encoding incongruent words elicited larger N400 responses than congruent words. However, incongruent words were less well recognized than congruent words. Furthermore, they evoked equally large N400 peak amplitudes at study whether or not they were subsequently recognized. These data suggest that the nature of the physiological processes manifesting as N400 does not determine whether a word will or will not be remembered. In contrast, the amplitude at encoding of a late positive component predicted subsequent recognition. Neville and colleagues attributed their results to the idea that expected sentence endings lead to integrated cognitive units that are more elaborated and therefore better encoded.

Such data are intriguing. Statements such as "A type of insect: sun" bear some resemblance to sentences that typically elicit the bizarreness memory effect (e.g., "The child was eating a bear"). One might have expected that the cognitive operations stimulated by semantic incongruity (as indexed by N400) should lead to enhanced encoding and better subsequent memory. Possibly, the absence of "interactivity" (Wollen, Weber, & Lowry, 1972) explains the lack of mnemonic advantage for the incongruous sentences used by Neville and colleagues. Future research clearly is needed to clarify this issue.

The neural correlates of the N400

1. *Sentential incongruity.* Relatively little is known regarding the neural generators of the N400. Electrical field potential recordings in epilepsy patients undergoing pre-surgical assessment (Elger, Grunwald, Helmstaedter, & Kurthen, 1995; Guillem, N'Kaoua, Rougier, & Claverie, 1995; McCarthy, Nobre, Bentin, & Spencer, 1995) and magnetoencephalography (Helenius, Salmelin, Service, & Connolly, 1998) suggest that left temporal structures may be particularly important.

   Several recent fMRI studies have explored sentential incongruity (Kang, Constable, Gore, & Avrutin, 1999; Kiehl, Laurens, Duty, Forster, & Liddle, 2002; Kuperberg et al., 2000, 2003; Newman, Pancheva, Ozawa, Neville, & Ullman, 2001; Ni et al., 2001). In these studies, responses to semantic (e.g., "The man sailed the hotel to China") and syntactic (e.g., "The woman read the with letter attention") incongruities were compared. Although the aim of these studies was to dissociate semantic from syntactic processes, their use of semantically incongruous sentences provides interesting data related to our purpose. All studies reported functional anatomic differences in responses to semantic vs. syntactic anomalies. Across fMRI studies, activations specific to semantic anomalies were found mostly in temporal (BA 21, 22, 41, 42) and frontal (BA 9/46, 6 and 44/45/47) areas. It has been suggested that the search for a meaning in response to reading incongruous sentences localizes to this temporal-frontal language network (Kuperberg et al., 2003).

Interestingly, Ni et al. (2000) manipulated the frequency of the semantically anomalous sentences. In a first experiment, blocks containing half normal sentences and half incongruous sentences were used. Subjects monitored sentences for incongruity (semantic or syntactic depending on the block). Regions activated by semantic incongruity included prefrontal cortex (BA 9/46, 6, 44/45, and 47), cingulate gyrus, angular gyrus, basal ganglia as well as superior and middle temporal gyri. In a second experiment, to maximize the intensity of the signal associated with incongruity, each block contained 7 incongruous sentences among 37 normal sentences. Subjects judged whether each sentence contained a living object. Semantic incongruity activated the same regions as in the first experiment as well as additional ones in prefrontal (BA 8 and 10), subinsular and superior parietal cortex. Although the brain coverage in this study was incomplete and the different experiments used different tasks, it is interesting to note that, at the neural level, frequency effects (primary distinctiveness) can be somewhat differentiated from incongruity effects (secondary distinctiveness).

2. *Visual incongruity.* It has been shown that the N400 can be elicited by pictures as well as by words (Ganis, Kutas, & Sereno, 1996; West & Holcomb, 2002). Yet, very few neuroimaging studies have explored the neural correlates of visual incongruity. All studies that used geometrically impossible or nonsense figures as controls for meaningful images reported that such stimuli elicited either comparable (Schacter et al., 1995; Martin, Wiggs, & Weisberg, 1997) or less (Vuilleumier, Henson, Driver, & Dolan, 2002) activation of infero-temporal cortex in comparison to meaningful images. Thus, mere nonreality does not elicit physiological correlates of incongruity (see below).

Only two recent neuroimaging studies used incongruous visual material likely to confer a mnemonic advantage. In the study of Gerlach, Law, Gade, and Paulson (1999) participants judged whether images depicted real or nonreal objects. The nonreal images were of two types: (1) semantically unidentifiable nonsense objects or (2) chimeric figures—for example, head of panda on body of bull. Comparing chimeric figures to real objects led to greater blood flow in infero-temporal cortex than comparing nonsense objects to real objects. These data suggest that incongruous stimuli evoke more activity than ordinary stimuli in regions involved in processing visual attributes of objects. Such activity could reflect deeper encoding processing. One problem interpreting these data is that dependency on incongruity was confounded by the task. Specifically, the chimeric vs. real judgment was more difficult than the nonsense vs. real judgment as indexed by response time. Another problem is that, as it was not an objective of their study, Gerlach et al. (1999) did not test memory for the objects they used. As a result, it is not known whether these chimeric objects induced a bizarreness memory effect.

To get a better understanding of the neural correlates of visual incongruity we recently conducted an fMRI study using incongruous pictures incorporating semantic violations concerning artifacts and living things (Michelon, Snyder, Buckner, & Zacks, 2003). Incongruous stimuli were generated by combining semantically unrelated parts (e.g., head of wrench fused onto the body of a sheep). Our specific aim was to test whether such stimuli elicit extra elaboration and/or a surprise response, two of the cognitive mechanisms proposed to explain the mnemonic advantage for incongruous material. In one condition (frequent incongruous condition) incongruous and ordinary pictures were presented with equal frequency. This condition allowed examination of encoding activity related to incongruity without contamination by frequency effects. Another condition (infrequent incongruous condition) was designed to examine the surprise response associated with the perception of incongruous pictures. We tried to maximize the possibility of a surprise response by (1) presenting only few incongruous pictures among several ordinary pictures and (2) always running this condition first so that these incongruous pictures were the first seen in the experiment. A small number of oddball stimuli (color inverted but otherwise ordinary pictures) were also included as a control for frequency effects. In both conditions, participants were instructed to detect upside down pictures. As the purpose of this task was to promote attention to the pictures, only one upside-down picture was presented at the very end of each run.

Three main findings emerged from this study. First, we observed functional responses to incongruity that were independent of the frequency of the incongruous pictures. A larger neural response to incongruous compared to ordinary pictures was observed, across conditions, in 26 regions. These regions covered a large portion of the occipital lobes bilaterally, including striate (BA 17) and extrastriate cortices (BA 18, 19) with bilateral extension to fusiform (BA 37) and parietal regions (BA 7). Similar results were observed bilaterally in frontal areas (BA 45/47, 6/9/44) and posterior thalamus and on the right only in the orbito-frontal cortex (BA 47 and 10).

A second finding was that a few regions were specifically sensitive to a combination of incongruity and surprise—that is, responded more to incongruous infrequent pictures than to all other types of pictures. The eight regions showing this pattern of activity included striate and extrastriate cortex on the left, intraparietal cortex on the right, thalamus bilaterally, supplementary motor area, and two inferior frontal regions. Our design deliberately confounded frequency and incongruity to examine the neural correlates of surprise. In an attempt to disentangle these two effects we included infrequent but not incongruous oddball stimuli distinguished by superficial visual features (color inversion). Larger responses for incongruous˘vs. oddball pictures occurred only in four regions: right fusiform, left ventral extrastriate cortex, peri-calcarine cortex, and right frontal operculum. These regions presumably respond specifically to secondary rather than primary incongruity.

A third finding was that all regions responding to frequent but not to infrequent incongruous pictures exhibited deactivation responses (greater for incongruous in comparison to ordinary pictures). These regions included right medial temporal cortex (BA 21), bilateral lateral parietal cortex (BA 39/40) and posterior cingulate cortex (BA 23/31).

In sum, certain findings provided by the study of visual incongruity are consistent with those provided by the study of sentential semantic violation. Indeed, both Ni et al. (2000) and Newman et al. (2001) reported left inferior frontal gyrus (probably BA 9/46) responses to semantic violations. Kuperberg et al. (2000) emphasized that semantic violations activate the left inferior temporal and fusiform cortex. Deactivations in parietal regions were reported by Kuperberg et al. (2003) in comparing anomalous vs. normal sentences. Such a convergence suggests that the neural response to incongruity is independent of the stimulus format (words or pictures). However, our study of visual incongruity also suggests that regions specific to the format—that is, visual regions—were also modulated by incongruity. We propose that incongruity or secondary distinctiveness modulates the activity of two types of neural networks: (1) a network that normally process semantic features of stimuli independently of the format and (2) modality specific regions whose activation depends on the stimulus format.

How do these results help us understand the memory advantage for incongruous material? Unfortunately, very few neuroimaging studies tested memory for the stimuli used during scanning. As far as we are aware, the only study of memory using the same incongruous stimuli used during scanning comes from our laboratory (Michelon et al., 2003). In this study, to exclude frequency effects, it was necessary to study a group of participants separate from those in the fMRI experiment. In the study phase, the stimuli were presented under conditions that closely matched the frequent incongruous fMRI condition. Participants performed the same task (upside-down picture detection) under the same instructions. They were asked to return in two weeks for recognition testing. In the recognition phase all participants viewed studied and non-studied pictures while performing a forced choice new vs. old discrimination task. The complete item set was randomly divided into screens of eight pictures. On each screen four pictures were old and four were new. Participants were asked to select by mouse click the four old pictures as quickly as possible.

Hit rates as well as false-recognition rates were higher for incongruous pictures than for ordinary pictures. Critically, recognition scores corrected for bias (hits minus false alarms) were higher for incongruous than for ordinary pictures. The sequential order of picture selection could be recorded, which allowed testing for a possible attentional bias toward one or the other type of stimuli. Participants picked incongruous pictures preferentially in the first and second positions. Moreover, corrected recognition scores were higher for incongruous than for ordinary pictures for stimuli picked in first and second position. No significant difference was observed between incongruous and ordinary pictures for stimuli picked in third position. Finally, in the fourth position, more ordinary pictures were correctly recognized than incongruous pictures.

In sum, we observed a robust bizarreness effect. The incongruous pictures used in our fMRI study did show a mnemonic advantage. This provides a basis for discussion of the physiological responses observed in the fMRI experiment in terms of recognition memory. In the following section, we will argue that the available data mainly support the attentional/processing explanation of the bizarreness memory effect, although, indirectly.

LINKING NEURAL RESPONSES TO MEMORY BENEFIT

Support for the Attentional or Processing Time Hypothesis

This account of the bizarreness memory effect proposes that enhanced elaboration processes elicited by incongruous items strengthens their memory trace. Functional imaging data seem to support this hypothesis.

First, previous studies have shown that specific frontal and temporal regions are associated with memory encoding. For example, numerous studies have noted increased responses in frontal cortex along the inferior frontal gyrus (near BA 45/47 extending into BA 44) during intentional encoding and also during deep incidental encoding (Buckner, Kelley, & Petersen, 1999; Fletcher, Shallice, & Dolan,1998; Tulving, Markowitsch, & Kapur, 1994). Responses in these regions can predict, even on a trial by trial basis, whether participants will remember individual stimuli (Brewer, Zhao, Desmond, Glover, & Gabrieli, 1998; Wagner et al., 1998). All neuroimaging studies mentioned earlier report responses to incongruous stimuli in cortical regions anatomically near to those associated with subsequent memory effects (Kang et al., 1999; Kuperberg et al., 2000, 2003; Michelon et al., 2003; Newman et al., 2001; Ni et al., 2001). In contrast to studies in which uncontrolled factors lead to variable encoding, secondary distinctiveness studies directly manipulate item processing by incorporating incongruity. The result is increased activity across a broad network of regions prominently including temporal and frontal regions previously implicated in the kinds of elaborative processing that lead to successful memory encoding.

Second, incongruity appears to modulate activity in right dorsolateral prefrontal cortex regions (Kang et al., 1999; Michelon et al., 2003), which are conventionally identified as central to processes used by working memory tasks (e.g., Barch et al., 1997; Courtney, Ungerleider, Keil, & Haxby 1997; D'Esposito et al., 1998; Smith & Jonides, 1999). It is possible that deep elaboration triggered by the need to resolve the cognitive inconsistency increases working memory load.

Finally, bilateral activations, larger for incongruous than ordinary stimuli, have been observed in the vicinity of the intra-parietal and lateral parietal sulci (Kuperberg et al., 2003; Michelon et al., 2003). This pattern may suggest differential activation by incongruous stimuli of systems mediating spatial attention and visual search (Shulman et al., 1997a, 1997b). Within this possibility, attentional factors may contribute to enhanced encoding.

In sum, neuroimaging results provide good evidence about the nature of the encoding of incongruous pictures. In particular, encoding processes as well as working memory and attentional processes seem to be enhanced by secondary distinctiveness. Such encoding factors have been shown in other studies to be related to memory performance, which allows us to conclude that increased physiological activity at encoding may account for at least part of the bizarreness effect. It is worth noting, however, that the relationship between encoding processes and later memory benefit is not clear given that no neuroimaging studies directly examined the correlation between neural activity at encoding and subsequent memory performance. Moreover, previous behavioral studies suggest that encoding factors such as encoding time or amount of attention allotted to ordinary and incongruous information do not reliably influence the memory performance (see Worthen, Garcia-Rivas, Green, & Vidos, 2000).

Previous research suggests that retrieval rather than encoding processes may be responsible for the bizarreness effect (see McDaniel et al., 2000; Riefer & LaMay, 1998; Riefer & Rouder, 1992). This idea is based principally on the fact that the bizarreness effect occurs more often in free recall than in recognition tasks in which retrieval processes are reduced. The fact that a robust bizarreness effect has sometimes been observed in a recognition task (Michelon et al., 2003; Worthen & Wood, 2001) may weaken this claim, suggesting that processes at encoding are also important. However, results suggest that retrieval stage processes may also play a role in some of the recognition performance characteristics. First, incongruous stimuli generally lead to substantially greater false recognition rates (Michelon et al., 2003; Worthen & Eller, 2002; Worthen & Wood, 2001). Second, when the recognition memory task involves the simultaneous presentation of several items, incongruous items tend to be selected first (Michelon et al., 2003). Enhanced orienting to incongruous pictures at retrieval would be expected to encourage more frequent and earlier selection of both false- and true-old incongruous pictures. Thus, it is possible that (1) processes engaged at retrieval rather than encoding account for the bizarreness effect and (2) that enhanced encoding and attention account for a response bias rather than for a memory advantage.

Support for the Distinctiveness and Surprise Hypotheses

The distinctiveness hypothesis proposes that primary distinctiveness plays a role in the bizarreness memory effect. This idea is based on the observation of enhanced memory regardless of stimulus type (incongruous or not) as long as items are isolated in the context of the experiment. The surprise hypothesis proposes that incongruous stimuli elicit a surprise response owing to the violation of expectations (secondary distinctiveness) that enhances contextual cues available for later recall.

Although these hypotheses are quite distinct, the available neuroimaging data do not allow testing them independently. Indeed, the only study to test the surprise hypothesis deliberately confounded surprise and primary distinctiveness (Michelon et al., 2003, described above). Among regions preferentially responding to the first few incongruous stimuli were right frontal operculum, right dorsal thalamus, and supplementary motor area. It was only in the right frontal operculum that the activity was greater for infrequent incongruous pictures than for infrequent ordinary (color-inverted) oddballs. This leads us to propose that processes represented in right frontal operculum may be closely related to the hypothesized surprise response (Hirshman et al., 1989).

Several studies have reported that unexpected or infrequent stimuli provoke activation of the right frontal operculum (Strange et al., 2000; Optitz, Mecklinger, Friederici, & von Cramon, 1999). This same region is activated by negative feedback in the Wisconsin Card Sorting task (WCST; Konishi et al., 2002; Monchi, Petrides, Petre, Worsley, & Dagher, 2001). Fink et al. (1999) observed similar responses in a slightly more dorsal region by creating (with mirrors) conflict between the visual and proprioceptive senses. Interestingly, Strange et al. (2000) reported frontal operculum activation specifically in response to emotional oddballs compared to perceptual and semantic oddballs. The common theme appears to be information at variance with the current subjective assessment of reality, which, in turn, reflexively leads to a shift or alteration in the mode of interaction with the environment.

In sum, the existence of physiological responses specific to infrequent (or unexpected) incongruous stimuli (Michelon et al., 2003) lends indirect support to the hypothesis that incongruous stimuli elicit a surprise response at encoding. The proposed relationship between such physiological response and subsequent memory effects (Hirshman et al., 1989) is not clear. It is worth noting that memory advantage for incongruous material is usually obtained using protocols designed to exclude frequency effects (Cornoldi et al., 1988; Hirshman et al., 1989; McDaniel & Einstein, 1986; Nicolas & Marchal, 1996; Riefer & Rouder, 1992; Worthen & Marshall, 1996). Therefore, although surprise may contribute to the memory phenomenon, it is not required. This is convergent with results from behavioral studies that directly tested the surprise hypothesis (e.g., Davidson et al., 2000; McDaniel et al., 1995). For instance, McDaniel and colleagues (1995) show that manipulations designed to augment or attenuate surprise in response to bizarre sentences had very little impact on subsequent memory for the bizarre sentences.

CONCLUSIONS

Studies of the neural correlates of incongruity reviewed here provide some answers to the question, Why is this type of information better remembered? Neuroimaging studies of secondary distinctiveness indirectly support the elaboration hypothesis, which states that incongruous percepts lead to the formation of more robust memory traces, in part, due to additional processing at the time of encoding. Structures differentially activated by incongruous materials include regions associated with object identification (fusiform cortex), working memory (prefrontal cortex), and spatial attention (parietal cortex). Little support can be found for the surprise hypothesis, which proposes that incongruous materials are better recalled because of enhanced availability of episodic cues triggered by surprise. A physiological response possibly related to surprise can be observed during the encoding of incongruous information. However, behavioral data demonstrate that enhanced memory for incongruous stimuli can be obtained under study conditions in which such items are not infrequent, conditions that do not elicit the neural correlates of surprise.

ACKNOWLEDGMENTS

Part of this research has been presented at the 49th Annual Meeting of the Southwestern Psychological Association, New Orleans, LA, April 2003.

REFERENCES

Adolphs, R. (2002). Neural systems for recognizing emotion. *Current Opinion in Neurobiology*, 12, 169–177.

Barch, D. M., Braver, T. S., Nystrom, L. E., Forman, S. D., Noll, D. C., & Cohen, J. D. (1997). Dissociating working memory from task difficulty in human prefrontal cortex. *Neuropsychologia, 35*, 1373–1380.

Bartholow, B., Fabiani, M., Gratton, G., & Bettencourt, A. (2001). A psychophysiological analysis of the processing time course of social expectancy violations. *Psychological Science, 12*, 197–204.

Brewer, J. B., Zhao, Z., Desmond, J. E., Glover, G. H., Gabrieli, J. D. E. (1998). Making memories: Brain activity that predicts how well visual experience will be remembered. *Science, 281*, 1185–1187.

Buckner, R. L., Kelley, W. M., & Petersen, S. E. (1999). Frontal cortex contributes to human memory formation. *Nature Neuroscience, 2*, 311–314.

Cabeza, R., & Nyberg, L. (2000). Imaging cognition II: An empirical review of 275 PET and fMRI studies. *Journal of Cognitive Neuroscience, 12*, 1–47.

Cardinal, R. N., Parkinson, J. A., Hall, J., & Everitt, B. J. (2002). Emotion and motivation: the role of the amygdala, ventral striatum, and prefrontal cortex. *Neuroscience Biobehavioral Review, 26*, 321–352.

Cornoldi, C., Cavedon, A., De Beni, R., & Pra Baldi, A. (1988). The influence of the nature of material and of mental operations on the occurrence of the bizarreness effect. *The Quarterly Journal of Experimental Psychology, 40*, 73–85.

Courchesne, E., Hillyard, S. A., & Galambos, R. (1975). Stimulus novelty, task relevance and the visual evoked potential in man. *Electroencephalography & Clinical Neurophysiology, 39*, 131–143.

Courtney, S. M., Ungerleider, L. G., Keil, K., & Haxby, J. V. (1997). Transient and sustained activity in a distributed neural system for human working memory. *Nature, 386*, 608–611.

Craik, F. I., & Lockhart, R. S. (1972). Levels of processing: A framework for memory research. *Journal of Verbal Learning and Behavior, 11*, 671–684.

Craik, F. I., & Tulving, E. (1975). Depth of processing and the retention of words in episodic memory. *Journal of Experimental Psychology: General, 104*, 268–294.

D'Esposito, M., Aguirre, G. K., Zarahn, E., Ballard, D., Shin, R. K., & Lease, J. (1998). Functional MRI studies of spatial and nonspatial working memory. *Cognitive Brain Research, 7*, 1–13.

Eichenbaum, H. (2001). The hippocampus and declarative memory: cognitive mechanisms and neural codes. *Behavioral Brain Research, 127*, 199–207.

Elger, C. E., Grunwald, T., Helmstaedter, C., & Kurthen, M. (1995). Cortical localization of cognitive functions. In T. A. Pedley & B. S. Meldrum (Eds.), *Recent advances in epilepsy* (No. 6, pp. 79–95). New York : Churchill Livingstone.

Engelkamp, J., Zimmer, H. D., & Biegelmann, U. E. (1993). Bizarreness effects in verbal tasks and subject-performed tasks. *European Journal of Cognitive Psychology, 5*, 393–415.

Fabiani, M., Karis, D., & Donchin, E. (1986). P300 and recall in an incidental memory paradigm. *Psychophysiology, 23*, 298–308.

Fink, G. R., Marshall, J. C., Halligan, P. W., Frith, C. D., Driver, J., Frackowiak, R. S. J., & Dolan, R. J. (1999). The neural consequences of conflict between intention and the senses. *Brain, 122*, 497–512.

Fletcher, P. C., Shallice, T., & Dolan, R. J. (1998). The functional roles of prefrontal cortex in episodic memory. I. Encoding. *Brain, 121*, 1239–1248.

Ganis, G., Kutas, M., & Sereno, M. I. (1996). The search for "common sense": An electrophysiological study of the comprehension of words and pictures in reading. *Journal of Cognitive Neuroscience, 8*, 89–106.

Gerlach, C., Law, I., Gade, A., & Paulson, O. B. (1999). Perceptual differentiation and category effects in normal object recognition. A PET study. *Brain, 122*, 2159–2170.

Guillem, F., N'Kaoua, B., Rougier, A., & Claverie, B. (1995). Intracranial topography of event-related potentials (N400/P600) elicited during a continuous recognition memory task. *Psychophysiology, 32*, 382–392.

Hagoort, P. (2003). Interplay between syntax and semantics during sentence comprehension: ERP effects of combining syntactic and semantic violations. *Journal of Cognitive Neuroscience, 15*, 883–899.

Hamann, S. (2003). Nosing in on the emotional brain. *Nature Neuroscience, 6*, 106–108.

Helenius, P., Salmelin, R., Service, E., & Connolly, J. F. (1998). Distinct time courses of word and context comprehension in the left temporal cortex. *Brain, 121*, 1133–1142.

Hirshman, E. (1988). The expectation-violation effect: Paradoxical effects of semantic relatedness. *Journal of Memory & Language, 27*, 40–58.

Hirshman, E., Whelley, M. M., & Palij, M. (1989). An investigation of paradoxical memory effects. *Journal of Memory and Language, 28*, 594–609.

Holcomb, P. J. (1988). Automatic and attentional processing: An event-related brain potential analysis of semantic priming. *Brain and Language, 35*, 66–85.

Hunt, R. (1995). The subtlety of distinctiveness: What von Restorff really did. *Psychonomic Bulletin & Review, 2*, 105–112.

Jacobs, L. F., & Schenk, F. (2003). Unpacking the cognitive map: the parallel map theory of hippocampal function. *Psychological Review, 110*, 285–315.

Johnson, R. (1986). A triarchic model of P300 amplitude. *Psychophysiology, 23*, 367–384.

Johnson, R. (1993). On the neural generators of the P300 component of the event-related potential. *Psychophysiology, 30*, 90–97.

Johnson, R., Pfefferbaum, A., & Kopell, B. S. (1985). P300 and long-term memory: Latency predicts recognition performance. *Psychophysiology, 22*, 497–507.

Kang, A. M., Constable, R. T., Gore, J. C., & Avrutin, S. (1999). An event-related fMRI study of implicit phrase-level syntactic and semantic processing. *Neuroimage, 10*, 555–561.

Karis, D., Fabiani, M., & Donchin, E. (1984). "P300" and memory: Individual differences in the von Restorff Effect. *Cognitive Psychology, 16*, 77–216.

Kiehl, K. A., Laurens, K. R., Duty, T. L., Forster, B. B., & Liddle, P. F. (2001). Neural sources involved in auditory target detection and novelty processing: An event-related fMRI study. *Psychophysiology, 38*, 133–142.

Kirino, E., Belger, A., Goldman-Rakic, P., & McCarthy, G. (2000). Prefrontal activation evoked by infrequent target and novel stimuli in a visual target detection task: An event-related functional magnetic resonance imaging study. *The Journal of Neuroscience, 20*, 6612–6618.

Knight, R. T. (1984). Decreased response to novel stimuli after prefrontal lesions in man. *Electroencephalography & Clinical Neurophysiology, 59*, 9–20.

Knight, R. T. (1996). Contribution of human hippocampal region to novelty detection. *Nature, 383*, 256–259.

Knight, R. T., & Nakada, T. (1998). Cortico-limbic circuits and novelty: A review of EEG and blood flow data. *Reviews in the Neurosciences, 9*, 57–70.

Knight, R. T., & Scabini, D. (1998). Anatomic bases of event-related potentials and their relationship to novelty detection in humans. *Journal of Clinical Neurophysiology, 15*, 3–13.

Knight, R. T., Scabini, D., Woods, D. L., & Clayworth, C. C. (1989). Contributions of temporal/parietal junction to the human auditory P3. *Brain Research, 502*, 109–116.

Konishi, S., Hayashi, T., Uchida, I., Kikyo, H., Takahashi, E., & Miyashita, Y. (2002). Hemispheric asymmetry in human lateral prefrontal cortex during cognitive set shifting. *Proceedings for the National Academy of Science, 99*, 7803–7808.

Kuperberg, G. R., McGuire, P. K., Bullmore, E. T., Brammer, M. J., Rabe-Hesketh, S., Wright, I. C., Lythgoe, D. J., Williams, S. C. R., & David, A. S. (2000). Ordinary and distinct neural substrates for pragmatic, semantic, and syntactic processing of spoken sentences: An fMRI study. *Journal of Cognitive Neuroscience, 12,* 321–341.

Kuperberg, G. R., Holcomb, P. J., Sitnikova, T., Greve, D., Dale, A. M., & Caplan, D. (2003). Distinct patterns of neural modulation during the processing of conceptual and syntactic anomalies. *Journal of Cognitive Neuroscience, 15,* 272–293.

Kutas, M., & Hillyard, S. A. (1983). Event-related brain potentials to grammatical errors and semantic anomalies. *Memory & Cognition, 11,* 539–550.

LeDoux, J. E. (2000). Emotion circuits in the brain. *Annual Review of Neuroscience, 23,* 155–184.

Liebenthal, E., Ellingson, M. L., Spanaki, M. V., Prieto, T. E., Ropella, K. M., & Binder, J. R. (2003). Simultaneous ERP and fMRI of the auditory cortex in a passive oddball paradigm, *Neuroimage, 19,* 1395–1404.

Martin, A., Wiggs, C. L., & Weisberg, J. (1997). Modulation of human medial temporal lobe activity by form, meaning, and experience. *Hippocampus, 7,* 587–593.

Matt, J., Leuthold, H., & Sommer, W. (1992). Differential effects of voluntary expectancies on reaction times and event-related potentials: Evidence for automatic and controlled expectancies. *Journal of Experimental Psychology: Learning, Memory, and Cognition, 18,* 810–822.

McCarthy, G., Nobre, A. C., Bentin, S., & Spencer, D. D. (1995). Language-related field potentials in the anterior-medial temporal lobe: I. Intracranial distribution and neural generators. *Journal of Neuroscience, 15,* 1080–1089.

McCarthy, G. Luby, M., Gore, J., & Goldman-Rakic, P. (1997). Infrequent events transiently activate human prefrontal and parietal cortex as measured by functional MRI. *Journal of Neurophysiology, 77,* 1630–1634.

McDaniel, M. A., & Einstein, G. O. (1986). Bizarre imagery as an effective memory aid: The importance of distinctiveness. *Journal of Experimental Psychology: Learning Memory and Cognition, 12,* 54–65.

McDaniel, M. A., DeLosh, E. L., & Merritt, P. S. (2000). Order of information and retrieval distinctiveness: Recall of common versus bizarre material. *Journal of Experimental Psychology: Learning Memory and Cognition, 26,* 1045–1056.

McDaniel, M. A., Einstein, G. O., DeLosh, E. L., May, C. P., et al. (1995). The bizarreness effect: It's not surprising, it's complex. *Journal of Experiment Psychology: Learning, Memory and Cognition, 21,* 422–435.

McPherson, W. B., & Holcomb, P. J. (1999). An electrophysiological investigation of semantic priming with pictures of real object. *Psychophysiology, 36,* 53–65.

Merry, R. (1980). Image bizarreness in incidental learning. *Psychological Reports, 46,* 427–430.

Michelon, P., Snyder, A. Z., Buckner, L. R., & Zacks, J. M. (2003). Neural correlates of incongruity: an fMRI study. *NeuroImage, 19,* 1612–1626.

Monchi, O., Petrides, M., Petre, V., Worsley, K., & Dagher, A. (2001). Wisconsin card sorting revisited: Distinct neural circuits participating in different stages of the task identified by event related magnetic resonance imaging. *The Journal of Neuroscience 21,* 7733–7741.

Naatanen, R. (1992). *Attention and brain function.* Hillsdale, NJ: Lawrence Erlbaum Associates.

Neville, H. J., Kutas, M., Chesney, G., & Schmidt, A. L. (1986). Event-related brain potentials during initial encoding and recognition memory of congruous and incongruous words. *Journal of Memory and Language, 25,* 75–92.

Newman, A. J., Pancheva, R., Ozawa, K., Neville, H., & Ullman, M. T. (2001). An event-related fMRI study of syntactic and semantic violations. *Journal of Psycholinguistic Research, 30,* 337–361.

Ni, W., Constable, R. T., Mencl, W. E., Pugh, K. R., Fulbright, R. K., Shaywitz, B. A., Gore, J. C., & Shankweiler, D. (2001). An event-related neuroimaging study distinguishing form and content in sentence processing. *Journal of Cognitive Neuroscience, 12,* 120–133.

Nicolas, S., & Marchal, A. (1996). Picture bizarreness effect and word association. *Current Psychology of Cognition, 15,* 629–643.

Optitz, B., Mecklinger, A., Friederici, A. D., & von Cramon, D. Y. (1999). The functional neuroanatomy of novelty processing: Integrating ERP and fMRI results. *Cerebral Cortex, 9,* 379–391.

Otten, L. J., & Donchin, E. (2000). Relationship between P300 amplitude and subsequent recall for distinctive events: Dependence on type of distinctiveness attribute. *Psychophysiology, 37,* 644–661.

Paller, K. A. (1990). Recall and stem-completion priming have different electrophysiological correlates and are modified differentially by directed forgetting. *Journal of Experimental Psychology: Learning Memory and Cognition, 16,* 1021–1032

Riefer, D. M., & LaMay, M. L. (1998). Memory for common and bizarre stimuli: A storage-retrieval analysis. *Psychonomic Bulletin & Review, 5,* 312–317.

Riefer, D. M., & Rouder, M. L. (1992). A multinomial modeling analysis of the mnemonic benefits of bizarre imagery. *Memory & Cognition, 20,* 601–611.

Rugg, M. D., Schloerscheidt, A. M., & Doyle, M. C. (1996). Event-related potentials and the recollection of associative information. *Cognitive Brain Research, 4,* 297–304.

Schacter, D. L., Reiman, E., Uecker, A., Polster, M. R., Yun, L. S., & Cooper, L. A. (1995). Brain regions associated with retrieval of structurally coherent visual information. *Nature, 376,* 587–590.

Schmidt, S. R. (1991). Can we have a distinctive theory of memory? *Memory & Cognition, 19,* 523–542.

Shulman, G. L., Corbetta, M., Buckner, R. L., Fiez, J. A., Miezin, F. M., Raichle, M. E., & Petersen, S. E. (1997a). Common blood flow changes across visual tasks: I.: Increases in subcortical structures and cerebellum but not in nonvisual cortex. *Journal of Cognitive Neuroscience, 9,* 624–647.

Shulman, G. L., Fiez, J. A., Corbetta, M., Buckner, R. L., Miezin, F. M., Raichle, M. E., & Petersen, S. E. (1997b). Common blood flow changes across visual tasks: II.: Decreases in cerebral cortex. *Journal of Cognitive Neuroscience, 9,* 648–663.

Small, S. A. (2002). The longitudinal axis of the hippocampal formation: its anatomy, circuitry, and role in cognitive function. *Review Neuroscience, 13,* 183–194.

Smith, E. E., & Jonides, J. (1999). Storage and executive processes in the frontal lobes. *Science, 283,* 1657–1661.

Sokolov, E. N. (1963). Higher nervous functions: The orienting reflex. *Annual Review of Physiology, 25,* 545–580.

Strange, B. A., Henson, R. N. A., Friston, K. J., & Dolan, R. J. (2000). Brain mechanisms for detecting perceptual, semantic and emotional deviance. *NeuroImage, 12,* 425–433.

Tulving, E., Markowitsch, H. J., & Kapur, S. (1994). Novelty encoding networks in the human brain: Positron emission tomography data. *Neuroreport, 5,* 2525–2528.

Von Restorff, H. (1933). Uber die Wirkung von Bereichsblidungen in Spurenfeld. *Psychologishe Forschung, 18,* 299–342.

Vuilleumier, P., Henson, R. N., Driver, J., & Dolan, R. J. (2002). Multiple levels of visual object constancy revealed by event-related fMRI of repetition priming. *Nature Neuroscience, 5,* 491–499.

Wagner, A. D., Schacter, D. L., Rotte, M., Koustaal, W., Maril, A., Dale, A. M., Rosen, B. R., & Buckner, R. L. (1998). Building memories: Remembering and forgetting of verbal experiences as predicted by brain activity. *Science, 281,* 1188–1191.

West, W. C., & Holcomb, P. J. (2002). Event-related potentials during discourse-level semantic integration of complex pictures. *Cognitive Brain Research, 13,* 363–375.

Williams, L. M., Brammer, M. J., Skerrett, D., Lagopolous, J., Rennie, C., Kozek, K., Olivieri, G., Peduto, T., & Gordon, E. (2000). The neural correlates of orienting: An integration of fMRI and skin conductance orienting. *NeuroReport, 11,* 3011–3015.

Wollen, K. A., & Cox, S. (1981). Sentence cuing and the effectiveness of bizarre imagery. *Journal of Experimental Psychology: Human Learning and Memory, 7,* 386–392.

Wollen, K. A., Weber, A., & Lowry, D. H. (1972). Bizarreness versus integration of mental images as determinants of learning. *Cognitive Psychology, 3,* 518–523.

Worthen, J., B., & Eller, L. S. (2002). A test of competing explanations of the bizarre response bias in recognition memory. *The Journal of General Psychology, 129,* 36–48.

Worthen, J., B., Garcia-Rivas, G., Green, C. R., & Vidos, R. A. (2000). Tests of a cognitive-resource-allocation account of the bizarreness effect. *The Journal of General Psychology, 127*, 117–144.

Worthen, J., B., & Marshall, P. H. (1996). Intralist and extralist distinctiveness and the bizarreness effect: The importance of contrast. *American Journal of Psychology, 109*, 239–263.

Worthen, J. B., & Wood, V. V. (2001). Memory discrimination for self-performed and imagined acts: Bizarreness effects in false recognition. *The Quarterly Journal of Experimental Psychology, 54*, 49–67.

17

Stimulus Novelty Effects on Recognition Memory: Behavioral Properties and Neuroanantomical Substrates

MARK M. KISHIYAMA AND ANDREW P. YONELINAS

Why are some events remembered while others are doomed to be forgotten? The answer to this question has to do, in part, with the relative novelty of different events—those that are unusual or distinctive are remembered better than those that are less distinct (e.g., Hunt, 1995; Kinsbourne & George, 1974; Parker, Wilding, & Ackerman, 1998; Tulving & Kroll, 1995; von Restorff, 1933). Although the beneficial effects of novelty on memory are now well established, significant challenges remain in determining precisely how novelty influences memory and in delineating the brain regions involved in producing novelty effects. In this chapter, we investigate the effects of stimulus novelty on two different processes known to support recognition memory (i.e., recollection and familiarity), and we examine how the temporal lobes and prefrontal cortex contribute to novelty effects seen in recognition memory by assessing memory in patients with damage to these regions.

USING THE VON RESTORFF PARADIGM TO EXAMINE THE EFFECTS OF STIMULUS NOVELTY ON MEMORY

Types of Stimulus Novelty

There are several ways in which items and events can be novel, and various experimental paradigms have been developed to assess the effects of novelty on subsequent memory (for reviews, see Schmidt, 1991; Wallace, 1965). In this chapter we examine the effects of stimulus novelty, or *distinctiveness*, on subsequent memory. By *stimulus novelty* we mean cases in which an item is isolated, or made distinctive, relative to some other set of items (see Hunt, chapter 1 this volume, for further discussion). Two general types of stimulus novelty or distinctiveness have been identified (Schmidt, 1991). First, *primary distinctiveness* refers to cases in which items are considered to be unusual relative to other items in their immediate or local context. The von Restorff (1933) paradigm (e.g., a single yellow word presented in a list of red words) capitalizes on this form of novelty (e.g., Hunt, 1995; Kinsbourne & George, 1974). In itself, a yellow word is no more novel than a red word, but it is relatively distinctive within the immediate context of several red words. In contrast, *secondary distinctiveness* refers to cases in which an item is unusual compared to other items from a category or class. For example, low-frequency words are novel relative to medium- and high-frequency words. In this case, distinctiveness is defined globally and is determined by subjects' past experience with different types of items.

Another method of examining the effects of novelty is the repetition paradigm. This paradigm is commonly used in neuroimaging studies of novelty, whereby items that are encountered for the first time in an experimental session are contrasted to those that have been repeated several times (e.g., Gabrieli, Brewer, Desmond, & Glover, 1997; Kirchhoff, Wagner, Maril, & Stern, 2000; Menon, White, Eliez, Glover, & Reiss, 2000; Tulving, Markowitsch, Craik, Habib, & Houle, 1996). Brain regions that are more active during the initial presentation of an item than for subsequent presentations are considered sensitive to stimulus novelty.

Advantages of Using the von Restorff Paradigm

In studying the effects of novelty on memory, we have focused on primary distinctiveness, using the von Restorff paradigm. One advantage of using this paradigm is that it allows us to counterbalance stimuli across the novelty manipulation (i.e., an item that is made novel for one subject will be made nonnovel for another). Thus, if we find effects of novelty, we can be confident that they are due to the novelty manipulation, rather than to other potential differences between the stimulus classes. For example, high- versus low-frequency words may differ not only with respect to how frequently they have been experienced by the subject but also in a number of other ways that are difficult to control, such as syntactic class, salience, semantic category, or the age at which the words were acquired. Another important property of the von Restorff paradigm is that subsequent memory for novel and nonnovel items can be directly contrasted, which is critical if we wish to understand the effects of novelty on memory. Although repetition paradigms can be used to look for differences between the brain regions that are sensitive to novelty, examining the effects of this form of novelty on subsequent memory is complicated by the fact that the nonnovel items are by definition studied more frequently than the novel items (see Dobbins, Kroll, Yonelinas, & Liu, 1998).

An important question is whether findings from studies that manipulate primary distinctiveness using the von Restorff paradigm will generalize to other forms of novelty. As we discuss below, there are some subtle differences among the effects produced by different novelty manipulations, but there are important generalizations that can be made about the effects of novelty on memory, and a relatively consistent story is emerging regarding the brain regions that are critically involved in various forms of novelty processing.

THE EFFECTS OF STIMULUS NOVELTY ON RECOLLECTION AND FAMILIARITY

Although the beneficial effects of stimulus novelty on free recall have been studied extensively (e.g., Hunt, 1995; Saltz & Newman, 1959; von Restorff, 1933; Wallace, 1965), relatively little is known about how novelty influences the processes supporting recognition memory. In this chapter, we focus on recognition memory, and we examine the effects of stimulus novelty on the two recognition subcomponents (i.e., recollection and familiarity). Recognition memory judgments can be based on recollection of qualitative information about previous study events or on assessments of episodic familiarity. Results from behavioral, neuroimaging, patient studies, and studies of rats and nonhuman primates have indicated that recollection and familiarity are functionally distinct and rely on partially distinct brain regions (for reviews, see Aggleton & Brown, 1999; Eichenbaum, Otto, & Cohen, 1994; Rugg & Yonelinas, 2003; Yonelinas, 2002). For example, recollection is a relatively slow retrieval process dependent on the hippocampus and the prefrontal cortex, whereas familiarity is a relatively fast retrieval process dependent on regions in the temporal cortex such as the parahippocampal gyrus.

Although stimulus novelty has been found to increase overall recognition memory accuracy (e.g., Fabiani & Donchin, 1995; Parker et al., 1998; von Restorff, 1933), it is less clear whether novelty influences recollection or familiarity-based recognition judgments. Addressing this issue is important because it has been suggested that one way of differentiating between recollection and familiarity is the extent to which they are sensitive to stimulus novelty. Two conflicting hypotheses have been proposed: the recollection-distinctiveness and familiarity-novelty hypotheses.

The Recollection-Distinctiveness Hypothesis

Rajaram (1996, 1998; also see Dobbins et al., 1998) suggested that the analysis of salient or distinctive aspects of items leads to recognition memory responses accompanied by the subjective experience of remembering, whereas variations in the processing fluency of items gives rise to feelings of familiarity in the absence of recollection (i.e., knowing). Although Rajaram (1996, 1998) did not make claims about recollection and familiarity processes per se, but rather focused exclusively on the subjective experiences of remembering and knowing (cf. Tulving, 1985), it is possible that this distinction also holds for the processes of recollection and familiarity that give rise to these subjective experiences (see Dobbins et al., 1998).

Support for the recollection-distinctiveness hypothesis comes from two sources. First, because robust stimulus novelty effects using the von Restorff paradigm have been observed in free recall (e.g., Hunt, 1995; Saltz & Newman, 1959; von Restorff, 1933; Wallace, 1965), and recollection is expected to be functionally similar to the search process involved in free recall (Mandler, 1980), it follows that recollection should be sensitive to stimulus novelty. Second, Rajaram (1998) found that orthographically distinctive words (e.g., *subpoena*) led to better recognition memory than orthographically common words (e.g., *sailboat*). Most important, in that study, recognition was measured using Tulving's (1985) remember/know procedure, and the distinctiveness advantage was observed in recognized items associated with remember responses, but not with items accepted as familiar in the absence of recollection (i.e., know responses).

The Familiarity-Novelty Hypothesis

There is reason to question the recollection-distinctiveness hypothesis, however, and to suspect that familiarity rather than recollection is selectively sensitive to novelty. The motivation for this familiarity-novelty hypothesis is that novelty and familiarity might reflect two extremes of the same continuum, and that the same mechanism that leads an item to appear novel might also be used as a basis for familiarity-based recognition judgments (e.g., "If it appears to be novel and I don't remember studying the item, then it probably was not studied"). This hypothesis is supported by a study that examined novelty using the von Restorff paradigm (Parker et al., 1998), in which human and nonhuman primates exhibited better recognition memory for the novel items (i.e., visual shapes were presented in a novel color, compared to shapes presented in a color that was more common in the experiment). Although the study did not include separate measures of recollection and familiarity, lesions in the nonhuman primates designed to isolate the hippocampal formation did not disrupt the novelty effects on memory, whereas lesions that included the surrounding parahippocampal gyrus eliminated the novelty effects. In light of previous studies indicating that the hippocampus supports recollection, whereas the parahippocampal gyrus supports familiarity-based recognition responses (e.g., Aggleton & Brown, 1999; Eichenbaum et al., 1994; Yonelinas, 2002; Yonelinas et al., 2002), these results suggest that stimulus novelty influences familiarity-based recognition, but not recollection-based recognition.

Examining the Effects of Primary Novelty Using the von Restorff Paradigm

In order to assess these two competing hypotheses, we examined the effects of stimulus novelty on recollection and familiarity-based recognition (Kishiyama & Yonelinas, 2003). For example, in experiment 2 in that study, subjects were presented with a study list containing a majority of nonnovel items (e.g., red thumbnail object images) mixed with a small number of novel items (e.g., yellow thumbnail object images). Note that experiment 1 used slightly different stimuli but led to similar conclusions. The objects and their colors were counterbalanced across subjects to control for possible effects of stimulus color and item differences. At the time of test, subjects were presented with a list of studied and new items and were required to make recognition judgments. Note that the color of the items did not change between study and test, and the test contained an equal number of new items in red and yellow. Recognition memory was measured using the remember/know procedure (Gardiner, 1988; Tulving, 1985), in which subjects were instructed to make a remember response if they could recollect some qualitative information about the study event in which that item was earlier presented, a know response if the item was familiar but they could not recollect anything specific about the study event, or a new response if they thought the item was not studied.

The remember and know responses were used to derive estimates of recollection and familiarity. Because subjects were instructed to respond "remember" whenever an item was recollected, the probability of a remember response was used as an estimate of recollection (i.e., R = remember). Because subjects were instructed to respond "know" when an item was familiar in the absence of recollection (i.e., know = $F(1 - R)$), familiarity was estimated as the probability of a know response given that an item was not recollected (i.e., F = know/$(1 - R)$; Yonelinas & Jacoby, 1995). To incorporate false-alarm rates the estimates of recollection and familiarity for old and new items were used as hits and false alarms to derive d' estimates of accuracy (MacMillan & Creelman, 1991). Note that we also measured recollection and familiarity using hits-minus-false-alarm measures of accuracy, and this led to the same pattern of results.

Two groups of subjects were tested. One group studied items under intentional encoding instructions in which they were told to try to remember the items for a later memory test, and the other group encoded the items under incidental encoding conditions in which they were told to count the number of symmetrical items in the list. The two encoding conditions were selected to produce approximately equivalent levels of recognition, and were included in order to test the generalizability of the novelty effects across different encoding conditions. Note that previous studies using tests of free recall have shown that novelty effects are observed under conditions of intentional (Koyanagi, 1957), but not incidental encoding (Gleitman & Gillett, 1957; Postman & Phillips, 1954; Saltzman & Carterette, 1959; but see Hunt & Lamb, 2001). If recollection involves a retrieval process that is similar to that involved in recall (e.g., Mandler, 1980), then one would expect the novelty effects on recollection to be reduced under incidental encoding conditions. Whether the novelty effects on familiarity would also be influenced by this manipulation was not clear.

Figure 17.1 presents the estimates of recollection and familiarity for novel and nonnovel items encoded under intentional and incidental encoding conditions. For the intentional group, both recollection and familiarity were greater for the novel than for the nonnovel items, indicating that both processes increased with stimulus novelty. This pattern has been observed in two other experiments (Kishiyama & Yonelinas, 2003, Experiment 1; Kishiyama, Yonelinas, & Lazzara, 2004) and was observed in the vast majority of subjects tested, indicating that it is quite robust. In contrast, for the incidental group, novelty effects were observed only in familiarity. Moreover, direct comparisons indicated that incidental compared to intentional encoding led to a significant reduction in the novelty effects seen on recollection, but that the encoding conditions did not affect the extent to which familiarity was sensitive to stimulus novelty. The former findings are consistent with results from tests of free recall (e.g., Gleitman & Gillett, 1957; Postman & Phillips, 1954; Saltzman & Carterette, 1959) in showing that novelty effects on recollection were reduced under incidental compared to intentional encoding conditions. Before interpreting these results, we briefly discuss related studies that have examined the effects of novelty on recollection and familiarity using different types of novelty manipulations.

Examining the Effects of Secondary Novelty

Do recollection and familiarity benefit from secondary forms of novelty (i.e., cases in which items are infrequent or unusual relative to other items of the same type)? An examination of the existing literature suggests that

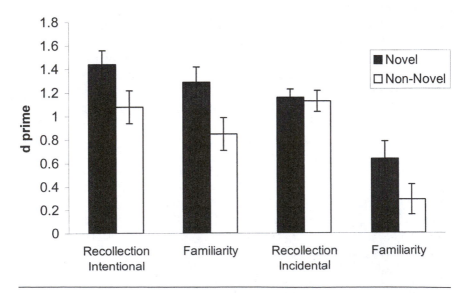

FIGURE 17.1 Estimates of recollection and familiarity for novel and nonnovel items following intentional and incidental encoding instructions.

they do. For example, Figure 17.2 presents the effects of orthographic distinctiveness, word frequency, and face typicality on recollection and familiarity, and indicates that all three of these forms of secondary distinctiveness lead to increases in both recollection and familiarity. The orthographic distinctiveness results are from the remember-know study by Rajaram (1998). As with the von Restorff experiment described above, we estimated recollection as the probability of a remember response, whereas familiarity was estimated as the probability of a know response given the item was not remembered. To account for response bias, false-alarm rates were subtracted from hits. This method was used because d' estimates could not be easily derived based on the experimental procedures in some of the studies described below. Figure 17.2a shows that orthographically distinctive items led to similar increases in both recollection and familiarity, compared to orthographically common words.

Word frequency is also found to influence both processes, such that recollection and familiarity are greater for low- compared to high-frequency words. Figure 17.2b presents the average estimates across a large number of studies using a variety of methods of measuring recollection and familiarity. The same pattern is seen across studies using Tulving's (1985) remember-know procedure (Bowler, Gardiner, & Grice, 2000; Gardiner & Java, 1990; Gardiner, Richardson-Klavehn, & Ramponi, 1997; Guttentag & Carroll, 1997; Hirshman, Fisher, Henthorn, Arndt, & Passannante, 2002; Joordens & Hockley, 2000; Kinoshita, 1995; Reder et al., 2000; Strack & Foerster, 1995), Jacoby's (1991) process-dissociation procedure (Guttentag & Carroll, 1997; Komatsu, Graf, & Uttl, 1995), and Yonelinas's (1994) receiver operating characteristic (ROC) procedure (Arndt & Reder, 2002). In every case, there was a low-frequency advantage for recollection and a smaller but consistent advantage for familiarity.

Finally, faces judged to be atypical are associated with greater recollection and familiarity than those judged to be typical. That is, Brandt, Macrae, Schloerscheidt, and Milne (2003) had subjects study typical and atypical faces under full or divided-attention conditions, then tested recognition memory using the remember-know procedure. Based on the remember and know responses, we estimated recollection and familiarity using the same procedure employed in the previous studies. Figure 17.2c shows that for faces encoded under full attention, atypical faces were associated with greater recollection and familiarity-based responses than were typical faces, indicating that both processes were sensitive to novelty. Moreover, the figure also indicates that for faces encoded under divided-attention conditions, the novelty effect on familiarity was still present, whereas the novelty effect on recollection was largely reduced. These effects are similar to those we saw with intentional versus incidental encoding in the von Restorff paradigm (i.e., the manipulation did not influence the familiarity-based novelty effects but did disrupt the recollection-based novelty effects). We return to this point later.

a.

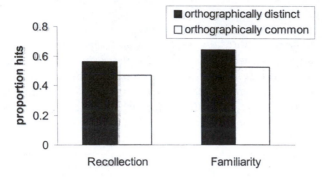

b.

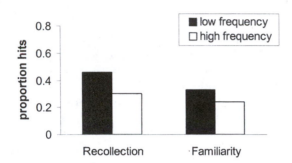

c.

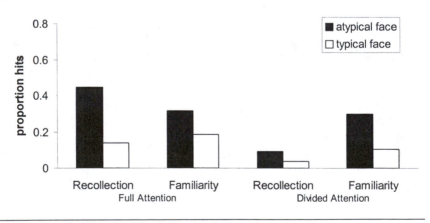

FIGURE 17.2 Estimates of recollection and familiarity across manipulations of orthographic distinctiveness (a), word frequency (b), and face typicality (c).

The results of these behavioral studies indicate that both primary novelty, as manipulated in the von Restorff paradigm, and secondary novelty, as manipulated by orthographic distinctiveness, word frequency, and face typicality, can lead to increases in recollection and familiarity. Thus, both memory processes benefit from different types of stimulus novelty. Note, however, that there were subtle differences in the degree to which each process was affected by these different types of novelty. For example, the extent to which recollection was affected by the von Restorff manipulation was dependent on whether the encoding was intentional or incidental. In contrast, the extent to which recollection and familiarity were influenced by word frequency does not appear to be much different in experiments that used intentional encoding (e.g., Gardiner & Java, 1990; Guttentag & Carroll, 1997) compared to those that used incidental encoding instructions (e.g., Kinoshita, 1995; Komatsu et al., 1995). Moreover, in all of the word-frequency experiments, the low- versus high-frequency advantage on recollection was numerically larger than that seen on familiarity, indicating that recollection might be more sensitive to this form of novelty than familiarity. In contrast, the von Restorff effects on familiarity were slightly larger and more consistent across encoding conditions than those seen on recollection (e.g., Kishiyama & Yonelinas, 2003). Future studies that more directly assess the relative sensitivity of recollection and familiarity to different forms of novelty will be useful, but it is now quite clear that both processes can benefit from both primary and secondary distinctiveness.

The existing results indicate that sensitivity to novelty does not provide a simple way of differentiating between recollection and familiarity. Thus, the results do not support the recollection-distinctiveness hypothesis in which novelty effects are expected to be driven primarily by recollection (e.g., Dobbins et al., 1998; Rajaram, 1998). Moreover, the results are also problematic for the familiarity-novelty hypothesis in which the effects are expected to be driven primarily by familiarity (e.g., Parker et al., 1998). Although previous studies have indicated that these two processes are differentially sensitive to a number of manipulations, such as levels of processing and response speeding (for a review, see Yonelinas, 2002), the current results indicate that they are not as easily separated on the basis of their sensitivity to stimulus novelty.

Two Distinct Effects of Novelty

Although both recollection and familiarity can benefit from stimulus novelty, the existing results suggest that the two processes differ in the manner in which they are influenced by these manipulations. That is, although the novelty effects seen on familiarity were not influenced by the intentional/incidental encoding manipulation, the novelty effects seen on recollection were (e.g., Kishiyama & Yonelinas, 2003). Similarly, the novelty effects on familiarity were not sensitive to the attentional encoding manipulation, whereas the novelty effects on recollection were (e.g., Brandt et al., 2003). These results indicate that the novelty effects on recollection and familiarity are functionally distinct and that the mechanisms that produce novelty effects on these two processes may therefore be different. Exactly what those different mechanisms are is not yet clear, but there are several possibilities.

Automatic versus Controlled Responses to Novelty

One possible account for the different effects of novelty on recollection and familiarity is that there may be separate controlled and automatic responses to novel items that differentially influence these processes. This possibility is suggested by the work of Jacoby and colleagues (e.g., Jacoby, 1991; Jacoby & Dallas, 1981; Jacoby & Witherspoon, 1982; Kelley & Jacoby, 2000) that indicates that recollection reflects a consciously controlled process, whereas familiarity is relatively automatic. Thus, novel items may lead to an automatic orienting response (Knight, 1996; Knight & Nakada, 1998; Schmidt, 1991) that may preferentially enhance subsequent familiarity-based recognition. In addition, novelty may lead to further elaborative or controlled processing (e.g., Karis, Fabiani, & Donchin, 1984; Schmidt, 1991), and this elaborative processing may preferentially benefit recollection. Consistent with this possibility is the observation that novelty effects on recollection, but not familiarity, were reduced by incidental encoding and divided attention—two manipulations known to have differential effects on automatic and controlled processes (e.g., Hasher & Zacks, 1979; Schneider & Shiffrin, 1977).

As a preliminary test of the automatic/controlled explanation, we examined the effects of novelty on perceptual implicit memory. We reasoned that if the novel items elicited an automatic orienting response that was responsible for an increase in memory, then the von Restorff effects should be observed in implicit measures of memory that are generally regarded as relatively automatic (e.g., Jacoby, Toth, & Yonelinas, 1993). We used the same materials and study procedures as in the incidental condition in the recognition memory experiment described above (i.e., Kishiyama & Yonelinas, 2003, Experiment 2), but at the time of test, subjects received a perceptual identification test rather than a recognition test. That is, the test objects were presented at a rapid rate intermixed with visually scrambled nonobjects, and subjects were required to make object/nonobject decisions for each item. After the test, an awareness questionnaire based on that used by Bowers and Schacter (1990) was administered to determine if subjects used explicit memory on the implicit test. Five of the 20 subjects claimed to have used explicit memory on the test, but their performance did not differ from the other subjects so they were not excluded from the analysis.

The results of the study indicated that there were significant priming effects, but that stimulus novelty did not influence performance (see Fig. 17.3). In fact, the priming effects are numerically slightly larger for the non-novel than the novel items. The results are consistent with prior studies indicating that perceptual implicit memory is not typically sensitive to or-

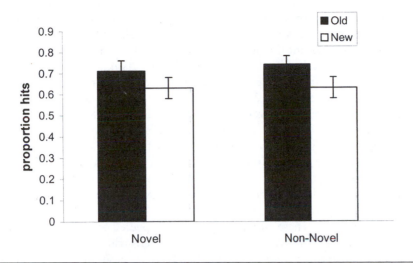

FIGURE 17.3 Proportions of correct object/nonobject decisions to old and new items for novel and nonnovel items.

thographic distinctiveness (Geraci & Rajaram, 2002; Kinoshita & Miller, 2000; but see Hunt & Toth, 1990) or manipulations of bizarreness (Nicolas & Marchal, 1996, 1998).

To the extent that novelty does not influence implicit memory, the results argue against the view that the von Restorff effects reflect an automatic orienting response to novel items. Thus, the results do not provide support for the claim that the von Restorff effects we observed in familiarity reflect an automatic orienting response. It should be noted, however, that more direct tests of the claim that the novelty effects on familiarity reflect an automatic response to novelty are needed. For example, it is important to determine whether more conceptual forms of implicit memory are sensitive to these novelty manipulations before one can rule out the automatic orienting explanation.

Effects of Novelty on Encoding versus Retrieval

Another possible account of the different novelty effects seen on recollection and familiarity is that the effects on recollection may reflect enhanced encoding of novel items, whereas the effects on familiarity may reflect reduced interference at the time of retrieval. Evidence that the effects of novelty seen on recollection but not familiarity were encoding-related comes from the observation that the novelty effects on recollection were modulated by encoding manipulations like intentional/incidental learning and full/divided attention whereas the novelty effects on familiarity were not modulated by these encoding manipulations (e.g., Brandt et al., 2003; Kishiyama & Yonelinas, 2003). Conversely, evidence that the effects of novelty on familiarity might arise at the time of retrieval comes from an examination of false-alarm rates. In general, false-alarm rates are lower for the novel items than for the nonnovel items. Given that the new items were not studied, it would seem that these novelty effects might be due, at least in part, to retrieval effects (e.g., reduced interference for the novel items; but see Worthen & Wood, 2001a, 2001b). That is, for a novel test item (e.g., a yellow item), there were far fewer interfering novel items (i.e., yellow studied items) than for a nonnovel test item (e.g., red items; for discussion of encoding and retrieval accounts of the von Restorff effect: see Fabiani & Donchin, 1995; Hunt & Lamb, 2001; Karis et al., 1984; Schmidt, 1991). In studies examining the von Restorff, word frequency, orthographic distinctiveness, and face distinctiveness effects, the novelty effect in false-alarm rates was carried largely by the know responses rather than the remember responses. These findings might be expected if one assumes that novelty effects on familiarity occur at time of retrieval.

In sum, the existing studies indicate that both recollection and familiarity-based recognition benefit from stimulus novelty. These effects are observed for both primary and secondary forms of novelty across a wide variety of experiments. The results thus argue against simple theoretical distinctions that align either recollection or familiarity alone with sensitivity to stimulus novelty. Although novelty can influence both recollection and familiarity, it does have dissociative effects on these two processes, indicating that there are at least two different responses to novelty observed in recognition. Whether these dissociations reflect distinct automatic and controlled or separate encoding- and retrieval-based responses to novelty is still largely unanswered. Future studies that address this issue will be critical in fully understanding why stimulus novelty leads to improvements in recollection and familiarity.

The Neuroanatomical Substrates of Novelty Processing

Neuroanatomical Theories of Novelty and Human Memory

Several anatomically motivated theories have been proposed to account for the effects of novelty on recall and recognition (e.g., Metcalfe, 1993, 1994; Tulving & Kroll, 1995; Tulving, Markowitsch, Kapur, Habib, & Houle, 1994). Although these theories differ in important ways, they are in agreement in the sense that novelty advantages in memory are assumed to reflect the interaction of episodic memory storage mechanisms in the medial temporal lobes and monitoring mechanisms supported by the prefrontal cortex. For example, Metcalfe (1993, 1994) developed a computational model that includes an episodic memory system that relies on the medial temporal lobes and a monitoring system that relies on the prefrontal cortex. The medial temporal lobes are assumed to be involved in assessing the degree of novelty for each item by comparing the item to information currently stored in memory. A prefrontal monitoring mechanism then differentially weights events to be encoded into memory on the basis of their relative novelty, such that novel events receive higher weights than familiar events. Similarly, Tulving and colleagues (Tulving & Kroll, 1995; Tulving et al., 1994) have argued that cortical and subcortical neural networks of the limbic system and the temporal lobes assess information for novelty and adaptive significance. Redundant or familiar information is screened from further processing, while relevant novel information is transmitted to the prefrontal cortex for higher elaborative or meaning-based encoding operations. On the basis of these models, one expects both the medial temporal lobes and the prefrontal cortex to be directly involved in producing novelty-related enhancements in memory.

Neuroimaging and Animal Studies of Novelty

A variety of brain regions are sensitive to stimulus novelty, including the prefrontal cortex, the thalamus, and various temporal lobe regions such as the hippocampus and the surrounding parahippocampal gyrus (for a review, see Ranganath & Rainer, 2003). For example, human brain imaging studies have shown that visually distinctive items and items that are presented for the first time (compared with repeated items), elicit greater activation throughout the temporal lobes as well as the thalamus and prefrontal cortex (e.g., Gabrieli et al., 1997; Kirchhoff et al., 2000; Martin, 1999; Menon et al., 2000; Stern et al., 1996; Tulving et al., 1996). Novelty responses have also been observed in the human medial temporal lobes using intracerebral recordings (Fried, MacDonald, & Wilson, 1997; Halgren et al., 1995, 1980). Furthermore, the P3a event-related scalp potential that is associated with unexpected stimuli is significantly reduced in human patients with medial temporal (Knight, 1996) or prefrontal cortex damage (Daffner et al., 2000; Knight, 1984; Knight & Scabini, 1998). A thorough review of the P3a is provided in Chapter 15, this volume. Moreover, single-unit recording studies in rats and nonhuman primates have identified novelty-sensitive neurons in the hippocampus (Rolls, Cahusac, Feigenbaum, & Miyashita, 1993), the parahippocampal gyrus (Brown, Wilson, & Riches, 1987; Fahy, Riches, & Brown, 1993; Riches, Wilson, & Brown, 1991), and the thalamus (Aggleton & Brown, 1999; Fahy et al., 1993).

These studies, however, do not indicate which structures are critical in producing novelty-related enhancements in memory because subsequent memory was typically not measured. Moreover, the activation studies indicate only which regions are sensitive to novelty; they do not show which regions play a necessary role in producing the novelty advantage in memory. For example, because repetition leads items to be more rapidly processed (i.e., repetition priming), reductions in activation related to repeated items may reflect priming effects rather than the enhanced encoding of novel stimuli (Wiggs & Martin, 1998). Thus, studies that examine novelty effects in patients with damage to these regions are essential for determining which regions play a critical role in producing novelty-related enhancements in memory.

We previously mentioned a lesion study that examined the von Restorff effect in nonhuman primates (Parker et al., 1998). Evidence from that study indicated that the hippocampus does *not* play a critical role in producing novelty effects, but that other brain regions, including the frontal lobes, the thalamus, and the anterior portion of the parahippocampal gyrus, are directly involved. In particular, Parker et al. found that lesions designed to isolate the hippocampus (i.e., bilateral amygdala and fornix lesions) did not disrupt the novelty effects, whereas lesions disconnecting the anterior parahippocampal gyrus and either the frontal lobes or medial dorsal thalamus eliminated the novelty effects. Given that the hippocampus is assumed to play a central role in the medial temporal lobe memory system, these results present a serious challenge to the existing memory models of novelty. However, it is not known whether comparable effects are observed in humans.

Novelty Effects in Human Amnesia

In a recent study, we examined whether the regions damaged in temporal lobe amnesic patients were necessary for the novelty-related memory enhancements seen in the von Restorff paradigm (Kishiyama et al., 2004). Although amnesics are expected to have lower levels of recognition memory than controls, whether or not they would exhibit a memory advantage for novel compared with nonnovel items was unknown. We tested 10 amnesic patients with damage to the medial temporal lobe system and 10 age-matched control subjects in the same von Restorff recognition test procedure described earlier.

The results were surprising in showing that the novelty effects seen in the control subjects were significantly reduced, and essentially eliminated, in the amnesic patients. Because the amnesics performed more poorly than the controls, we conducted an additional analysis that included only the lowest performing half of the control group. Note that this did not influence the magnitude of the novelty effect in the control group. The results—presented separately for three different patient subgroups—indicate that in contrast to the control group, none of the patient subgroups showed any evidence of a novelty effect (see Fig. 17.4). The H+ group consisted of 6 patients with damage to the hippocampus and surrounding parahippocampal gyrus, and included posterior cerebral artery infarct patients and temporal lobectomy patients. The H group consisted of 3 post-hypoxic cardiac arrest patients expected to have selective hippocampal atrophy. One additional patient was included who had bilateral thalamic infarcts (Th) (this patient is described in more detail in Kishiyama et al., in press). For each patient, the damage was verified on the basis of magnetic resonance

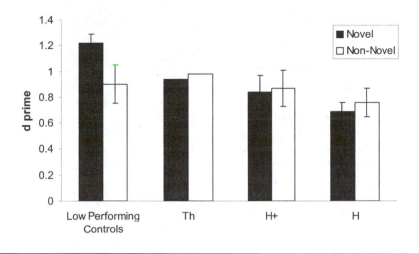

FIGURE 17.4 Overall recognition performance for novel and nonnovel items for controls, patients with hippocampal damage (H), patients with damage to the hippocampus and parahippocampal gyrus (H+), and a patient with thalamic damage (Th).

imaging, with the exception of the hypoxic patients, who could not be scanned because they had defibrillators. However, histological studies have indicated that mild hypoxic patients of this type exhibit damage limited primarily to the hippocampus (Cummings, Tomiyasu, Read, & Benson, 1984; Rempel-Clower, Zola, Squire, & Amaral, 1996).

Recollection and familiarity estimates were derived on the basis of remember and know responses. As in the previous experiments (e.g., Kishiyama & Yonelinas, 2003), both recollection and familiarity increased for novel compared to nonnovel items in the control subjects. In contrast, in the amnesic patients, neither recollection nor familiarity was sensitive to novelty. These results indicate that the regions damaged in the amnesic patients were necessary for producing novelty-related enhancements in both recollection- and familiarity-based recognition.

The finding that temporal lobe amnesia eliminated the novelty effects provides direct support for the existing memory models of novelty by demonstrating the importance of this region in novelty-related memory enhancements. Moreover, the fact that the novelty effects were eliminated in the hypoxic patients and in the thalamic patient indicates that the human hippocampus and thalamus play critical roles in producing the novelty advantage in memory. Whether or not the parahippocampal gyrus plays a critical role in these novelty effects cannot be determined on the basis of the current results. The H+ patients showed no evidence of a novelty effect, but they suffered damage to the parahippocampal gyrus as well as the hippocampus, either of which may have been responsible for the reduced novelty effects.

The current results are consistent with previous studies showing that the hippocampus and thalamus are involved in novelty processing (e.g., Gabrieli et al., 1997; Halgren et al., 1995; Kirchoff et al., 2000; Knight, 1996; Stern et al., 1996; Tulving et al., 1996). The results, however, are not consistent with Parker et al.'s (1998) finding that the hippocampus was not involved in producing von Restorff effects in nonhuman primates. Because of the many differences between the two studies, it is not possible to determine with certainty why this discrepancy arose. One possibility is that there may be inherent differences in how human and nonhuman primates respond to novelty in the von Restorff paradigm. Another possibility is that the discrepancy may be due to the different lesion locations in the two studies. The H group in the current study consisted of hypoxic patients who are known to suffer damage to the hippocampus, whereas the group in the Parker et al. study underwent amygdala and fornix resections. Although the fornix represents one major output of the hippocampus, the hippocampus may still be able to support novelty detection and encoding through interactions via reciprocal connections with other temporal lobe structures such as the entorhinal, perirhinal, and parahippocampal cortices (Suzuki, 1996; Suzuki & Amaral, 1994). In any case, the current results indicate that, at least in humans, the hippocampus does appear to be necessary for producing normal novelty effects in recognition memory. Whether it plays a similar role in nonhuman primates is less clear.

If recollection and familiarity are supported by the hippocampus and parahippocampal gyrus, respectively, then why did hippocampal damage disrupt the novelty effect on familiarity? One possibility is that during the time of encoding, these two regions interact to produce increases in subsequent memory for novel items. For example, the temporal lobes, including the parahippocampal gyrus, may be involved in identifying the abstract identity of each object independent of its specific perceptual characteristics (e.g., see Rolls, 2000). As such, this region would not be sensitive to the novelty manipulation used in the present study. However, the detection of novelty in the hippocampus may trigger additional processing in the surrounding temporal lobe regions that are involved in identifying that object. This may lead to increases in familiarity for novel items at time of retrieval.

Whether the hippocampus plays a critical role in other forms of novelty-related memory effects, such as secondary distinctiveness, is not known. However, the existing literature suggests that this region may be involved in processing a variety of types of novelty. For example, orienting responses to novel events are reduced in patients with hippocampal damage (Knight, 1996), and the hippocampus responds preferentially to a number of different novelty manipulations including perceptual, semantic, and emotionally distinctive items (e.g., Kirchhoff et al., 2000; Stern et al., 1996; Strange & Dolan, 2001).

Novelty Effects After Damage to the Prefrontal Cortex

To examine whether the prefrontal cortex plays a necessary role in novelty effects, we are currently examining patients with damage to the lateral prefrontal cortex. These patients have unilateral dorsolateral lesions resulting from a single infarction of the precentral branch of the middle cerebral artery (see Sylvester & Shimamura, 2002). Preliminary results from 2 patients with left hemisphere damage and 2 patients with right hemisphere damage, as well as from age-matched control subjects, are presented in Figure 17.5. Although the study is not yet complete, the results suggest that the patients with left prefrontal lobe damage exhibit normal novelty effects whereas patients with right hemisphere damage show no evidence of novelty effects. The finding that the right hemisphere alone seems to be critical is intriguing because previous studies have suggested that it may be particularly critical for novelty detection (e.g., Martin, 1999). At a minimum, the results provide preliminary support for models assuming that the frontal lobes play a critical role in producing novelty-related enhancements in memory (e.g., Metcalfe, 1993, 1994; Tulving & Kroll, 1995; Tulving et al., 1994).

Evaluation of the Neuroanatomical Models of Novelty and Human Memory

The models of novelty and memory (e.g., Metcalfe, 1993; Tulving et al., 1994) have proved useful in guiding research, and the current results verify the core assumptions of those models in showing that the hippocampus

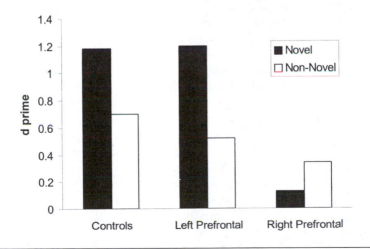

FIGURE 17.5 Overall recognition performance for novel and nonnovel items for controls, patients with left prefrontal damage, and patients with right prefrontal damage.

and frontal lobes play central roles in producing the novelty effects on memory. It is important to note that the roles of these regions go beyond the traditional role of encoding and retrieval in long-term episodic memory. For example, if this were the sole function of the hippocampus, then recognition of novel and nonnovel items should have been equally affected in amnesic patients. However, the differential reduction of memory for novel items in these patients indicates that the hippocampus plays a direct role in novelty detection.

There are, however, several important limitations to these models. First, they do not currently differentiate between recollection and familiarity or between hippocampal and parahippocampal functions. Given the behavioral dissociations that we observed between recollection and familiarity with respect to their responses to stimulus novelty, further modifications of these models would seem necessary. Second, these models treat novelty effects as arising solely as a function of enhanced processing at time of encoding. To the extent that the current results suggest that at least part of the novelty advantage arises because of a reduction in interference at time of retrieval, the models may not accurately describe why these novelty effects are observed.

CONCLUSION

Recognition memory is enhanced for novel compared to nonnovel items. This effect occurs because novelty increases the likelihood that items will be later recollected and because it increases the likelihood that they will be recognized on the basis of familiarity. These effects are observed for primary distinctiveness, in which items are made unusual in an immediate context (e.g., the von Restorff paradigm), and for secondary distinctiveness, in which items are unusual in a more global context (e.g., orthographic distinctiveness, word frequency, and face atypicality effects). These results indicate that simple theoretical distinctions aligning either recollection or familiarity alone with sensitivity to stimulus novelty are not generally viable. Nonetheless, the effects of novelty on recollection and familiarity can be dissociated, suggesting that there are at least two different responses to novelty observed in recognition memory (e.g., automatic/controlled or encoding/retrieval-related responses). The results of our patient investigations join a growing body of research indicating that regions in the medial temporal and frontal lobes are sensitive to stimulus novelty, but also indicate that they play a necessary role in producing novelty-related enhancements in recognition memory. Moreover, these results support existing memory models of novelty by indicating that the novelty enhancements in memory may reflect the contribution of episodic memory storage mechanisms supported by the hippocampus and monitoring mechanisms supported by the prefrontal cortex.

ACKNOWLEDGMENTS

We are grateful to Kilianne Kimball, Alexandra Velasquez, and Amber Whitney for their comments on an earlier version of this manuscript. Research in this chapter was supported by NIMH MH 59352 and P01 NS40813 (A.Y.). Portions of this chapter were presented to the Southwestern Psychological Association, New Orleans, LA 2003.

REFERENCES

Aggleton, J. P., & Brown, M. B. (1999). Episodic memory, amnesia and the hippocampal-anterior thalamic axis. *Behavioral and Brain Sciences, 22,* 425–489.

Arndt, J., & Reder, L. M. (2002). Word frequency and receiver-operating characteristic curves in recognition memory: Evidence for a dual-process interpretation. *Journal of Experimental Psychology: Learning, Memory, and Cognition, 28,* 830–842.

Bowers, J. S., & Schacter, D. L. (1990). Implicit memory and test awareness. *Journal of Experimental Psychology: Learning, Memory, and Cognition, 16,* 404–416.

Bowler, D. M., Gardiner, G. M., & Grice, S. J. (2000). Episodic memory and remembering in adults with Asperger syndrome. *Journal of Autism & Developmental Disorders, 30* (4), 295–304.

Brandt, K. R., Macrae, C. N., Schloerscheidt, A. M., & Milne, A. B. (2003). Remembering or knowing others? Person recognition and recollective experience. *Memory, 11*(4), 89–100.

Brown, M. W., Wilson, F. A. W., & Riches, I. P. (1987). Neuronal evidence that inferomedial temporal cortex is more important than hippocampus in processing underlying recognition memory. *Brain Research, 409,* 158–162.

Cummings, J. L., Tomiyasu, U., Read, S., & Benson, D. F. (1984). Amnesia with hippocampal lesions after cardiopulmonary arrest. *Neurology, 34,* 679–681.

Daffner, K. R., Mesulam, M. M., Scinto, L. F. M., Acar, D., Calvo, V., Faust, R., et al. (2000). The central role of the prefrontal cortex in directing attention to novel events. *Brain, 123,* 927–939.

Dobbins, I. G., Kroll, N. E. A., Yonelinas, A. P., & Liu, Q. (1998). Distinctiveness in recognition and free recall: The role of recollection in the rejection of the familiar. *Journal of Memory and Language, 38,* 381–400.

Eichenbaum, H., Otto, T., & Cohen, N. J. (1994). Two functional components of the hippocampal memory system. *Behavioral and Brain Sciences, 17,* 449–518.

Fabiani, M., & Donchin, E. (1995). Encoding processes and memory organization: A model of the von Restorff effect. *Journal of Experimental Psychology: Learning, Memory, and Cognition, 21,* 224–240.

Fahy, F. L., Riches, I. P., & Brown, M. W. (1993). Neuronal activation related to visual recognition memory: Long-term memory and the encoding of recency and familiarity information in the primate anterior and medial inferior temporal and rhinal cortex. *Experimental Brain Research, 96*, 457–472.

Fried, I., MacDonald, K. A., & Wilson, C. L. (1997). Single neuron activity in human hippocampus and amygdala during recognition of faces and objects. *Neuron, 18*, 753–765.

Gabrieli, J., Brewer, J. B., Desmond, J. E., & Glover, G. H. (1997). Separate neural bases of two fundamental memory processes in the human medial temporal lobe. *Science, 276*, 264–266.

Gardiner, J. M. (1988). Functional aspects of recollective experience. *Memory & Cognition, 16*, 309–313.

Gardiner, J. M., & Java, R. I. (1990). Recollective experience in word and nonword recognition. *Memory & Cognition, 18*, 23–30.

Gardiner, J. M., Richardson-Klavehn, A., & Ramponi, C. (1997). On reporting recollective experiences and "direct access to memory systems". *Psychological Science, 8(5)*, 391–394.

Geraci, L., & Rajaram, S. (2002). The orthographic distinctiveness effect on direct and indirect tests of memory: Delineating the awareness and processing requirements. *Journal of Memory and Language, 47*, 273–291.

Gleitman, H., & Gillett, E. (1957). The effect of intention upon learning. *Journal of General Psychology, 57*, 137–149.

Guttentag, R. E., & Carroll, D. (1997). Recollection-based recognition: Word frequency effects. *Journal of Memory & Language, 37(4)*, 502–516.

Halgren, E., Baudena, P., Clarke, J. M., Heit, G., Marinkovic, K., Devaux, B., et al. (1995). Intracerebral potentials to rare target and distractor stimuli: 2. Medial, lateral, and posterior temporal lobe. *Electroencephalography and Clinical Neurophysiology, 94*, 229–250.

Halgren, E., Squires, N. K., Wilson, C. L., Rohrbaugh, J. W., Babb, T. L., & Crandall, P. H. (1980). Endogenous potentials generated in the human hippocampal formation and amygdala by infrequent events. *Science, 210*, 803–805.

Hasher, L., & Zacks, R. T. (1979). Automatic and effortful processes in memory. *Journal of Experimental Psychology: General, 108*, 356–388.

Hirshman, E., Fisher, J., Henthorn, T., Arndt, J., & Passannante, A. (2002). Midazolam amnesia and dual-process models of the word-frequency mirror effect. *Journal of Memory and Language, 47*, 499–516.

Hunt, R. R. (1995). The subtlety of distinctiveness: What von Restorff really did. *Psychonomic Bulletin and Review, 2(1)*, 105–112.

Hunt, R. R., & Lamb, C. A. (2001). What causes the isolation effect? *Journal of Experimental Psychology: Learning, Memory, and Cognition, 27(6)*, 1359–1366.

Hunt, R. R., & Toth, J. P. (1990). Perceptual identification, fragment completion, and free recall: Concepts and data. *Journal of Experimental Psychology: Learning, Memory, and Cognition, 16(2)*, 282–290.

Jacoby, L. L. (1991). A process dissociation framework: Separating automatic from intentional uses of memory. *Journal of Memory and Language, 30*, 513–541.

Jacoby, L. L., & Dallas, M. (1981). On the relationship between autobiographical memory and perceptual learning. *Journal of Experimental Psychology: General, 110,* 306–340.

Jacoby, L. L., Toth, J. P., & Yonelinas, A. P. (1993). Separating conscious and unconscious influences of memory: Measuring recollection. *Journal of Experimental Psychology: General, 122*(2), 139–154.

Jacoby, L. L., & Witherspoon, D. (1982). Remembering without awareness. *Canadian Journal of Psychology, 36,* 300–324.

Joordens, S., & Hockley, W. E. (2000). Recollection and familiarity through the looking glass: When old does not mirror new. *Journal of Experimental Psychology: Learning, Memory, and Cognition, 26,* 1534–1555.

Karis, D., Fabiani, M., & Donchin, E. (1984). "P300" and memory: Individual differences in the von Restorff effect. *Cognitive Psychology, 16,* 177–216.

Kelley, C. M., & Jacoby, L. L. (2000). Recollection and familiarity: Process-dissociation. In E. Tulving & F. I. M. Craik's (Eds.), *The Oxford handbook of memory* (pp. 215–228). New York: Oxford University Press.

Kinoshita, S. (1995). The word frequency effect in recognition memory versus repetition priming. *Memory & Cognition, 23*(5), 569–580.

Kinoshita, S., & Miller, M. (2000). The orthographic distinctiveness effect on fragment completion: Not implicit. *Australian Journal of Psychology, 52,* 63–68.

Kinsbourne, M., & George, J. (1974). The mechanism of the word-frequency effect on recognition memory. *Journal of Verbal Learning & Verbal Behavior, 13,* 63–69.

Kirchhoff, B. A., Wagner, A. D., Maril, A., & Stern, C. E. (2000). Prefrontal-temporal circuitry for episodic encoding and subsequent memory. *The Journal of Neuroscience, 20,* 6173–6180.

Kishiyama, M. M., & Yonelinas, A. P. (2003). Novelty effects on recollection and familiarity in recognition memory. *Memory & Cognition, 31,* 1045–1051.

Kishiyama, M. M., Yonelinas, A. P., Kroll, N. E. A., Lazzara, M. M., Jones, E.G., & Jagust, W. J. (in press). Bilateral anteromedial thalamic lesions affect recollection and familiarity-based recognition memory judgments. *Cortex.*

Kishiyama, M. M., Yonelinas, A. P., & Lazzara, M. M. (2004). The von Restorff effect in amnesia: The contribution of the hippocampal system to novelty-related memory enhancements. *Journal of Cognitive Neuroscience, 16,* 15–23.

Knight, R. T. (1984). Decreased responses to novel stimuli after prefrontal lesions in man. *Electroencephalography and Clinical Neurophysiology, 59,* 9–20.

Knight, R. T. (1996). Contribution of the human hippocampal region to novelty detection. *Nature, 383,* 256–259.

Knight, R.T., & Nakada, T. (1998). Cortico-limbic circuits and novelty: A review of EEG and blood flow data. *Reviews in the Neurosciences, 9,* 57–70.

Knight, R. T., & Scabini, D. (1998). Anatomic bases of event-related potentials and their relationship to novelty detection in humans. *Journal of Clinical Neurophysiology, 15,* 3–13.

Komatsu, S., Graf, P., & Uttl, B. (1995). Process dissociation procedure: Core assumptions fail, sometimes. *European Journal of Cognitive Psychology, 7*(1), 19–40.

Koyanagi, K. (1957). Studies in incidental learning: II. Interaserial interference. *Tohoku Psychologica Folia, 15,* 1–12.

MacMillan, N. A., & Creelman, C. D. (1991). *Detection theory: A user's guide.* New York: Cambridge University Press.

Mandler, G. (1980). Recognizing: The judgment of previous occurrence. *Psychological Review, 87,* 252–271.

Martin, A. (1999). Automatic activation of the medial temporal lobe during encoding: Lateralized influences of meaning and novelty. *Hippocampus, 9,* 62–70.

Menon, V., White, C. D., Eliez, S., Glover, G. H., & Reiss, A. L. (2000). Analysis of a distributed neural system involved in spatial information, novelty, and memory processing. *Human Brain Mapping, 11,* 117–129.

Metcalfe, J. (1993). Monitoring and gain control in an episodic memory model: Relation to the P300 event-related potential. In A. F. Collins, S. E. Gathercole, M. A. Conway, & P. E. Morris (Eds.), *Theories of memory* (pp. 327–353). Hillsdale, NJ: Lawrence Erlbaum Associates.

Metcalfe, J. (1994). A computational modeling approach to novelty monitoring, metacognition, and frontal lobe dysfunction. In J. Metcalfe & A. P. Shimamura (Eds.), *Metacognition: Knowing about knowing* (pp. 137–156). Cambridge, MA: MIT Press.

Nicolas, S., & Marchal, A. (1996). Picture bizarreness effect and word association. *Current Psychology of Cognition, 15,* 629–643.

Nicolas, S., & Marchal, A. (1998). Implicit memory, explicit memory and the picture bizarreness effect. *Acta Psychologica, 99,* 43–58.

Parker, A., Wilding, E., & Ackerman, C. (1998). The von Restorff effect in visual object recognition memory in humans and monkeys: The role of frontal/perirhinal interaction. *Journal of Cognitive Neuroscience, 10,* 691–703.

Postman, L., & Phillips, L. W. (1954). Studies in incidental learning: I. The of crowding and isolation. *Journal of Experimental Psychology, 48,* 48–56.

Rajaram, S. (1996). Perceptual effects on remembering: Recollective processes in picture recognition memory. *Journal of Experimental Psychology: Learning, Memory, and Cognition, 22*(2), 365–377.

Rajaram, S. (1998). The effects of conceptual salience and perceptual distinctiveness on conscious recollection. *Psychonomic Bulletin & Review, 5*(1), 71–78.

Ranganath, C., & Rainer, G. (2003). Neural mechanisms for detecting and remembering novel events. *Nature Reviews. Neuroscience, 4*(3), 193–202.

Reder, L. M., Nhouyvanisvong, A., Schunn, C. D., Ayers, M. S., Angstadt, P., & Hiraki, K. (2000). A mechanistic account of the mirror effect for word frequency: A computational model of remember-know judgments in a continuous recognition paradigm. *Journal of Experimental Psychology: Learning, Memory, & Cognition, 26*(2), 294–320.

Rempel-Clower, N. L., Zola, S. M., Squire, L. R., & Amaral, D. G. (1996). Three cases of enduring memory impairment after bilateral damage limited to the hippocampal formation. *Journal of Neuroscience, 16*, 5233–5255.

Riches, I. P., Wilson, F. A. W., & Brown, M. W. (1991). The effects of visual stimulation and memory on neurons in the hippocampal formation and the neighboring parahippocampal gyrus and inferior temporal cortex of the primate. *Journal of Neuroscience, 11*, 1763–1779.

Rolls, E. T. (2000). Functions of the primate temporal lobe cortical visual areas in invariant visual object and face recognition. *Neuron, 27*, 205–218.

Rolls, E. T., Cahusac, P. M. B., Feigenbaum, J. D., & Miyashita, Y. (1993). Responses to single neurons in the hippocampus of the macaque related to recognition memory. *Experimental Brain Research, 93*, 299–306.

Rugg, M. D., & Yonelinas, A. P. (2003). Human recognition memory: A cognitive neuroscience perspective. *Trends in Cognitive Sciences, 7*, 313–319.

Saltz, E., & Newman, S. E. (1959). The von Restorff isolation effect: Test of the intralist association assumption. *Journal of Experimental Psychology, 58*, 445–451.

Saltzman, I. J., & Carterette, T. (1959). Incidental and intentional learning of isolated and crowded items. *American Journal of Psychology, 72*, 230–235.

Schmidt, S. R. (1991). Can we have a distinctive theory of memory? *Memory & Cognition, 19*(6), 523–542.

Schneider, W., & Shiffrin, R. M. (1977). Controlled and automatic human information processing: I. Detection, search, and attention. *Psychological Review, 84*(1), 166.

Stern, C. E., Corkin, S., Gonzalez, R. G., Guimaraes, A. R., Baker, J. R., Jennings, P. J., et al. (1996). The hippocampal formation participates in novel picture encoding: Evidence from functional magnetic resonance imaging. *Proceedings of the National Academy of Sciences USA, 93*, 8660–8665.

Strack, F., & Foerster, J. (1995). Reporting recollective experiences: Direct access to memory systems? *Psychological Science, 6*(6), 352–358.

Strange, B. A., & Dolan, R. J. (2001). Adaptive anterior hippocampal responses to oddball stimuli. *Hippocampus, 11*, 690–698.

Suzuki, W. A. (1996). The anatomy, physiology and functions of the perirhinal cortex. *Current Opinion in Neurobiology, 6*, 179–186.

Suzuki, W. A., & Amaral, D. G. (1994). Topographic organization of the reciprocal connections between the monkey entorhinal cortex and the perirhinal and parahippocampal cortices. *Journal of Neuroscience, 14*, 1856–1877.

Sylvester, C. C., & Shimamura, A. P. (2002). Evidence for intact semantic representations in patients with frontal lobe lesions. *Neuropsychology, 16*, 197–207.

Tulving, E. (1985). Memory and consciousness. *Canadian Psychologist, 26*, 1–12.

Tulving, E., & Kroll, N. (1995). Novelty assessment in the brain and long-term memory encoding. *Psychonomic Bulletin & Review, 2*(3), 387–390.

Tulving, E., Markowitsch, H. J., Craik, F. I. M., Habib, R., & Houle, S. (1996). Novelty and familiarity activations in PET studies of memory encoding and retrieval. *Cerebral Cortex, 6,* 71–79.

Tulving, E., Markowitsch, H. J., Kapur, S., Habib, R., & Houle, S. (1994). Novelty encoding networks in the human brain: Positron emission tomography data. *NeuroReport, 5,* 2525–2528.

von Restorff, H. (1933). Uber die wirkung von bereichsbildungen im spurenfeld. *Psychologische Forschung, 18,* 299–342.

Wallace, W. P. (1965). Review of the historical, empirical, and theoretical status of the von Restorff phenomenon. *Psychological Bulletin, 63*(6), 410–424.

Wiggs, C. L., & Martin, A. (1998). Properties and mechanisms of perceptual priming. *Current Opinion in Neurobiology, 8,* 227–233.

Worthen, J. B., & Wood, V. V. (2001a). Memory discrimination for self-performed and imagined acts: Bizarreness in false recognition. *Quarterly Journal of Experimental Psychology: Human Experimental Psychology, 54A,* 49–67.

Worthen, J. B., & Wood, V. V. (2001b). A disruptive effect of bizarreness on memory for relational and contextual details of self-performed and other-performed acts. *American Journal of Psychology, 114,* 535–546.

Yonelinas, A. P. (1994). Receiver operating characteristics in recognition memory: Evidence for a dual-process model. *Journal of Experimental Psychology: Learning, Memory, and Cognition, 20,* 1–14.

Yonelinas, A. P. (2002). The nature of recollection and familiarity: A review of 30 years of research. *Journal of Memory & Language, 46,* 441–517.

Yonelinas, A. P., & Jacoby, L. L. (1995). The relation between remembering and knowing as bases for recognition: Effects of size congruency. *Journal of Memory and Language, 34,* 622–643.

Yonelinas, A. P., Kroll, N. E. A., Quamme, J. R., Lazzara, M. M., Sauve, M., Widaman, K. F., & Knight, R. T. (2002). Effects of extensive temporal lobe damage or mild hypoxia on recollection and familiarity. *Nature Neuroscience, 5,* 1236–1241.

VII

DENOUEMENT

18

What Do Explanations of the Distinctiveness Effect Need to Explain?

Endel Tulving and R. Shayna Rosenbaum

What do explanations of the distinctiveness effect need to explain? What a silly question this is. Surely what needs to be explained is the *distinctiveness effect*, the phenomenon that items or events that stand out from others in a collection or series are usually more readily recalled than items that do not stand out in the same way.[1] It does not matter much how these special items or events stand out or how we label them—distinct, isolated, salient, vivid, novel, incongruent, surprising, affect-laden, or whatever. For our present purposes, we treat these forms of distinctiveness as the same, and ask instead: What do explanations of the enhanced recall of these outstanding items need to explain?[2]

In one sense, of course, as Reed Hunt has argued in his introductory chapter as well as elsewhere (e.g., Hunt & Lamb, 2001), the superior memorability of distinctive events needs no explanation at all because, according to what Hunt calls the *intuitive theory*, it is obvious. Events that stand out are salient—they catch attention—and attention, as everyone knows, facilitates memory. The distinctiveness effect—the superior memorability of distinctive items—may therefore be thought of as what the philosopher Stephen Toulmin (1961) classified as a "natural given," a kind of happening in the world that every thinking individual knows and understands, a kind about which there is no felt urge to raise questions (e.g., Why is water wet?). Only happenings that deviate from the general norm, those that do not make immediate sense—or "phenomena," in Toulmin's terms—need exploration and explanation (e.g., Why does water turn into ice?).

Now, as frequently happens in science, when one takes a closer look, things may turn out to be more complex than they appeared to be initially. There are problems with the intuitive theory, and as Hunt has pointed out, the problems do not have to do only with the fit between data and theory but also with some of the basic concepts and terms that are used in attempts to create such fits.

Given the problems with the intuitive theory, a search for a better account, or better accounts, of the distinctiveness effect is called for. In this volume, one finds a variety of ways of framing the issues to be explored, a variety of approaches to problems that arise, and a variety of explanations of the phenomena that are seen as requiring explanation. Our chapter is meant to contribute to the ongoing debate by presenting and elaborating a variation on an idea that, although well known to the researchers, has not been popular in the past and has not been seriously explored. It represents a minority view in the present collection of papers.

SUPERIOR, SPECIAL OR INFERIOR, STANDARD ITEMS?

The popular framing of the issue is stated in terms of the *superior recall* of more distinctive over less distinctive stimuli or events. This tradition began with Mary Calkins's (1896) approach to the study of the effects of vividness on memory. What we need to understand, according to this approach, is why more distinctive items of experience are more readily recallable than less distinctive ones. What needs explanation is the superior memorability of distinctive items.

This superior-recall approach appears repeatedly in the contributions to this volume. Geraci and Rajaram (Chapter 10 this volume), for example, maintain the theme of superior recall throughout their chapter and conclude, "As several contributions in this volume as well as findings from our work show, distinctiveness ubiquitously *aids* explicit memory performance. In this chapter, we have shown that it can also aid implicit memory (p. 228)." Fabiani (Chapter 15 this volume), in her review of event-related potential components sensitive to distinctiveness, nicely demonstrates how "the processing of distinctive events is underlined by multiple phenomena, each of which may contribute, directly or indirectly, to the *enhanced* memory performance that often accompanies distinctive events (p. 340)." Kishiyama and Yonelinas (Chapter 17 this volume) refer to superior recall when they talk about "the relative novelty of different events" those that are unusual or distinctive are remembered *better* than those that are less distinct (p. 381)." Schacter and Wiseman (Chapter 5 this volume) discuss how a distinctiveness heuristic serves to *benefit* subsequent memory by helping to reduce or suppress false recognition of novel items (see also Schacter, Israel, & Racine, 1999).

The logical alternative to the superior-recall approach could be called the *inferior-recall* approach. It is stated in terms of the inferior recall of less distinctive in comparison with more distinctive items. What needs to be explained, according to this view, is not the superior recall of the special events (distinctive, salient, isolated, incongruous, surprising, etc.) but, rather, the impoverished recall of the standard events (nondistinctive, regular, massed, congruous, nonsurprising).

These two logical possibilities are well known to all researchers: The recall of the special items in a collection is enhanced *in relation to* the recall of standard items in the same collection. We are talking about relative rather than absolute values. Enhanced recall of special items does not imply any spectacularly superior achievement by some superhuman standard, the kind of "Wow! Look at that!" performance that characterizes the memory expert.[3]

But, at this point, the skeptical reader will ask, What difference does merely changing the wording of the *description* of the phenomenon make for its explanation? If a theory explains why the bottle is half full, it also explains why it is half empty, and vice versa, does it not? Surely we are only caviling about words and not talking about the ways of nature. Surely the words one uses cannot possibly make any difference to the facts or to the theoretical ideas that one may wish to express about those facts. One can, of course, choose to say that the bottle is half empty rather than half full, or vice versa, but the choice serves only to tell the pessimists from the optimists. Both logically and pragmatically, the two expressions mean the same thing. One can say, as we have done, that the memorability of nondistinctive items is low when compared with that of distinctive items, but both logically and pragmatically, this expression does not tell us anything that is not there in the proposition that memorability of distinctive items is high. If A is superior to B, then of course by logic and by definition B is inferior to A, and whatever one says about the superiority of A also automatically applies to the inferiority of B.

As long as we speak rather generally, the critical reader is correct. But when we delve into the matter a bit more deeply, we find that some subtlety is called for. Even in the half-full/half-empty analogy the two alternatives are, strictly speaking, not logically interchangeable. When a bottle is half full, we know what it is half full *of*; when it is half empty, we do *not* know what it half empty *of*. We can *assume* that what is missing in the upper half is the same stuff that is present in the lower, but that is merely a guess. The guess, as all guesses, may or may not be correct. A similar situation arises when we compare the superior recall of special items with the inferior recall of standard items.

Although the logic of the comparison is impeccable, there is more to the game of science than logic. Sometimes words do make a difference, as Hunt and Lamb (2001) have pointed out in discussing this very issue. In the present case, we think that they make a difference that counts. We thus beg the skeptical reader to bear with us and to withhold judgment until after we have told our story.

We prefer the inferior-recall approach because, as it turns out, it can help us to understand a wider range of phenomena than superior recall of distinctive items in the von Restorff-type experiments. We will list and briefly discuss these other phenomena presently.

In the story we tell here, the von Restorff-type distinctiveness effect, and other members of the same conceptual family, can be seen as a special instance of a general category. This is a category of instances in which impoverished recall of one particular subset of items makes recall of items in another subset appear to be superior by comparison, even if it is not superior in any absolute sense. In all the instances in this category, according to our story, the superior recall of the special events becomes a natural given, about which no (further) questions need be asked, and the inferior recall of the standard items becomes the phenomenal happening that requires study and explanation.

Another distinctive feature here is a new concept (*camatosis*) that figures prominently in our story. It can be defined and discussed abstractly, as a hypothetical construct whose sole purpose is to help tie together otherwise unrelated phenomena, but it is also reasonable to assume that something corresponding to the term actually exists as a part of the physiologic operations of the brain. The introduction of a physiological concept, as we will see, also helps us to overcome circular reasoning necessarily inherent in some of the purely psychological explanations of the distinctiveness effect (see Baddeley, 1978; Schmidt, 1991).

What Needs Explanation?

Our thesis here is that there is nothing especially noteworthy about the memorability—recognition, recall, recollection—of the special (outstanding) items in distinctiveness paradigms and, accordingly, nothing much to be explained. Special items are encoded "normally," as might happen in a neutral "cognitive environment" (Tulving, 1983; Watkins, 1979), or in the presence of a (hypothetical) "default mode of brain function" (Raichle et al., 2001; Gusnard, Akbudak, Shulman, & Raichle, 2001). Recall of special (distinctive, isolated, incongruous) items reflects what subjects' memory systems are capable of encoding for long-term storage, by virtue of their evolved physical structure and by virtue of the consequences of accumulated past experiences, in the absence of any situational constraints, whether physiological or psychological. Such "normal" or "baseline" recall requires no explanation. Instead, what does need explanation is the inferior recall of standard (nondistinctive, massed, congruous) events. Once we understand why standard events are so poorly recalled, the "distinctiveness effect" also becomes clear.

In situations under scrutiny, the reasons for impaired recall of standard items do not lie inherent in the identity of these items. We could take any one of the standard items and, by manipulating the composition of the list, have them serve the role of a distinctive item. Standard and special items in a collection are perfectly interchangeable. In a string of letters, a digit is special and every one of the letters is standard. But any such letter would be special in a string of digits. Thus, as conceptualized by von Restorff

(1933) and elaborated by Reed Hunt in this volume (Chapter 1) and else-where: what makes items distinctive (or special as we have been referring to them) is not the nominal identity of the item as such, but rather the way they are organizationally and distinctively processed (Hunt & McDaniel, 1993).

If any standard item could in principle serve as a special item and be recalled "normally," at a level that the capability of the memory system al-lows, then it must be something in the situation in which it is processed that keeps its recall suboptimal. There must be something that does not al-low the processing of the standard items to reach their natural potential, the kind of potential that they, too, would readily demonstrate if they were special items in the collection. What is that something?

The textbook answer is that what constrains, or puts the brakes on, the execution of the full potential of processing of an event is interference. Von Restorff (1933) called the relevant determinant *interference* and, for her time, quite appropriately so. Now, more than 70 years later, things are a bit more complicated. For one, the term *interference* has suffered the same fate as many others in the science of memory (Tulving, 2000): it has ac-quired a number of rather different meanings. It could refer to a hypo-thetical process, an observed reduction in memory performance, a relation between two associations, a block that prevents effective learning or recall; it has thus become unacceptably vague. For another, in its purely descrip-tive sense, it readily leads to circular reasoning. Thus, if we ask what causes the poor recall of massed items in a list, we could say that it is interfer-ence. But if we then ask how we know it is interference, there is not much else to do but point to poor recall as evidence.

THE CAMATOSIS HYPOTHESIS

We propose that what is responsible for poor recall of standard items is something that we call *camatosis*. The term is derived from *kamatos*, a word in classical Greek that can be translated into English as "tiredness" or "weariness."[4] We introduce this term partly to escape the circularity of reasoning inherent in most existing ideas, but mostly in order to relate the distinctiveness effect to other memory-based phenomena.

Camatosis is a (hypothetical) physiological process in the brain: a spe-cific activity-dependent fatigue or weariness of a neuronal network or en-semble that results from the execution of a particular behavioral/cognitive task. It is analogous to the fatigue that many biological systems incur as a consequence of their operations. Camatosis manifests itself in the diminu-tion of the operational or functional efficacy of a particular neural ensem-ble to do again at time T2 what it did at an earlier time T1. It is closely related to the concept of *neural fatigue* that has occasionally been used in discussions of a variety of phenomena, such as adaptive filtering (Desimone, 1992), stimulus specific adaptation (Ringo, 1996), and neuronal habituation (Sohal & Hasselmo, 2000), as well as various kinds of sensory adaptation (Carandini, 2000; Clifford, 2002; Toppino, Long, & Mondin, 1992). We give it a distinctive name in order to discuss it specifically as a process that plays a role, possibly a crucial role, in memory by influencing encoding of information for long-term storage, a key process in memory (Tulving, 1983).

Although camatosis of a given neuronal ensemble can be defined with respect to a single event, such as the presentation of an item in a list of to-be-remembered items, behavioral analysis of its putative role in encoding requires two events (or occurrences of stimuli) that are processed sequentially. The typical situation in which such processing occurs is one of temporal succession: event 1 occurs at time T1, and event 2 at a subsequent time T2, either immediately or after an interval. (The same analysis applies to situations in which two items are physically presented simultaneously but psychologically processed sequentially). The pair-based analysis can be extended to longer sequences of successive events by redefining event 1 in terms of a string of events.

We propose the camatosis hypothesis as an aid to understanding the distinctiveness effect, as well as related phenomena that we will describe: The processing of later events in a series suffers to the extent that it is affected by the camatosis of the neuronal ensembles subserving the processing of earlier events. We designate the earlier events collectively as event 1 and the subsequent events as event 2.

The processing of event 1 causes camatosis in the corresponding neuronal ensemble. If the processing of event 2 requires the recruitment of components of the neuronal ensemble that is camatotic as a result of its participation in the earlier act of processing event 1, this processing will be impaired, unless additional (compensatory) neural resources can be recruited for that purpose. The extent of such camatotic impairment depends on the extent of neurocognitive similarity between events 1 and 2. The greater the similarity, the greater the overlap between the neuronal ensembles corresponding to events 1 and 2, the greater the need of the (camatotic) neuronal ensemble of event 1 for the processing of event 2, and hence the greater the likelihood of the reduction in the efficacy of such processing.

Consider the extreme case of massed repetition: complete nominal identity between two events that immediately follow each other in time. Their corresponding neuronal activity would be expected to be highly similar. (Not identical, of course.) After event 1 is processed for long-term storage, the corresponding ensembles are camatotic for a while and the processing of event 2 remains incomplete as a result. Under such conditions of massed repetition, the recall of the repeated item suffers. In some cases, massed repetition can be totally useless and the resulting recall may be no higher than that of an item presented just once (Waugh, 1970).

If we assume that camatosis is (at least usually) transitory, it would be reasonable to expect that when repetition is distributed, in the sense that other items intervene between the successive appearances of a given target item, the effectiveness of repetition increases, as indeed it does (Madigan, 1969; Waugh, 1970). Waugh (1970) accounted for the striking effect of distributed repetition in her study in terms of *displaced rehearsal*, which was a perfectly fine explanation for the time. Today, we can also say that her data very nicely reflect the operation of camatosis. The memory system, like many other cognitive systems, can well encode change—alteration of the stimulating conditions—but cannot encode constancy. From the point of evolution, such systems make good sense: nonchange is evolutionarily irrelevant (see also Fabiani, Chapter 15 this volume, for a related idea).

In the more typical case in which successive events are not nominally identical, camatosis of event 1 affects encoding of event 2 to the extent of their neurocognitive similarity (as well, of course, as a function of other variables, such as the temporal relations between the events). Any two events always are similar to each other because they always share some features, thereby calling for the engagement of partly overlapping neuronal ensembles. Thus, the feature of visualness, wordness, or printedness may require the involvement of partially overlapping neuronal ensembles and are thereby potentially subject to camatosis, even if the printed words are different graphemically and semantically. One of the major sources of camatosis is the environmental "context" in which the events occur, which is almost invariably the same.

Consider some illustrative examples of the operation of camatosis in experimental situations in which successive events (appearances of to-be-remembered items) are different instances of one and the same category. All the examples are of the well-known phenomenon called the primacy effect. The primacy effect is defined by the higher recall of the first, in comparison to the second, of two successively presented items. It has been shown in laboratory experiments on list learning, such as free recall of unrelated words (e.g., Murdock, 1962; Craik, 1971) as well as in paired-associate recall (e.g., Tulving & Arbuckle, 1963; Madigan & McCabe, 1972). Prominent primacy effects are also shown by people suffering from amnesia (e.g., Baddeley & Warrington, 1970). Primacy effects are found in experiments on delayed recognition of visual patterns by humans, monkeys, and pigeons (Wright, Santiago, Sands, Kendrick, & Cook, 1985). Rats, too, seem to have a special fondness for the first happening in a series (e.g., Bouton, 1993). There is a large literature on young human infants' proclivity for primacy, under the label of the so-called A-not-B paradigm, a proclivity shared by monkeys (e.g., Diamond, 1988; Diamond & Goldman-Rakic, 1989) and adult human amnesics (e.g., Schacter, Moscovitch, Tulving, McLachlan, & Freedman, 1986). Even in a minimal paired-associate task in which the subjects are shown only two pairs of simple verbal items and a few seconds later are tested for one or the other pair, the first pair is retained better than the second. And there is nothing much that either the subject or the experimenter can do about changing this inferiority of recall of the second pair (Peterson & Peterson, 1962). By a small stretch of the imagination, one can even conceive of an affinity between the clinically well-known perseveration effect in patients with damage to their frontal lobes (Stuss & Benson, 1986) and the patients' difficulty or inability to learn the second of two successively presented facts (e.g., Lezak, Howieson, & Loring, 2004).

We suggest that all these varied instances of the primacy effect make as much sense in light of the camatosis hypothesis as do the various distinctiveness effects seen in von Restorff-type experiments.

Related Empirical Facts

We have suggested that the understanding of massed versus distributed repetition effects, as well as various kinds of primacy effects, can benefit from the concept of camatosis and, more specifically, from the camatosis hypothesis, as does the understanding of the distinctiveness effect. We next list some additional facts and findings reported in the memory literature that can be thought of as candidates for analysis in terms of camatosis. Because of the scope of our chapter, we cannot describe any of them at length and can only recommend that interested readers consult the original sources.

One phenomenon that can be accounted for in terms of the camatosis hypothesis is the buildup of proactive interference (PI) in short-term memory (e.g., Keppel & Underwood, 1962) and its release. The release from PI occurs either as a result of waiting a minute or two (e.g., Loess & Waugh, 1967) or by shifting the materials to a new category (e.g., Wickens, 1970). Increasing the interval between the presentations of successive sets of items presumably works because of random episodic silent thoughts (REST; Andreasen et al., 1995), or endogenous mental activity occurring during the interval. In either case, however, one can imagine that the psychological phenomenon of a buildup of PI signals the increasing effect of camatosis, and release from PI signals the lessened dependence of the processing of shifted target items on the camatotic neuronal ensembles subserving the PI buildup items.

In a paired-associate study of negative transfer and retroactive interference, Bower, Thompson-Schill, & Tulving (1994) found that categorical similarity of pairs within a list greatly retarded learning. Holding constant everything else, including the nominal identity of the members of a to-be-learned pair, and varying only the conceptual categories of other pairs in the list, the researchers found that the memorability of a given pair was drastically changed. We assume that category-dependent camatosis resulted in impaired encoding and hence impaired recall of categorically homogeneous lists.

Camatosis might provide one basis for detection or assessment of novelty. In an earlier paper (Tulving & Kroll, 1995) it was suggested that "familiar items are less well recognized than novel items because the novelty-assessment system screens out familiar items from further processing for subsequent recognition at an early stage of encoding" (p. 389). Instead of screening out familiar items, such items would be encoded less efficaciously because of camatosis.

The concept of camatosis may also be relevant to the understanding of some other cognitive phenomena of attention, perception, and memory. These might include, but need not be limited to, attentional blink (e.g., Raymond, Shapiro, & Arnell, 1992), negative priming (e.g., Tipper, 1985), inhibition of return (e.g., Spence & Driver, 1998), habituation in infants (e.g., Trehub, 2001) and animals (e.g., Sokolov, 1963), flashbulb memories (e.g., Conway et al., 1994), and "repetition suppression" (e.g., Desimone, 1996). Even the understanding of phenomena such as negatively accelerated learning curves and the advantage of subject-performed tasks (Nilsson, 2000) may benefit from the inclusion of camatosis in theoretical accounts of these phenomena.

We could provide further examples, but the selection above, we trust, makes the intended point: when other conditions are held constant, negative transfer frequently occurs. That is, the processing of one item presented in a collection is impaired by virtue of the processing of *other* items. Such negative transfer can be interpreted in terms of the camatosis hypothesis. The general underlying principle is that no event in the brain, or in the mind, ever occurs, nor can it be understood, in isolation of other events.

RELATED THEORETICAL IDEAS

Apart from the novel terminology, there is little that is original about the concept of camatosis, or the camatosis hypothesis. We referred earlier to physiological concepts such as habituation and adaptation that are closely related to what we call camatosis. But camatosis is also closely related to several purely psychological concepts that have been proposed to account for phenomena of learning and memory that come under the general rubric of interference, as well as those that are treated under the label of inhibition. Experimental studies of these phenomena can be traced back to Müller and Pilzecker (1900) and indeed for a period in history, phenomena and theories of interference occupied the center stage of learning and memory (McGeoch & Irion, 1952; Underwood & Postman, 1960; Waugh & Norman, 1965).

The inferior-recall approach appears in von Restorff's original work. She attributed inferior recall of massed items to interference among them. The same approach was also taken by Hunt and Lamb (2001): "We shall also assume that the isolation effect is due to impoverished conditions for the control item, but our particular hypothesis about the disadvantage is different from von Restorff's" (p. 1360). Whereas von Restorff, more than 70 years ago, ascribed the interference among the homogeneous items to the nature of the to-be-remembered materials (inter-item similarity), Hunt and Lamb, operating within the Zeitgeist of today's processing views of memory (Craik & Lockhart, 1972; Foster & Jelicic, 1999), derive the inferiority of recall of massed items from their hypothesized deficiency of organizational and distinctive processing (see also Hunt & McDaniel, 1993). Our proposal is that at least part of this inferiority is attributable to camatosis.

The idea of similarity has always occupied the center stage in interference-based phenomena of memory. In interference theories, impoverished retention of the standard items is accounted for in terms of their similarity to one another, and the consequent interference in their processing (von Restorff, 1933). Concepts such as associative interference, retroactive interference, (response) competition, proactive inhibition (PI), release from PI, cue overload, the fan effect, and others sharing family resemblance with these, define the boundaries of the domain within which the implications of the camatosis hypothesis, and the concept of similarity, can be explored. In the development of the camatosis hypothesis, we have assumed, as a basic given, that in addition to the specification of the nominal identity of the target events or items, similarity requires the specification of the processing of the events at the time of their original occurrence, the principle of encoding specificity, and the context (neurocognitive environment) in which the to-be-remembered event occurs.

Let us try to be clear about what the camatosis hypothesis can do and what it cannot do. It postulates the physiological existence of camatosis (multifaceted fatigue of specific neuronal ensembles) that, under certain conditions, leads to suboptimal processing of perceived events for long-term memory storage. And it offers suggestions as to how this hypothetical construct may work in situations where such suboptimal processing comes about. If one accepts at least the general line of reasoning that the camatosis hypothesis represents, one can understand why some events in a collection of events are encoded more effectively than others and, hence, exhibit higher recall. The camatosis hypothesis, if accepted, renders unnecessary any specific theoretical accounts of the superior recall of distinctive events because the principles governing such recall are no different from those governing recall of all events under camatosis-free conditions. Finally, the camatosis hypothesis holds that the distinctiveness effect represents only one particular, methodologically defined instance of a larger class of similar phenomena, each of which can be seen as reflecting the operations of the hypothetical camatotic process.

The camatosis hypothesis leads to a number of expected consequences of presentation of items. A couple of examples are mentioned here.

1. *Temporal context effects.* To the extent that two items, A and B, are similar and draw upon overlapping neural processing resources, their processing is subject to camatosis. This means that when the two items are presented in sequence, the specific encoding of A (and of B) varies depending upon whether it is presented first or second in the sequence. To the extent that the nature of the specific encoding

of an item determines the effectiveness of retrieval cues for A (and B)—the so-called encoding specificity principle—the camatosis hypothesis predicts that the effectiveness of a particular cue for a target A would differ depending on the position of A (and B) in the encoding sequence.

2. *Spatial context effects.* To the extent that two items, A and B, are similar, drawing upon overlapping neural processing resources, their processing is subject to camatosis. When the two items are presented side by side at the same time, the specific encoding of A (and of B) differs from what it would have been in the absence of camatosis, for example, had it been presented alone. Following such encoding, therefore, a copy cue, A' (or B'), as in a yes/no recognition test, is less effective when it appears alone than when it appears as a member of the original pair.

3. *Encoding variability.* If a given item A is presented twice, the encoding of the second presentation is subject to camatosis produced by the first presentation. This camatosis reduces the effectiveness of the encoding of the second presentation of A to the extent that the encoding processes are similar on the two occasions. When the second presentation follows the first immediately (at lag 0), such similarity is likely to be greater than it is with larger interpresentation distances, and hence the effectiveness of the second presentation is likely to increase with such distance.

Although the camatosis hypothesis leads to certain expectations, as we have just seen, it alone of course cannot explain specific findings that can be obtained in experimental situations in which camatosis may be present and in which its consequences affect the findings. It is seldom that a single-factor hypothesis can account for the detailed outcomes of experiments or happenings in real life, in which large numbers of variables and their interactions are at work, and the camatosis hypothesis is no exception to the rule.

The camatosis hypothesis claims a sufficiency relation—if A, then B—between a hypothesized entity (camatosis) and the efficacy of a hypothetical process (encoding of perceptual information for long-term storage). As such, it is necessarily silent on other sufficiency relations. Specifically, it does not rule out the possibility (near certainty, perhaps) that other variables and experimental conditions produce behavioral outcomes of experiments or happenings in real life that look like distinctiveness effects. Indeed, Schmidt, in Chapter 3 this volume, urges that it is essential to distinguish between novelty and significance, both of which can produce what may appear as distinctiveness effects. We agree.

There is no reason to doubt that other variables and other processes (other than camatosis) can selectively influence the recall of individual items of a collection. These other processes may include those known under terms such as strategic processing, or distinctive processing that Hunt writes about. After all, *any* specific item in a collection or a series can always be *selected*, wittingly or unwittingly, for special cognitive treatment and, as a consequence, encoded for storage more efficaciously than nonselected items. Whether the instructions for such special treatment are provided by the experimenter or self-generated by the subject is presumably not of primary importance. Even such a trivial feature as the color of a printed word may be used to thus set apart some items in an otherwise homogeneous list that are then recalled better than the nonselected or massed items. But that does not necessarily mean that camatosis is at the root of such differentiation. It may turn out to be true, of course, but such a conclusion cannot yet be safely drawn against the backdrop of the evidence currently available.

The other relevant factors may also include conditions such as those designated as novelty, as discussed by Kishiyama and Yonelinas in Chapter 17, this volume. There is a good deal of evidence that novel events are better retained than are less novel ones. One can argue that novelty operates like distinctiveness—novel events stand out in a collection in which other events are less novel. It is always possible, of course, that what makes strategic processes, or novelty, effective turns out to be some camatosis-like process. But it is too early to tell.

Conclusion

In this chapter we adopt what we refer to as the inferior-recall approach to the problem of explaining the distinctiveness effect. We propose a hypothetical but possibly real physiological process, camatosis, and use it to account for suboptimal processing and hence suboptimal subsequent recall of standard events in a collection. The camatosis hypothesis holds that specific neural ensembles (or pathways, or circuits, or systems) that correspond to specific cognitive processes become weary as a result of their activity and are therefore less readily available for the support of identical or similar processes. As a consequence, the encoding of similar items is impaired, and recall is impaired, while recall of nonsimilar or distinctive items, by comparison, appears to be superior.

The camatosis hypothesis applies not only to the von Restorff-type isolation and distinctiveness effects but also to a number of other kindred phenomena that include primacy effects, massed versus distributed repetition effects, buildup and release from proactive inhibition, rapid learning of heterogeneous lists, novelty detection, latent inhibition, and so on. Such a wider applicability of the hypothesis will be further explored in future research.

The concept of camatosis is closely related to psychological concepts such as habituation and interference, but they are not identical. Camatosis is a hypothesized physiological process or mechanism that is postulated as one of the *causes* of habituation and interference. It provides a possible way out of the circular reasoning involved in, say, attributing reduced or less than optimal execution of memory-related tasks to interference while at the same time inferring the operation of interference from the reduced performance.

In any case, at the very least, the concept of camatosis can serve as a foundation for an alternative theoretical perspective within which one can characterize the distinctiveness effect. It provides another way of thinking about the problem, and thereby presents as a major contrast with existing theories that look for psychological explanations of the superior memorability of distinctive events. We readily admit, of course, that ours is a rather speculative account, even if the ideas are directly testable. We also concede that camatosis cannot tell the whole story, and in no way can explain everything about distinctiveness effects and the many other phenomena that we have suggested could be considered to lie in the domain to which camatosis is relevant. Future research will separate the speculative chaff from the theoretical wheat, as always.

ACKNOWLEDGMENTS

Preparation of this chapter was supported by a foundation of Anne and Max Tanenbaum in support of research in cognitive neuroscience and by a Natural Sciences and Engineering Research Council of Canada grant awarded to E.T. R.S.R. is supported by a Heart and Stroke Foundation of Canada/Canadian Institutes of Health Research postdoctoral fellowship.

NOTES

1. For the sake of convenience, we will use the term recall throughout this essay as a collective designator for all types of measured retrieval that have been used in demonstrations of distinctiveness effects. The nonuse of other relevant terms carries no hidden theoretical message.
2. The *ceteris paribus* clause ("other things being equal"), of course, applies in this case as it does in all psychological theories. Many other variables may produce patterns of data that can be described in terms of distinctiveness of particular items and that may have little to do with camatosis. We claim that the camatosis hypothesis holds under conditions in which all other variables, including materials (Jenkins, 1979), are held constant. We also take it for granted, without discussion, that other well-known and accepted facts about memory processes, such as levels of processing, encoding specificity, and the like, hold for the recall of distinctive items as they do for all others.
3. Like, say, the performance of the chess master who can play 50 games, against 50 opponents simultaneously without looking at any of the 50 chessboards at any time during any game and who still wins most of the games. Very few people who play chess are capable of playing even a single game in this "blindfolded" fashion.
4. We are grateful to Professor Jaan Puhvel of UCLA for suggesting the term to us for the intended purpose.

REFERENCES

Andreasen, N. C., O'Leary, D. S., Cizadlo, T., Arndt, S., Rezai, K., Watkins, G. L., Ponto, L. L., & Hichwa, R. D. (1995). Remembering the past: two facets of episodic memory explored with positron emission tomography. *Americal Journal of Psychiatry, 152,* 1576–1585.

Baddeley, A. D. (1978). The trouble with levels: A reexamination of Craik and Lockhart's framework for memory research. *Psychological Review, 85,* 139–152.

Baddeley, A. D., & Warrington, E. K. (1970). Amnesia and the distinction between long- and short-term memory. *Journal of Verbal Learning and Verbal Behavior, 9,* 176–189.

Bower, G. H., Thompson-Schill, S., & Tulving, E. (1994). Reducing retroactive interference: An interference analysis. *Journal of Experimental Psychology: Learning, Memory, and Cognition, 20,* 51–66.

Bouton, M. E. (1993). Context, time, and memory retrieval in the interference paradigms of Pavlovian learning. *Psychological Bulletin, 114,* 80–99.

Calkins, M. W. (1896). Association: An essay analytic and experimental. *Psychological Monographs, 1,* 1–56.

Carandini, M. (2000). Visual cortex: Fatigue and adaptation. *Current Biology, 10,* 605–607.

Clifford, C.W.G. (2002). Perceptual adaptation: Motion parallels orientation. *Trends in Cognitive Sciences, 6,* 136–143.

Conway, M. A., Anderson, S. J., Larsen, S. F., Donnelly, C. M., McDaniel, M. A., McClelland, A. G., Rawles, R. E., & Logie, R. H. (1994). The formation of flashbulb memories. *Memory and Cognition, 22,* 326–343.

Craik, F. I. (1971). Primary memory. *British Medical Bulletin, 27,* 232–236.

Craik, F. I. M., & Lockhart, R. S. (1972). Levels of processing: A framework for memory research. *Journal of Verbal Learning and Verbal Behavior, 11,* 671–684.

Desimone, R. (1992). The physiology of memory: recordings of things past. *Science, 258,* 245–246.

Desimone, R. (1996). Neural mechanisms for visual memory and their role in attention. *Proceedings of the National Academy of Sciences, 93,* 13494–13499.

Diamond, A. (1988). Abilities and neural mechanisms underlying AB performance. *Child Development, 59,* 523–527.

Diamond, A., & Goldman-Rakic, P. S. (1989). Comparison of human infants and rhesus monkeys on Piaget's AB task: evidence for dependence on dorsolateral prefrontal cortex. *Experimental Brain Research, 74,* 24–40.

Foster, J. K., & Jelicic, M. (1999). *Memory: Systems, process, or function?* Oxford, UK: Oxford University Press.

Gusnard, D. A., Akbudak, E., Shulman, G. L., & Raichle, M. E. (2001). Medial prefrontal cortex and self-referential mental activity: relation to a default mode of brain function. *Proceedings of the National Academy of Sciences, 98,* 4259–4264.

Humphreys, M. S. (1976). Relational information and the context effect in recognition memory. *Memory & Cognition, 4,* 221–232.

Hunt, R. R. (1995). The subtlety of distinctiveness: What von Restorff really did. *Psychonomic Bulletin & Review, 2,* 105–112.

Hunt, R. R., & McDaniel, M. A. (1993). The enigma of organization and distinctiveness. *Journal of Memory and Language, 32,* 421–445.

Hunt, R. R., & Lamb, C. A. (2001). What causes the isolation effect? *Journal of Experimental Psychology: Learning, Memory, and Cognition, 27,* 1359–1366.

Jenkins, J. J. (1979). Four points to remember: A tetrahedral model of memory experiments. In L. S. Cermak & F. I. M. Craik (Eds.), *Levels of processing and human memory* (pp. 429–446). Hillsdale, NJ: Lawrence Erlbaum Associates.

Keppel, G., & Underwood, B. J. (1962). Proactive inhibition in short-term retention of single items. *Journal of Verbal Learning and Verbal Behavior, 1,* 153–161.

Lezak, M. D., Howieson, D. B., & Loring, D. W. (2004). *Neuropsychological assessment,* 4th Ed. New York: Oxford University Press.

Loess, H., & Waugh, N. C. (1967). Short-term memory and inter-trial interval. *Journal of Verbal Learning and Verbal Behavior, 6,* 455–460.

Long, G. M., Toppino, T. C., & Mondin, G. W. (1992). Prime time: Fatigue and set effects in the perception of reversible figures. *Perception & Psychophysics, 52,* 609–616.

Madigan, S. A. (1969). Intraserial repetition and coding processes in free recall. *Journal of Verbal Learning and Verbal Behavior, 8,* 828–835.

Madigan, S., & McCabe, L. (1972). Perfect recall and total forgetting: A problem for models of short-term memory. *Journal of Verbal Learning and Verbal Behavior, 10,* 101–106.

McGeogh, J. A., & Irion, A. L. (1952). *The psychology of human learning.* New York: MacKay.

Metcalfe, J. (1993). Monitoring and gain control in an episodic memory model: Relation to the P300 event-related potential. In A. F. Collins, S. E. Gathercole, M. A. Conway, & P. E. Morris (Eds.), *Theories of memory* (pp. 327–353). Hillsdale, NJ: Lawrence Erlbaum Associates.

Müller, G. E., & Pilzecker, A. (1900). Experimentelle Beiträge zur Lehre vom Gedächtnis. *Zeitschrift für Psychologie Ergänzungsband, 1,* 1–300.

Murdock, B. B. (1962). The serial position effect of free recall. *Journal of Experimental Psychology, 64,* 482–488.

Nilsson, L.-G. (2000). Remembering actions and words. In E. Tulving & F. I. M. Craik (Eds.), *The Oxford handbook of memory* (pp. 137–148). New York: Oxford University Press.

Peterson, L. R., & Peterson, M. J. (1962). Minimal paired-associate learning. *Journal of Experimental Psychology, 63,* 521–527.

Raichle, M. E., MacLeod, A. M., Snyder, A. Z., Powers, W. J., Gusnard, D. A., & Shulman, G. L. (2001). A default mode of brain function. *Proceedings of the National Academy of Sciences, 98,* 676–682.

Raymond, J. E., Shapiro, K. L., & Arnell, K. M. (1992). Temporary suppression of visual processing in an RSVP task: An attentional blink? *Journal of Experimental Psychology: Human Perception and Performance, 18,* 849–860.

Ringo, J. L. (1996). Stimulus specific adaptation in inferior temporal and medial temporal cortex of the monkey. *Behavioural Brain Research, 76,* 191–197.

Schacter, D. L., Israel, L., & Racine, C. A. (1999). Suppressing false recognition in younger and older adults: The distinctiveness heuristic. *Journal of Memory and Language, 40,* 1–24.

Schacter, D. L., Moscovitch, M., Tulving, E., McLachlan, D. R., & Freedman, M. (1986). Mnemonic precedence in amnesic patients: An analogue of the AB error in infants? *Child Development, 57,* 816–823.

Schmidt, S. R. (1991). Can we have a distinctive theory of memory? *Memory and Cognition, 19,* 523–542.

Sohal, V. S., & Hasselmo, M. E. (2000). A model for experience-dependent changes in the responses of inferotemporal neurons. *Network, 11,* 169–190.

Sokolov, E. N. (1963). Higher nervous functions: The orienting reflex. *Annual Review of Physiology, 25,* 545–580.

Spence, C., & Driver, J. (1998). Auditory and audiovisual inhibition of return. *Perception and Psychophysics, 60,* 125–139.

Stuss, D. T., & Benson, D. F. (1986). *The frontal lobes.* New York: Raven Press.

Tipper, S. P. (1985). The negative priming effect: Inhibitory priming by ignored objects. *Quarterly Journal of Experimental Psychology, 37A,* 571–590.

Toulmin, S. E. (1961). *Foresight and understanding: An enquiry into the aims of science.* Bloomington: Indiana University Press.

Trehub, S. E. (2001). Musical predispositions in infancy. *Annals of the New York Academy of Sciences, 930,* 1–16.

Tulving E. (1983). *Elements of episodic memory.* Oxford, UK: Clarendon Press.

Tulving, E. (1985). Memory and consciousness. *Canadian Psychology, 26,* 1–12.

Tulving, E. (2000). Concepts of memory. In E. Tulving & F. I. M. Craik (Eds.), *The Oxford handbook of memory* (pp. 33–44). New York: Oxford University Press.

Tulving, E., & Arbuckle, T. Y. (1963). Sources of intratrial interference in immediate recall of paired associates. *Journal of Verbal Learning and Verbal Behavior, 1,* 321–334.

Tulving, E., & Kroll, N. (1995). Novelty assessment in the brain and long-term memory encoding. *Psychonomic Bulletin & Review, 2,* 387–390.

Tulving, E., Markowitsch, H. J., Kapur, S., Habib, R., & Houle, S. (1994). Novelty encoding networks in the human brain: Positron emission tomography data. *NeuroReport, 5,* 2525–2528.

Underwood, B. J., & Postman, L. (1960). Extraexperimental sources of interference in forgetting. *Psychological Review, 67,* 73–95.

von Restorff, H. (1933). Uber die Wirkung von Bereichsbildungen im Spurenfeld. *Psychologische Forschung, 18,* 299–342.

Watkins, M. J. (1979). Engrams as cuegrams and forgetting as cue overload: A cueing approach to the structure of memory. In C. R. Puff (Ed.), *Memory organization and structure* (pp. 347–372). New York: Academic Press.

Waugh, N. C. (1970). On the effective duration of a repeated word. *Journal of Verbal Learning and Verbal Behavior, 9,* 587–595.

Waugh, N. C., & Norman, D. A. (1965). Primary memory. *Psychological Review, 72,* 89–104.

Wickens, D. D. (1970). Encoding categories of words: An empirical approach to meaning. *Psychological Review, 77,* 1–15.

Wright, A. A., Santiago, H. C., Sands, S. F., Kendrick, D. F., & Cook, R. G. (1985). Memory processing of serial lists by pigeons, monkeys, and people. *Science, 229,* 287–289.

19

Distinctiveness and Memory: Comments and a Point of View

Fergus I. M. Craik

Reed Hunt opened the present debate by remarking that whereas it seems intuitively obvious that distinctive events are well remembered simply because we pay more attention to them, this commonsense analysis may conceal more complex truths. One purpose of this final chapter is to weigh Hunt's remark in light of the data and arguments presented in the book. It is immediately clear that the authors responded gladly to the call for greater complexity, so a second purpose of the present chapter is to survey the various points of view and assess the degree to which there is agreement on the role of distinctiveness in memory. Third, given that I have been mulling over the role of distinctiveness in memory for some time in my own work (e.g., Jacoby & Craik, 1979; Moscovitch & Craik, 1976), I will take the opportunity to relate the authors' ideas and findings to my own point of view.

One factor contributing to the complexity (or richness) of the debate is the profusion of terms used to refer to the central point of interest. As well as examining distinctiveness, the authors analyze isolation, inconsistency, incongruity, novelty, salience, bizarreness, and significance, among others. Do these terms all converge on a common concept or are several distinguishable factors involved? If so, what are their different effects and how do they relate to each other? One point of agreement is the distinction between events that stand out because they differ from other events that are nearby in space and/or time, and events that stand out because they differ from our general knowledge of such events. This is the useful distinction between primary and secondary distinctiveness (Schmidt, 1991) invoked by many of present authors. As I understand it, primary distinctiveness includes isolation effects (also known as the von Restorff effect)—in general, situations in which expectancy for the next event is violated. Since expectancy is typically established by the local context, there is general agreement that distinctiveness is a *relative* concept (e.g., Hunt, Chapter 1 this volume). It is important to note, however, that the features that distinguish the distinctive event from its context may take a wide variety of forms; the isolate may be a tone of a different pitch, a word presented in a different color or typescript, a word in a series of pictures, or a word drawn from a different semantic class than its neighbors. That is, the isolated event may be distinctive perceptually or semantically, and I for one would like to believe that the consequences for subsequent memory will be rather different in these two cases (Craik & Tulving, 1975).

Secondary distinctiveness includes cases in which the event is incongruent relative to a person's general knowledge or beliefs about that class of events. Bizarreness fits this description—more or less grotesque violations of learned concepts or scripts—as does novelty in the sense of a completely new type of event, as opposed to novelty in the primary distinctive sense of a violation of locally induced expectancy. It seems to me that significance (Schmidt, Chapter 3 this volume) is different from both primary and secondary distinctiveness, in that *significance* implies some important consequence for the person. Thus, a significant event will attract attention, reflection, and elaborate processing regardless of whether it is anomalous in the local context, and regardless of whether it was expected. Significant events may also invoke an emotional reaction and feelings of surprise or shock depending on such factors as expectancy and emotional consequences.

Thus, an event can be distinctive and attract attention for several different reasons; it may differ perceptually from its neighbors and so violate locally induced expectancy; it may differ semantically from its neighbors and so again be seen as incongruous; it may be incongruous relative to the general case for such events; and finally it may be an event with significant consequences for the person.

With regard to the effect of distinctiveness on memory, my tentative view (to be scrutinized in light of the present chapters) is that good memory performance is very largely dependent on the formation of a representation that is (1) congruent with some well-established body of schematic knowledge in the learner, but also (2) well differentiated from other similar events in the dimensions that are relevant to that schematic knowledge. Most cases that are reliably associated with excellent memory can be described in such terms. For example, deep semantic processing in the levels of processing (LOP) sense is associated with good subsequent memory because (1) deep analysis of the event results in an encoded representation that is well differentiated from other similar events, (2) the differentiation is in the terms of some well-established and highly accessible aggregation of schematic knowledge, and (3) this body of organized knowledge enables and facilitates the processes of reconstructive retrieval. In my opinion, the self-reference effect (excellent memory following encoding that relates an event to the participant personally) is a prime example of an effect reflecting the involvement of a highly developed and well-integrated body of knowledge, beliefs, and attitudes that serves, first, to differentiate a newly encoded event; second, to relate that newly formed representation to existing schematic knowledge; and third, to facilitate retrieval. In general, expertise in any domain of knowledge appears to function in this way (Bartlett, 1932; Bransford, Franks, Morris & Stein, 1979).

As I see it, the following four cases of distinctiveness will all be associated with good subsequent memory, but for somewhat different reasons:

1. Isolated events that differ from their neighbors perceptually but are similar in other respects will simply attract attention and therefore more elaborate processing. Crucially they will also be tagged with a distinctive descriptor (e.g. "the red one") that will serve as a cue in the retrieval phase.

2. Events that differ from their neighbors semantically or in kind—for example, one animal name in a list of vegetables or one picture in a list of words—will attract attention and more processing, but in this case the tagged description will be more fully differentiated from other descriptions when used as a cue.

3. Cases of secondary distinctiveness (e.g., bizarreness and novelty) will attract attention, but will typically require substantial amounts of analytic processing to comprehend the event and relate it to current knowledge structures. Interestingly, there appears to be an optimal amount of anomaly or departure from known instances for bizarre (and perhaps also novel) events. As the event differs from the norm it will engender progressively more analytic processing to resolve and comprehend the anomaly, but if the event differs too much it will simply be disregarded. There is therefore an inverted-U relation between degree of anomaly and later memory, arguably as a function of the amount of analytic processing necessary and also perhaps as a function of how well (or poorly) current structures can act to facilitate retrieval. That is, a very bizarre or atypically novel event will be tagged with a description that cannot be utilized readily in the course of reconstructive retrieval (see Howe, Chapter 11 this volume; Davidson, Chapter 8 this volume).

4. Significant events are well remembered because they attract attention and processing resources (sometimes to the detriment of neighboring events; Schmidt, Chapter 3 this volume). They are meaningful by definition and so receive the benefit of deep processing; they may also give rise to an emotional reaction—an additional factor in boosting subsequent memory (Schmidt, Chapter 3 this volume). Finally, significant events often call for some action to be made, and the encoded intention to act will enrich the encoded record and so further enhance memory.

The remainder of the chapter is devoted to an examination of these ideas in light of the current evidence.

DISTINCTIVENESS AND TYPES OF MEMORY

The effects of distinctiveness on memory have usually been considered in the context of episodic memory, with the basic ideas being that a distinctive event will be well recollected at some future time. It seems likely, however, that distinctiveness should also play a part in the acquisition of new knowledge—that is, in additions to semantic memory. Clearly, highly emotional and significant events will be well processed and add to the person's general world knowledge as well as to his or her episodic recollection of the event. I have previously suggested that the distinction between episodic and semantic memory be thought of in terms of a hierarchy of generality to specificity rather than in terms of two separate systems (Craik, 2002). The notion of grain size (Goldsmith & Koriat, 1999; Schmidt, Chapter 3 this volume) has a similar flavor. In those terms, a significant event may be thought of as adding both specific (episodic) and general (semantic) representations. Highly emotional events typically give rise to particularly rich and vivid encodings at specific levels—the "flashbulb effect" (Brown & Kulik, 1977); interestingly, the specific and general aspects can dissociate, in that after months or years the person still claims to have a "vivid recollection" of the events, despite the fact that the remembered details may have changed substantially over the intervening period (see, e.g., Winograd & Neisser, 1992).

The interplay between episodic and semantic memory is well illustrated by Davidson's (Chapter 8 this volume) work on scripts. Bizarre sentences and atypical scripted actions are better recalled than common sentences or typical actions at short delays, but schema-appropriate sentences and actions are better recalled at longer intervals. This result highlights the importance of reconstructive retrieval in this whole area. At longer intervals, episodic detail is less available and/or accessible; there is correspondingly greater reliance on schematic representations of "the usual case," leading to a benefit for common as opposed to atypical events; and there is a heightened liability to make false-positive recognition responses to common as opposed to unusual stimuli (Davidson, Chapater 8 this volume; Roediger & McDermott, 1995). Interestingly, Davidson also reports that older adults are apparently more reliant on schema-based recall.

Schacter and Wiseman (Chapter 5 this volume) invoke two further types of memory in their discussion of the distinctiveness heuristic. Metamemory is involved in the assessment of what people feel they *should* remember when presented with an item for recognition. If the item is unusual or distinctive in some way, yet not accompanied by feelings of familiarity, it will be rejected confidently; the person reasons that "I would have remembered something that distinctive." This notion also gives a good account of the low false-positive rate for low-frequency words (Brown, 1976). Schacter and Wiseman also discuss the role of distinctiveness in prospective memory. In this context, distinctiveness plays a role in connection with the reminders that people construct for themselves to cue the recollection that some action should be performed. The prospective memory cue may be more or less well associated with the planned intention (it will be more effective if it *is* well associated), but the crucial characteristic of such cues is that they should be distinctive and unexpected in their context, so that the person's routine is interrupted by the thought "Why is this here?"

Does distinctiveness affect implicit memory? This question is posed by several authors in the present volume and given a tentative yes answer, although the effects are limited to rather special circumstances, it seems. At first the evidence appears to be clearly negative. Mulligan (Chapter 9 this volume) quotes studies that manipulate the difficulty of initial processing, present items as pictures as opposed to words (Weldon & Coyote, 1996), present concrete as opposed to abstract words (Hamilton & Rajaram, 2001), or have words processed deeply as opposed to shallowly (Jacoby & Dallas, 1981); in all cases the manipulation had strong effects on explicit recall but none on implicit memory tests. Mulligan concludes that implicit tests rely heavily on relational information and are therefore not sensitive to the foregoing manipulations that largely boost item-specific information.

Geraci and Rajaram (Chapter 10 this volume) argue that distinctiveness often prompts conceptual, evaluative processing ("Why is that anomalous or unexpected item present?"), and that the benefit of this extra processing can be shown, *provided* that the initial context is reinstated at the time of retrieval. I find this an interesting and attractive argument; distinctiveness (more generally, unexpectedness) triggers conceptual-relational processing that presumably alters the participant's schematic knowledge base in some small ways. These changes, in turn, can be detected in the absence of awareness of the initial episode provided that the principle of transfer-appropriate processing is observed. The combination of need for contextual reinstatement yet absence of conscious recollection suggests that the representations tapped are midway between highly specific episodic traces and completely abstract acontextual representations, in line with the notion that knowledge is represented hierarchically at various levels of specificity to generality (see Craik, 2002). Kishiyama and Yonelinas (Chapter 17 this volume) also discuss the effects of distinctiveness (or in their case, novelty) on general schematic knowledge (or in their case, familiarity judgments). Their conclusions are in agreement with those of Geraci and Rajaram: novelty promotes more extensive processing of the event, and this extra processing will be evident at the time of retrieval provided that the test requires the type of processing that was initially carried out (see Jacoby, 1983). One final example of the effects of distinctiveness on implicit retrieval comes from the domain of social psychology; Coats and Smith (Chapter 14 this volume) make the good point that social stereotypes are strongly affected by salient experiences, and that such implicit attitudes may exist alongside more socially acceptable views that the holders express publicly.

DISTINCTIVENESS AND TYPES OF PROCESSING

The positive effects of distinctiveness on memory are attributable to a number of factors that (with one interesting exception) are generally agreed upon by the present set of authors. This suggests the hopeful possibility that here is at least one phenomenon in cognitive psychology that is reasonably well understood; the alternative, though not mutually exclusive, hypothesis is that the authors were selected for their amiability as well as for their erudition! The authors of the dissenting opinion (Tulving & Rosenbaum, Chapater 18 this volume), while no less amiable, take a radically different perspective to be discussed later. In any event, the components of the more generally held view are, first, the point that distinctiveness is not an explanation; its effects must be understood in terms of underlying processes and representations. Second, distinctiveness is a *relative* term; the item or event is distinctive against a particular background, which ideally should be present (in terms of ongoing processing operations) at both encoding and retrieval (Hunt, Chapter 1 this volume; Jacoby & Craik, 1979). Third, the distinction between item and relational processing is made by Nairne (Chapter 2 this volume), Worthen (Chapter 7 this volume), and Burns (Chapter 6 this volume), among others. Fourth, whereas salience (or isolation) of an event is not a *necessary* precursor of distinctive processing (Hunt, Chapter 1 this volume), it does seem that these characteristics play a significant role in attracting attention and extra processing to the event. How do these factors translate into processing terms?

First, it seems clear that anomalous or unexpected items or events receive more attention and more extensive processing. This extra processing will yield a stronger mental representation of the event and, especially if the additional processing is evaluative or semantic in nature, it will yield a record that is deeper and more elaborated. Why do deeper levels of processing result in such high levels of recollection? My speculative answer is that processing in the semantic domain allows for greater differentiation of the event than is possible at shallower levels of processing, and this greater differentiation is amplified by more elaborate processing. Further, the organized nature of semantic schemas provides both a means of specifying the event precisely in relation to other events and also the structure that enables reconstructive retrieval. As an analogy, compare the efficiency of a library system that organizes books simply by size, weight, and by the color of their covers with one that organizes by topic, date, and author. The second system obviously provides a much more specific basis for storing books, for representing them in a catalogue, and for retrieving them in response to a well-specified cue. For example, compare "a book on memory by Endel Tulving in 1983" with "a book measuring $6^1/_2 \times 9^1/_2$ inches with a dark cover and weighing about a pound!"

Greater amounts of attention paid to an item, therefore, specifies it more exactly, and this in turn yields a more distinctive representation, but often at the cost of less attention being paid to neighboring items. Thus, Schmidt

(Chapter 3 this volume) describes an experiment in which a picture of a nude was well remembered, but at the expense of pictures of common objects before and after the attention-attracting item. Schmidt also points out that the recall benefit disappears if *all* pictures are of nudes—a clear case of "nude overload!" Bizarreness seems to work in the same way (Worthen, Chapter 7 this volume). That is, bizarre items attract attention, extra processing, and presumably some evaluative processing as the participant attempts to comprehend the item in terms of current schemas. This extra processing is "stolen" from neighboring items, whose memorability is correspondingly depressed. By this argument, a complete list of bizarre items would show little benefit over a list of common items. Worthen also makes the point that bizarreness boosts item-specific encoding, but at the expense of detailed intra-item processing. Finally, the depression of memory for items preceding and succeeding a distinctive item was also reported by Tulving (1969) and discussed by him as an experimental analogy of retrograde amnesia (EARA).

A number of authors stress the importance of the reinstatement of study context at the time of retrieval (e.g., Geraci & Rajaram, Chapter 10 this volume; Hunt, Chapter 1 this volume; McDaniel & Geraci, Chapter 4 this volume). The importance of such reinstatement makes sense in light of the ideas (1) that subjective encoding of both items and cues is flexible and context dependent, also (2) that distinctiveness is necessarily a relative concept. That is, for the encoded cue to effectively specify the wanted item, the original context must be reinstated so that both the cue and the sought-for item can be encoded distinctively (and similarly). As an example, the word *piano* may be encoded either as a musical instrument or as "a heavy object." If the list contains many other musical instruments, then the cue "a musical instrument" may not be effective, but if the other list members are words such as *flute, violin*, and *piccolo*, the cue "something heavy" may be quite powerful.

The work on buildup and release from proactive interference (PI) is relevant here. Many studies have shown that if four successive lists of 3–4 words are all drawn from one semantic category in the Brown-Peterson paradigm, recall declines markedly from list 1 to list 4. If the words on list 4 are switched to a different category, however, recall performance returns to a high level (Wickens, 1970). It may be said that the list 4 words are distinctive or discriminable against the background of lists 1–3. In a variant of this paradigm, Gardiner, Craik and Birtwistle (1972) conducted a study of this type in which list 4 words were from the same *general* category as list 1–3 words (e.g., *games*), but from a different subcategory (e.g., *indoor games* as opposed to *outdoor games*). When participants were not informed of this subtle switch, they showed no release from PI for list 4; when they were informed during presentation of list 4 they did show release, however—presumably the words were encoded differentially. Most interestingly, release was also shown by participants who were not informed of the subcategory until retrieval. They utilized the difference between list

4 and lists 1–3 despite the fact that they were unaware of any difference during presentation. One way to describe this result is to say that list 4 items were encoded with their specific attributes (e.g., darts and rugby have very different characteristics) and that the retrieval cue "indoor games" has its effect by changing mental set at retrieval, and so causing the "indoor" aspects of list 4 words to emerge distinctively against the background of "outdoor" aspects of list 1–3 words.

Locus of the Effect: Encoding or Retrieval?

One central question in this area concerns the mechanism of the distinctiveness advantage. Does it occur primarily during encoding or during retrieval? The most obvious answer is that it is essentially an encoding effect; distinctive items attract more attention, and this in turn yields an encoded representation that is well differentiated from neighboring items. Several authors point out difficulties with this account, however. For example, if an anomalous item in a list is presented first, it is not known to be anomalous until the rest of the list is presented and so should not attract any extra processing. Given that such items do show a distinctiveness advantage, this suggests a retrieval locus for the effect (McDaniel & Geraci, Chapter 4 this volume; Worthen, Chapter 7 this volume). McDaniel, De-Losh and Merritt (2000) also talk about "distinctiveness as a cue," but I find it difficult to know what is meant by that phrase. A slightly different way of putting it would be to say that the encoded representation of the distinctive event is discriminable from other recent events (this would be true even if the event in question was presented first), and so the appropriate cue would specify the wanted item precisely, but not specify other list items. That is, the cue would have a high diagnostic value (McDaniel & Geraci, Chapter 4 this volume) and cue overload would be minimal. This is what Nairne (Chapter 2 this volume) is arguing for, as I understand it, although it is important to point out that *both* encoding and retrieval are involved in such an account. Encoding provides the potential for good memory performance (either by virtue of the item itself being different from others, or by virtue of receiving extra processing for a variety of reasons), and the appropriate retrieval cue serves to realize that potential (Moscovitch & Craik, 1976).

When attempting to assign the locus of memory effects, it is important to specify the perspective taken. As one example, Endel Tulving and I once conducted a sort of genteel theoretical arm-wrestling contest about whether both levels of processing ideas and encoding specificity ideas were necessary to give an adequate account of memory phenomena, or whether encoding specificity was sufficient by itself (the astute reader can probably deduce whose view was which!). This debate went on for several years, until a bright young graduate student (initials D.S., now sufficiently evolved to be an author of one of the present chapters) pointed out that our perspectives were simply different; Craik was arguing about the recipe for good memory *before* the event occurred (therefore, deep processing plus transfer-appropriate cues) whereas Tulving's view was that once the event was encoded, all that was necessary was to specify how it had been encoded and then furnish the most appropriate cue. In the present context I stand by my view that distinctiveness effects necessarily involve *both* encoding and retrieval, and that the way forward is to understand the factors that are important at each stage. It is also possible to argue that the locus is storage (e.g., Howe, Chapter 11 this volume), and that distinctively encoded events are less vulnerable to interference from succeeding events (Nairne, Chapter 2 this volume), although I personally think of such effects as reflecting essentially a prolongation of encoding processes. That is, one set of factors determines how the event is represented relative to other encoded events, and a second set determines how the encoded event is retrieved.

A rather different type of encoding explanation is proposed by Tulving and Rosenbaum (Chapter 18 this volume). In their view, distinctive items do not receive especially beneficial processing and are not encoded differentially; rather, it is the other nondistinctive items in the list that (owing to the hypothesized neural phenomenon of camatosis) are processed *less well* than the distinctive item. As I understand the argument, the distinctiveness effect is in essence a type of "release from PI" effect—the distinctive item is represented by different neural circuits relative to its neighbors and is therefore relatively immune to camatosis. This account is somewhat similar to the notions of proactive inhibition and of cue overload, although it differs from these previous ideas in suggesting a neural basis for the effect. The discovery of a neural "fatigue" affect with the requisite characteristics will be crucial to the longevity of the camatosis suggestion. It is an attractive idea in many respects; one could speculate, for example, that the aging nervous system becomes increasingly camatotic, with the result that encodings generally are less precise and less well specified (e.g., Craik, 2002). Two questions that occur to me are:

1. How does the notion of camatosis deal with the indoor games/outdoor games experiment of Gardiner et al. (1972) described earlier? It seems necessary to invoke the notion of retrieval set to account for the good recall of the new subset, remembering that the subset does *not* show release from PI unless the subset cue is provided.
2. What would the camatosis notion predict for the recall of an identical word presented in the first serial position of a list in three lists of the following types?
   a. *CAMEL, table, chair, desk, carpet,* etc.
   b. *CAMEL, table, lawyer, cabbage, shark,* etc.
   c. *CAMEL, lion, donkey, hyena, giraffe,* etc.
   In my thought experiment, the probabilities of recalling *CAMEL* would be best for (a), the isolated list, poorer for (b), the unrelated

list, and worst for (c), the PI list, whereas the camatosis effects on the first word should be equivalent, should they not? We await further developments of this interestingly different way of approaching distinctiveness effects.

The work reported in the present volume makes it clear that the type of retrieval test is an important factor for understanding distinctiveness. For example, bizarreness has a strong effect on free-recall measures but typically less of an effect on recognition (Worthen, Chapter 7 this volume). It is again important to understand the interplay between encoding and retrieval processes in any specific situation before drawing conclusions that are too general. If the emphasis is on reconstructive retrieval (as in free recall), then the dominating factor may be how well the event fits with existing schemas, whereas if the retrieval environment is appropriate and complete (recognition in context for example), the critical factor may be how well differentiated the encoded event is from other similar representations. An instructive parallel may be drawn to word frequency effects; high-frequency words are better recalled, whereas low-frequency words are better recognized. It is reasonable to argue that high-frequency words are not very distinctive, but are well integrated with accessible schemas, whereas low-frequency words are less well integrated with schematic information but are more clearly differentiated. At one extreme, stimuli that we have no good schemas for are poorly remembered, even though they are perceptually quite distinctive. A nice example here concerns snowflake patterns that are perfectly well distinguishable perceptually, but are very poorly remembered, even in a recognition test (Goldstein & Chance, 1971). The corollary of this example is that a "snowflake expert" would find recognition trivially easy—as do wallpaper salesmen and whisky tasters in their respective domains of expertise.

The contrast between the relative advantages of well-differentiated representations on the one hand and congruity with highly integrated schemas on the other is clearly parallel to the distinction between item-specific and relational processing pointed out by Hunt (Chapter 1 this volume; Hunt & Einstein, 1981) and others. An additional consideration in this context is that whereas bizarreness typically boosts memory performance, if the event is too inconsistent with existing schemas it will not be well remembered simply because it cannot be integrated with the current knowledge base (Howe, Chapter 11 this volume; Coats & Smith, Chapter 14 this volume). A further link with previous work is Hunt's (Chapter 1 this volume) reference to the study by Epstein, Phillips, and Johnson (1975), who showed that when word pairs are already related (e.g., *apple-orange*) it is best to process them by emphasizing a difference between the words, whereas for unrelated word pairs (e.g., *apple-turkey*), memory performance is increased by finding some similarity between the words. The first case stresses differentiation of well-integrated events and the second stresses integration of well-differentiated events. See also Burns's useful account of the relations between types of processing and different memory tests (Chapter 6 this volume).

One final topic in this section is the notion of grain size—the idea that retrieval typically proceeds from general coarse-grained representations to specific fine-grained representations (Burns, Chapter 6 this volume; Mulligan, Chapter 9 this volume; Goldsmith & Koriat, 1999; Hunt & Einstein, 1981). The distinctiveness of an encoded representation is relative to the grain size under consideration, so yet again, retrieval processes must tap into the correct value of this dimension for the distinctiveness to be useful (Schmidt, Chapter 3 this volume). Schacter's notion of the distinctiveness heuristic (Schacter & Wiseman, Chapter 5 this volume) is also relevant here. If the participant retrieves an event at a very general level of representation, a similar (but nonpresented) event may be falsely recognized (cf., the false-memory effect illustrated by Roediger & McDermott, 1995). Deeper, more analytic, retrieval operations allow the distinctiveness heuristic to operate and lead to a reduction of false-positive errors.

DEVELOPMENTAL AND SOCIAL IMPLICATIONS

If memory mechanisms are essentially continuous between younger and older children, younger adults, and older adults, it is to be expected that such powerful factors as distinctiveness would affect memory at all ages. This indeed appears to be the case (Howe, Chapter 11 this volume; Smith, Chapter 12 this volume), although it is also true that the details of how distinctiveness affects memory vary as cognitive mechanisms change across the life span. One major factor is the growth of knowledge in young children. As Howe points out, anomalous items cannot be perceived as anomalous until organized schematic knowledge structures have been formed, along with their expectancies and boundaries. One interesting downside of knowledge formation is that false memories in the Deese-Roediger-McDermott (DRM) paradigm actually *increase* as children get older, presumably owing to the increased priming of items that are highly probable in that schematic context. This observation fits both the fuzzy-trace theory of Brainerd and Reyna (2001) and Howe's (2000) trace-integrity theory. Howe also points out that moderate discrepancies from the prevailing context provide the optimal boost to later memory; highly similar items do not attract especial attention, but highly discrepant items are simply rejected as irrelevant to current concerns. Howe concludes that whereas distinctiveness is important from the earliest days of life, what constitutes distinctiveness will necessarily change with the growth of knowledge.

Distinctiveness can also boost memory in older adults (Smith, Chapter 12 this volume), but again the specific effects vary as both item-specific and relational processing change with age. There is reasonable evidence that older adults rely more on general, abstract, gistlike representations than on specific, verbatim representations of events (cf. Brainerd & Reyna, 2001;

Craik, 2002). This change suggests that older adults should be more vulnerable to false memories in the DRM paradigm, and there is evidence to support this suggestion (e.g., Benjamin, 2001). Davidson (Chapter 8 this volume) also comments that older adults rely more on schema-based recall, and reports finding effects of both bizarreness and interruption in older adults. Thus, elderly participants are sensitive to secondary distinctiveness but interestingly they appear to be less sensitive to primary distinctiveness (Cimbalo & Brink, 1982; Fabiani, Chapter 15 this volume; McDaniel & Geraci, Chapter 4 this volume). McDaniel and Geraci argue that this result makes sense if primary distinctiveness is largely a retrieval effect and if retrieval processes are less efficient in older adults. I am personally skeptical of this conclusion, however. As previously mentioned, distinctiveness cannot operate at retrieval unless the encoded representation is distinctive, so my speculative suggestion is that older adults are simply less reactive to anomaly, pay less extra attention to anomalous items, and spend less effort in attempting to resolve violations of expectancy. The finding that divided attention at encoding reduces the effects of novelty and anomaly on later recollection (Kishiyama & Yonelinas, Chapter 17 this volume) is in line with this speculation, given that the effects of divided attention are similar to those of aging in many respects (Craik, 1982). Additionally, the observation that amnesic patients show reduced novelty effects (Kishiyama & Yonelinas, Chapter 17 this volume) may be a more extreme example of the same phenomenon. This is not to argue that older adults will *never* show effects of isolation or unexpectedness, but rather that they are less sensitive to these effects than their younger counterparts. Clearly this is a question that can be clarified by neurophysiological techniques (Fabiani, Chapter 15 this volume).

Memory is crucial for building up and maintaining our sense of who we are—our sense of self. It is equally central to constructing perceptions of other individuals and characterizations of our own and other groups. In turn, these perceptions and characterizations engender and support our attitudes—reasonable and balanced, or biased and prejudiced—toward other individuals and groups. The role of distinctiveness in these social interactions is explored and documented by Mullen and Pizzuto (Chapter 13 this volume) and by Coats and Smith (Chapter 14 this volume). As Coats and Smith point out, perceivers expect some degree of coherence and unity in the behaviors of both individuals and defined groups, although this expectation is stronger for individuals. Behaviors that violate our expectations are anomalous with the person or group schema, attract attention, and evoke attempts to understand the discrepancy. Presumably the degree to which the anomalous behavior modifies the perceiver's schema of the target will depend on the number of prior episodes that have been integrated and cumulated to form the schema and on whether the perceiver can generate a plausible rationale for the anomaly ("Not like Bill at all, he must be overstressed at work"). Coats and Smith also consider memory for information that is consistent or inconsistent with the target. As discussed in previous sections, the relative memorability of these two types of information will depend on (1) the degree to which the new information is differentiated from the background (schematic) information—its distinctiveness; and (2) the degree to which the memory test depends on reconstructive processes. Coats and Smith report that schema-consistent information is better *recalled* than schema-inconsistent information, but that the opposite relation holds for recognition memory. As discussed in this and other chapters, recall depends more on relational and reconstructive processing, whereas recognition depends more on item-specific and distinctive processing. In this sense, congruity and incongruity appear to function in the same way in social and in cognitive contexts. Coats and Smith provide other instructive examples from the social literature that are well handled by the relational/item-specific comparison.

Whereas Coats and Smith focus largely on explicit memory, Mullen and Pizzuto (Chapter 13 this volume) examine the effects of social distinctiveness on stereotypes, prejudice, and other implicitly held results of personal and cultural learning. Group size is important, with smaller groups generally considered more distinctive. Our own ingroup is felt to be more heterogeneous than contrasting outgroups whose members' characteristics tend to be viewed as "all alike"—cross-racial face recognition is a good example. The distinctiveness of small groups leads to enhanced memory for their characteristics and hence to an increase in perceived prevalence. Distinctiveness also leads to increased availability in memory of a group's salient features, and this "knee-jerk shorthand" (to mix my metaphors) is one of the main components of prejudice. A final, interesting conclusion is that information about the group that is more distinctive is remembered in terms of prototypes, whereas information about the less distinctive group is remembered in terms of exemplars (Mullen & Pizzuto, Chapter 13 this volume). In general, the chapters on social cognition extend the range of applicability of such concepts as distinctiveness, and show how its effects on memory are rather fundamental to our lives in society.

NEURAL BASES OF DISTINCTIVENESS

Both Fabiani (Chapter 16 this volume) and Michelon and Snyder (Chapter 15 this volume) point out the biologically adaptive value of novelty and incongruity. Departures from the normal state of affairs may signal danger, or perhaps reward; in either case it is worthwhile for the animal to process the anomalous event more completely, analyze its significance, and assess the consequences of various possible courses of action. It may also be advantageous to remember the anomalous stimulus, either implicitly or explicitly, so that appropriate action can be taken more rapidly on a subsequent occasion. Given that lower mammals probably do not possess episodic memory (in the sense of being able to recall the contextual details of previous events; Tulving, 1983), this suggests an adaptive advantage for registering "distinctive" anomalous events in implicit memory. In turn, the suggestion is in line with the findings of Geraci and Rajaram (Chapter 10 this volume), who conclude that distinctive events can boost memory in the absence of conscious awareness, provided that the retrieval situation recapitulates the encoding situation (which would typically be the case for animals other than humans). It may therefore be *novelty* and *anomaly* that are the triggers with survival value, rather than distinctiveness as such, although presumably novel and anomalous events result in distinctive encoded representations, either of the original event or of some adaptive stimulus-response sequence.

One major benefit of using neurophysiological methods in the study of distinctiveness is that evidence from ERPs and other neuroimaging techniques can shed light on such questions as the locus of the effect. By segregating those specific stimulus events that are recalled in the retrieval phase, it is possible to determine the neural commonalities among such events, and how they differ from events that are not subsequently recalled. The chapters by Fabiani, Michelon and Snyder, and Kishiyama and Yonelinas (Chapters 15, 16, and 17 this volume, respectively) provide converging evidence on these issues. The N100 wave and the mismatch negativity effect appear to signal sensory changes and may have little relevance for later memory. Semantic incongruity, signaled for example by an unexpected or bizarre final word or phrase in a sentence, is associated with an amplification of the N400 wave. I was surprised to learn that the N400 does *not* predict subsequent memory (Fabiani, Chapter 15 this volume; Michelon & Snyder, Chapter 16 this volume)—surprising in that I would expect semantic incongruity to lead to semantic processing in an attempt to resolve the anomaly, and thus to improved memory. It is possible, however, that such experiments involve incongruous endings that are just *too* far removed from the preceding sentence context to be integrated with it (cf. Howe, this volume; Coats & Smith, this volume). Alternatively, if the participant's task is to decide whether the complete sentence is "sensible," then clearly anomalous sentences will produce an N400 response, but little in the way of reflective processing; the sentence is simply classified as "not sensible" and left at that. Endings that are almost plausible might necessitate more reflection and therefore be associated with higher levels of subsequent memory.

The P300 wave is the one classically associated with anomaly and distinctiveness in perceptual sequences. Fabiani concludes that the P300 *does* predict later memory, but only in situations in which the anomalous event is followed by elaborative processing. That is, the anomalous event causes "surprise" experientially, and attracts attention experientially, behaviorally, and neurally, but the crucial factor for memory enhancement appears to be post-event reflective, semantic, elaborative processing—one more time! The temptation for the present reviewer is obviously to suggest the concept of "levels of distinctiveness," with early sensory discrepancies signaled by the N100 wave and by mismatch negativity, N400 signaling anomalies at a deeper cognitive level, and P300 signaling events that *may* be processed deeply and elaborately depending on their functional utility to the person. Fabiani suggests a scheme along such lines.

The brain regions associated with distinctiveness may, therefore, be separated into those signaling anomaly, novelty, and surprise on the one hand (right frontal regions, hippocampus, hippocampal gyrus, and thalamus, according to Kishiyama and Yonelinas, Chapter 17 this volume) and those involved in the types of processing that yield distinctive representations—possibly left prefrontal areas (Kapur et al., 1994) and various posterior regions (Michelon & Snyder, Chapter 16 this volume).

Kishiyama and Yonelinas (Chapter 17 this volume) survey the evidence on whether distinctiveness boosts the recollection (*R*) or familiarity (*F*) component of remembering. They conclude that both components may be affected, although by different mechanisms. One rather heretical personal suggestion here is that the remember/know distinction (see Gardiner & Richardson-Klavehn, 2000) reflects degrees of contextual specificity, rather than two separate memory systems. That is, "remember" aspects are represented with contextual detail and "know" aspects (yielding feelings of familiarity, but not specific recollection) are generalized, gistlike representations abstracted as commonalities from specific instances (see Craik, 2002). In these terms, distinctiveness would affect *R* and *F* processing to the extent that post-event processing emphasized either specific contextual detail or the general abstract meaning aspects of the event. Thus the suggestion again is that it is not anomaly, incongruity, isolation, bizarreness, or novelty as such that determines the memory outcome but, rather, that these aspects of the situation simply draw attention to the event, which is then processed according to current needs and demands. Subsequent memory effects are determined in turn by the type of processing that ensues, by the differentiation of the resulting representation from its neighbors, and by the integration of the representation with existing schematic knowledge.

SUMMING UP

Overall, I found the chapters uniformly interesting, informative, and impressively coherent in the picture they present. It is clear that distinctiveness plays a major role in memory, but it is also clear that we must look at the concept in a more sophisticated manner. That is, items can be "distinctive" for a variety of somewhat different reasons, and the "distinctiveness effect" is more accurately described as a set of related effects. It seems clear that *both* encoding and retrieval processes play a part; one way of summing it up is that encoding provides the *potential* for excellent performance, which will be realized provided that such retrieval factors as context reinstatement, appropriate set, and valid cues are also in place. In my opinion, distinctive events are well remembered either because they attract more attention and therefore more analytic processing, are discriminable from neighboring events on one or more of many possible dimensions, or have some personal significance for the person. Greater amounts of processing, especially of a meaningful type, will differentiate the distinctive event from others, perhaps resulting in a representation of finer grain size. Interestingly, these principles apply to social situations as well as to purely cognitive ones. Finally, it seems likely that current work in the cognitive neuroscience tradition will soon confirm, disconfirm, or (perhaps most likely) *change* our present understanding of how distinctiveness affects memory.

REFERENCES

Bartlett, F. C. (1932). *Remembering: An experimental and social study*. Cambridge, UK: Cambridge University Press.

Benjamin, A. S. (2001). On the dual effects of repetition on false recognition. *Journal of Experimental Psychology: Learning, Memory, and Cognition, 27*, 941–947.

Brainerd, C. J., & Reyna, V. F. (2001). Fuzzy-trace theory: Dual processes in memory, reasoning, and cognitive neuroscience. *Advances in Child Development and Behavior, 28*, 41–100.

Bransford, J. D., Franks, J. J., Morris, C. D., & Stein, B. S. (1979). Some general constraints on learning and memory research. In L. S. Cermak & F. I. M. Craik (Eds.), *Levels of processing in human memory* (pp. 331–354). Hillsdale, NJ: Lawrence Erlbaum Associates.

Brown, J. (1976). An analysis of recognition and recall and of problems in their comparison. In J. Brown (Ed.), *Recall and recognition* (pp. 1–35). London: Wiley.

Brown, R., & Kulik, J. (1977). Flashbulb memories. *Cognition, 5*, 73–99.

Cimbalo, R. S., & Brink, L. (1982). Aging and the von Restorff isolation effect in short-term memory. *The Journal of General Psychology, 106*, 69–76.

Craik, F. I. M. (1982). Selective changes in encoding as a function of reduced processing capacity. In F. Klix, J. Hoffman, & E. Van der Meer (Eds.), *Cognitive research in psychology* (pp. 152–161). Berlin: DVW.

Craik, F. I. M. (2002). Human memory and aging. In L. Bäckman & C. von Hofsten (Eds.), *Psychology at the turn of the millennium* (pp. 261–280). Hove, UK: Psychology Press.

Craik, F. I. M., & Tulving, E. (1975). Depth of processing and the retention of words in episodic memory. *Journal of Experimental Psychology: General, 104*, 268–294.

Epstein, M. L., Phillips, W. D., & Johnson, S. J. (1975). Recall of related and unrelated word pairs as a function of processing level. *Journal of Experimental Psychology: Human Learning and Memory, 1*, 149–152.

Gardiner, J. M., Craik, F. I. M., & Birtwistle, J. (1972). Retrieval cues and release from proactive inhibition. *Journal of Verbal Learning and Verbal Behavior, 11*, 778–783.

Gardiner, J. M., & Richardson-Klavehn, A. (2000). Remembering and knowing. In E. Tulving & F. I. M. Craik (Eds.), *The Oxford handbook of memory* (pp. 229–244). New York: Oxford University Press.

Goldsmith, M., & Koriat, A. (1999). The strategic regulation of memory reporting: Mechanisms and performance consequences. In D. Gopher & A. Koriat (Eds.), *Attention and performance XVII* (pp. 373–400). Cambridge, MA: MIT Press.

Goldstein, A. G., & Chance, J. E. (1971). Visual recognition memory for complex configurations. *Perception & Psychophysics, 9*, 237–241.

Hamilton, M., & Rajaram, S. (2001). The concreteness effect in implicit and explicit memory. *Journal of Memory and Language, 44*, 96–117.

Howe, M. L. (2000). *The fate of early memories: Developmental science and the retention of childhood experiences.* Washington, DC: American Psychological Association.

Hunt, R. R., & Einstein, G. O. (1981). Relational and item-specific information in memory. *Journal of Verbal Learning and Verbal Behavior, 20*, 497–514.

Jacoby, L. L. (1983). Remembering the data: Analyzing interactive processes in reading. *Journal of Verbal Learning and Verbal Behavior, 22*, 485–508.

Jacoby, L. L., & Craik, F. I. M. (1979). Effects of elaboration of processing at encoding and retrieval: Trace distinctiveness and recovery of initial context. In L. S. Cermak & F. I. M. Craik (Eds.), *Levels of processing in human memory.* Hillsdale, NJ: Lawrence Erlbaum Associates.

Jacoby, L. L, & Dallas, M. (1981). On the relationship between autobiographical memory and perceptual learning. *Journal of Experimental Psychology: General, 3*, 306–340.

Kapur, S., Craik, F. I. M., Tulving, E., Wilson, A. A., Houle, S., & Brown G. M. (1994). Neuroanatomical correlates of encoding in episodic memory: Levels of processing effect. *Proceedings of the National Academy of Sciences, 91*, 2008–2011.

McDaniel, M. A., DeLosh, E. L., & Merritt, P. S. (2000). Order information and retrieval distinctiveness: Recall of common versus bizarre material. *Journal of Experimental Psychology: Learning, Memory, and Cognition, 26*, 1045–1056.

Moscovitch, M., & Craik, F. I. M. (1976). Depth of processing, retrieval cues, and uniqueness of encoding as factors in recall. *Journal of Verbal Learning and Verbal Behavior, 15*, 447–458.

Roediger, H. L., & McDermott, K. B. (1995). Creating false memories: Remembering words not presented in lists. *Journal of Experimental Psychology: Learning, Memory, and Cognition, 21*, 803–814.

Schmidt, S. R. (1991). Can we have a distinctive theory of memory? *Memory & Cognition, 19*, 523–542.

Tulving, E. (1969). Retrograde amnesia in free recall. *Science, 164*, 88–90.

Tulving, E. (1983). *Elements of episodic memory.* New York: Oxford University Press.

Weldon, M. S., & Coyote K. C. (1996). Failure to find the picture superiority effect in implicit conceptual memory tests. *Journal of Experimental Psychology: Learning, Memory and Cognition, 22,* 670–686.

Wickens, D. D. (1970). Encoding categories of words: An empirical approach to meaning. *Psychological Review, 77,* 1–15.

Winograd, E., & Neisser, U. (Eds.). (1992). *Affect and accuracy in recall: Studies of "flashbulb" memories.* New York: Cambridge University Press.

Author Index

Note: Page numbers followed by f refer to figures.

Subject Index

Note: Page numbers followed by f and t refer to figures and tables, respectively.

461